Praise for *Conducting Hea...*

This text provides clear, detailed, student-focused explanations for critical concepts of research, appropriate for both undergraduate and graduate health sciences students.

—Janet Reid-Hector, Rutgers University

After reading this book, I know that my students will be on the correct path to starting a productive research career or project.

—Michelle Renee Chyatte, University of Cincinnati

This is very well written, with clear explanations of methods and concepts as well as tables and figures to assist in the learning processes. It's great for graduate students, and I would recommend this book to my colleagues.

—John R. Contreras, Westminster College

With its succinct style and broad coverage, this text provides an excellent platform upon which to build a research curriculum. It frees the instructor to provide in-depth coverage of preferred topics by providing the essentials in a readily digestible style.

—Robert Duval, West Virginia University

The textbook provides a good overview of research methods that allows students to develop skills in basic research needed for their careers. Definitely hang on to this book.

—Robert LaChausse, California Baptist University

Conducting Health Research

To Leona B. Kviz

Sara Miller McCune founded SAGE Publishing in 1965 to support the dissemination of usable knowledge and educate a global community. SAGE publishes more than 1000 journals and over 800 new books each year, spanning a wide range of subject areas. Our growing selection of library products includes archives, data, case studies and video. SAGE remains majority owned by our founder and after her lifetime will become owned by a charitable trust that secures the company's continued independence.

Los Angeles | London | New Delhi | Singapore | Washington DC | Melbourne

Conducting Health Research
Principles, Process, and Methods

Frederick J. Kviz
University of Illinois at Chicago

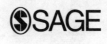

Los Angeles | London | New Delhi
Singapore | Washington DC | Melbourne

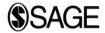

FOR INFORMATION:

SAGE Publications, Inc.
2455 Teller Road
Thousand Oaks, California 91320
E-mail: order@sagepub.com

SAGE Publications Ltd.
1 Oliver's Yard
55 City Road
London EC1Y 1SP
United Kingdom

SAGE Publications India Pvt. Ltd.
B 1/I 1 Mohan Cooperative Industrial Area
Mathura Road, New Delhi 110 044
India

SAGE Publications Asia-Pacific Pte. Ltd.
18 Cross Street #10-10/11/12
China Square Central
Singapore 048423

Acquisitions Editor: Helen Salmon
Content Development Editor: Chelsea Neve
Editorial Assistant: Megan O'Heffernan
Production Editor: Bennie Clark Allen
Copy Editor: Melinda Masson
Typesetter: C&M Digitals (P) Ltd.
Proofreader: Jennifer Grubba
Indexer: Jean Casalegno
Cover Designer: Anupama Krishnan
Marketing Manager: Shari Countryman

Copyright © 2020 by SAGE Publications, Inc.

All rights reserved. Except as permitted by U.S. copyright law, no part of this work may be reproduced or distributed in any form or by any means, or stored in a database or retrieval system, without permission in writing from the publisher.

All third party trademarks referenced or depicted herein are included solely for the purpose of illustration and are the property of their respective owners. Reference to these trademarks in no way indicates any relationship with, or endorsement by, the trademark owner.

Printed in the United States of America

Library of Congress Cataloging-in-Publication Data

Names: Kviz, Frederick J., author.

Title: Conducting health research : principles, process, and methods / Frederick J. Kviz.

Description: Los Angeles : Sage, [2020] | Includes bibliographical references and index.

Identifiers: LCCN 2018048862 | ISBN 9781483317588 (pbk. : alk. paper)

Subjects: | MESH: Biomedical Research—methods | Research Design

Classification: LCC R850 | NLM W 20.5 | DDC 610.72/4—dc23
LC record available at https://lccn.loc.gov/2018048862

This book is printed on acid-free paper.

19 20 21 22 23 10 9 8 7 6 5 4 3 2 1

• Brief Contents •

Preface	xxiii
Companion Website	xxviii
About the Author	xxix

Chapter 1	•	The Nature and Process of Research	xxx
Chapter 2	•	Conducting Ethically Responsible Research	24
Chapter 3	•	Variables and Relationships	48
Chapter 4	•	Research Design Diagrams and Components	82
Chapter 5	•	Research Design Validity	102
Chapter 6	•	Research Designs	134
Chapter 7	•	Random Sampling and Assignment	156
Chapter 8	•	The Measurement Process, Reliability, and Validity	190
Chapter 9	•	Developing a Measurement Instrument	220
Chapter 10	•	Developing a Structured Questionnaire	242
Chapter 11	•	Writing Survey Questions	270
Chapter 12	•	Survey Research Methods	304
Chapter 13	•	Qualitative Research Methods	338
Chapter 14	•	Secondary Analysis and Existing Data	370
Chapter 15	•	The Analysis Process and Reporting Results	390

Glossary	427
References	443
Index	451

Detailed Contents

Preface	xxiii
Companion Website	xxviii
About the Author	xxix
Chapter 1 • The Nature and Process of Research	xxx
Learning Objectives	1
Overview	1
The Nature of Research	2
Research Objectives	2
The Scientific Approach	2
Objectivity	3
Control	6
Replication	6
The Role of Theory	7
Reasoning	8
Inductive reasoning	8
Deductive reasoning	8
A holistic perspective	9
Inference	9
Research Validity	11
The Research Process	12
Problem Statement	12
Research Question	13
Conceptual Approach	14
Research Design	14
Subjects	15
Target population	15
Units of study	16
Inclusion/exclusion criteria	16
Selection procedure	17
Sample size	17
Data Collection	17
Key variables	17
Subjects	17
Method	18
Data Analysis	18
Conclusions	18
Next Study	18
Pilot Study	19
Plan and design	19
Subjects	20
Sites	20

Data	20
Assessment	21
Key Points	21
Review and Apply	22
Study Further	23

Chapter 2 • Conducting Ethically Responsible Research — 24

Learning Objectives	25
Overview	25
Ethical Principles of Research With Human Subjects	26
Respect for Persons	26
Self-determination	26
Vulnerable populations	27
Beneficence	27
Benefits	28
Risks	28
Assessing risks	28
Justice	28
Inclusion	28
Treatment	29
Federal Regulations and the IRB	29
The Common Rule	29
Institutional Review Board (IRB)	30
Purpose and composition	30
IRB protocol	30
IRB review	31
Training	32
Informed Consent	33
Process	33
Elements	33
Assessment	33
Documentation	35
Proposed Changes in Federal Regulations	38
Privacy Protection	39
Privacy	39
Anonymity	39
Not recording identifiers	40
Not collecting identifiers	40
De-identification	40
Uses of Identifiers	40
Prenotification	40
Scheduling	41
Follow-up	41
Data collection evaluation	41
Missing data recovery	42
Data verification/clarification	42
Payments	42
Linking data sets	42
Tracking	42
Sharing results	43

Maintaining Confidentiality	43
Subject identification codes	43
Security	43
Nondisclosure	44
Collect necessary information only	44
Limitations of confidentiality	45
Certificate of Confidentiality	45
Key Points	46
Review and Apply	47
Study Further	47

Chapter 3 • Variables and Relationships — 48

Learning Objectives	49
Overview	49
Types of Variables	50
Levels of Measurement	50
Discrete Variables	50
Continuous Variables	50
Attributes of Relationships	51
Contingency	51
Direction	52
Strength	54
Causal Concepts	54
Independent and Dependent Variables	54
Path Diagrams	55
Exogenous variables	55
Endogenous variables	56
Necessary and Sufficient Conditions	56
Noncausal Relationships	57
Risk factor	57
Common cause	57
Spurious relationship	58
Ecological fallacy	60
Inferring Causality	61
Covariation	61
Temporal precedence	62
Alternative explanations	62
Mechanism/process	62
Consistency	63
Guidelines for inferring causality	63
Multiple Causes and Multiple Effects	63
Reciprocal Causality	64
Mediated Causal Relationships	66
Basic mediation model	66
Complete mediation	68
Partial mediation	68
Analyzing mediated causal relationships	69
Multiple Mediator Models	71
Simultaneous/parallel multiple mediator model	71
Sequential/serial multiple mediator model	71

Mixed multiple mediator model	72
Multiple independent variable mediation	72
Moderated Causal Relationships	73
Basic moderation model	73
Analyzing moderated causal relationships	74
Multiple moderator models	75
Mediation and Moderation Combined	75
Mediated moderation	75
Moderated mediation	76
Does the sequence matter?	77
Complex Causal Models	77
Key Points	79
Review and Apply	80
Study Further	81

Chapter 4 • Research Design Diagrams and Components — 82

Learning Objectives	83
Overview	83
Research Design Diagrams	83
Research Design Components	85
Time Frame	86
Accessibility	86
Observations	86
Treatment implementation	86
Groups	87
Number	87
Composition	88
Conditions	89
One group	89
Multiple groups	90
Observation Points	95
Treatment designs	95
Observational designs	98
Key Points	99
Review and Apply	99
Study Further	100

Chapter 5 • Research Design Validity — 102

Learning Objectives	103
Overview	103
Observational Designs	104
Causal Designs	104
Internal Validity	104
External Validity	105
Internal Validity Threats and Strategies	106
Design Threats	106
Nonequivalent groups	106
History	108

Maturation	109
Attrition	109
Testing	110
Instrumentation	111
Regression toward the norm	112
Design Strategies	113
Nonequivalent groups	113
History	114
Maturation	115
Attrition	116
Testing	117
Instrumentation	118
Regression toward the norm	118
Nondesign Threats	119
Treatment diffusion/control group contamination	119
Treatment imitation	119
Compensatory equalization	120
Compensatory rivalry	120
Demoralization	120
Participant reactivity	120
Nondesign Strategies	120
Treatment diffusion/control group contamination	121
Treatment imitation	121
Compensatory equalization	122
Compensatory rivalry and demoralization	122
Participant reactivity	122
External Validity Threats and Strategies	123
Unrepresentative Units	123
Threats	123
Strategies	124
Unrepresentative Setting	125
Threats	125
Strategies	125
Unrepresentative Treatment	126
Threats	126
Strategies	126
Unrepresentative Outcome	127
Threats	127
Strategies	128
Balancing Internal and External Validity	129
Key Points	130
Review and Apply	132
Study Further	132
Chapter 6 • Research Designs	**134**
Learning Objectives	135
Overview	135
Observational Designs	136
Cross-sectional Designs	136

Longitudinal Designs	137
Trend study (sequential cross-sectional design)	137
Panel study	138
Causal Designs	140
Nonexperimental Designs	140
One-group posttest-only design	140
One-group pretest–posttest design	141
Nonequivalent-groups posttest-only design	142
Experimental Designs	143
Pretest–posttest control group design	143
Posttest-only control group design	143
Solomon four-group design	144
Separate-sample designs	145
Quasi-experimental Designs	146
Nonequivalent pretest–posttest control group design	146
Interrupted time-series designs	147
Case-control design	149
Cohort studies	149
Design Variations	150
Staggered starts	150
Switching replications	151
Counterbalancing	152
Key Points	152
Review and Apply	154
Study Further	155

Chapter 7 • Random Sampling and Assignment   156

Learning Objectives	157
Overview	157
Random Sampling	158
Reasons for Sampling	158
Random Sampling Concepts	159
Terms and notation	159
Random selection	160
Simple random sampling	160
Random Sampling Procedures	164
Sampling frame	164
Random selection	165
Stratified Random Sampling	169
Conditions	169
Impact	169
Specifying strata	170
Proportionate allocation	171
Disproportionate allocation	171
Cluster Random Sampling	173
Conditions	173
Specifying clusters	174
Selecting clusters	174
Selecting individuals within clusters	176
Impact	176

Sample Size	177
Population estimates	177
Difference between proportions	179
Statistical power analysis	179
Field sample size	180
Logistical aspects	180
Random Assignment	181
Separate Random Samples	182
Simple Random Assignment	182
Stratified Random Assignment	182
Block Randomization	182
Matching	183
Pairwise matching	183
Key Points	184
Review and Apply	187
Study Further	188

Chapter 8 • The Measurement Process, Reliability, and Validity   190

Learning Objectives	191
Overview	191
From Concepts to Data	192
Conceptualization	192
Operationalization	193
Instrumentation	193
An Example	193
Levels of Measurement	194
Nominal Level	195
Strategies	195
Ordinal Level	195
Strategies	196
Interval/Ratio Level	197
Strategies	197
Comparative Summary	198
Measurement Theory	199
Random Error	199
Measurement Reliability	200
Systematic Error	200
Measurement Validity	201
The Relationship Between Reliability and Validity	202
Assessing Measurement Reliability	202
Test–Retest Reliability	204
Limitations	204
Interrater Reliability	205
Kappa coefficient	205
Limitations	206
Parallel Forms Reliability	206
Limitations	207
Split-half reliability	207
Cronbach's coefficient alpha	207

Assessing Measurement Validity	209
Judgment-Based Validity	209
Face validity	209
Content validity	211
Performance-Based Validity	212
Concurrent criterion validity	212
Predictive criterion validity	213
Convergent and discriminant validity	213
Construct validity	214
Item Response Theory	215
Key Points	217
Review and Apply	218
Study Further	219

Chapter 9 • Developing a Measurement Instrument   220

Learning Objectives	221
Overview	221
The Instrument Development Process	222
Specifying Variables	222
Specifying Format	223
Drafting and Revising	223
Field Pretesting	223
Using Existing Instruments	225
Advantages	225
Disadvantages	226
Modifications	227
Developing a Rating Scale	227
Single-Item Scales	228
Bipolar scale	228
Unipolar scale	229
Branching	231
Item-specific scale	231
Number of points	232
Including a midpoint	232
Labeling	233
Multiple-Item Scales	236
Key Points	239
Review and Apply	240
Study Further	241

Chapter 10 • Developing a Structured Questionnaire   242

Learning Objectives	243
Overview	244
Key Concepts	244
Standardization	244
The Response Process	244
Satisficing	245
Questionnaire Development Process	246

  Outline   246
  Drafting   247
  Cognitive Interviewing   247
   Implementation   248
   Assessment   248
  Field Pretesting   248
   Sample   249
   Assessment   250

Questionnaire Design and Data Collection Mode   252
  Data Collection Modes Overview   252
  Understanding Questions   253
  Question Order Control   253
  Response Situation Control   254
  Recorded Response Quality   255
  Question Complexity   255
  Questionnaire Complexity   255
  Questionnaire Length   256
  Visual Aids   256
  Records Referral   257
  Sensitive Topics   257
  Open Questions   257
  Summary   258

Questionnaire Format   258
  Type   259
  Layout   259
  Instructions   262
  Web Questionnaires   262

Questionnaire Structure   263
  Question Order Overall   263
  Question Order Within a Topic   264
  Navigation   266
   Question numbering   266
   Filter questions and skip patterns   266

Key Points   267
Review and Apply   269
Study Further   269

Chapter 11 • Writing Survey Questions   270

Learning Objectives   271
Overview   271
Types of Questions   272
  Closed Questions   273
   Advantages   273
   Disadvantages   273
  Open Questions   274
   Advantages   274
   Disadvantages   275

Question Wording   275
  Vocabulary   276

Tone	277
Problem Words	278
Question Structure	**279**
Short and Simple	279
Use Complete Sentences	281
Ask One Question at a Time	281
Do Not Use Double Negatives	282
Specify Conditions at the Beginning	282
Do Not Ask Biased Questions	283
Response choices	283
Providing information	284
Citing authority	285
One-sided	285
Presenting examples	285
Assumptions	285
Sensitive Topics	285
Introduce the topic	286
Generalize negative conditions	286
Make responses acceptable	286
Provide an excuse	286
Ask for an opinion	287
Response Choices	**287**
General Guidelines	287
Be responsive to the question	288
Present one response at a time	288
Unidimensional	289
Exclusive	289
Exhaustive	290
Short and simple	290
Use "Don't know" cautiously	290
Nominal Level	291
Fill in the blank	291
Dichotomous choice	292
Multiple choice	292
Multiple response	293
Ordinal Level	294
Dichotomous choice	294
Multiple choice	294
Rating scales	294
Ranking	294
Interval/Ratio Level	296
Fill in the blank	296
Multiple choice	297
Key Points	**299**
Review and Apply	**300**
Study Further	**303**

Chapter 12 • Survey Research Methods — 304

Learning Objectives	305
Overview	305

Basic Concepts ... 306
    Survey Advantages ... 306
    Survey Disadvantages ... 307
    The Survey Process ... 307
Data Collection Modes ... 309
    Overview ... 309
    Comparison ... 310
        Costs ... 310
        Time ... 311
        Geographic distribution ... 311
        Anonymity ... 311
        Unit response rate ... 312
        Item nonresponse ... 312
        Summary ... 313
    Additional Considerations ... 313
    Mixed Modes ... 314
    Computer-Assisted Modes ... 315
        Advantages ... 316
        Disadvantages ... 317
Conducting a Survey ... 317
    Mail ... 317
        General protocol ... 317
        Options ... 320
        Sample ... 321
    Monitored ... 321
    Web ... 322
    Telephone Interviews ... 322
        General protocol ... 322
        Making contact ... 323
        Sample ... 324
    In-Person Interviews ... 324
        General protocol ... 324
        Making contact ... 325
        Sample ... 326
Interviewing ... 326
    General Guidelines ... 326
    Recording Responses ... 327
    Probing ... 328
        Encouragement ... 329
        Clarification ... 329
        Completeness ... 330
    Interviewer Characteristics ... 330
    Interviewer Training ... 331
    Interviewer Supervision ... 331
Key Points ... 332
Review and Apply ... 333
Study Further ... 337

Chapter 13 • **Qualitative Research Methods** ... **338**

Learning Objectives ... 339
Overview ... 340

Basic Concepts	340
Key Characteristics	340
Limitations	341
Qualitative Interview Methods	342
Unstructured Interviews	342
Semistructured Interviews	343
Structured Open-Ended Interviews	344
Focus Groups	345
Qualitative Interviewing Techniques	349
Observation Methods	351
Participant Observation	351
Nonparticipant Observation	354
Reactivity	356
Recording Observation Data	357
Sampling	359
Purposive Sample	359
Typical case sample	360
Atypical case sample	360
Homogeneous sample	360
Heterogeneous sample	360
Key Informants Sample	361
Referral Sample	361
Chain referral/snowball sample	361
Respondent-driven sample	361
Convenience Sample	361
Sample Size	362
Mixed Methods	362
Concurrent Designs	364
Exploratory Sequential Designs	365
Explanatory Sequential Designs	366
Confirmatory/Generalizability Sequential Designs	366
Monomethod Designs	366
Key Points	367
Review and Apply	368
Study Further	369

Chapter 14 • Secondary Analysis and Existing Data — 370

Learning Objectives	371
Overview	371
Basic Concepts	372
The Secondary Data Analysis Process	373
Advantages, Limitations, and Ethics	374
Advantages	374
Limitations	375
Ethics	376
Secondary Data Sources	376
Major Sources	376
Qualitative Data	378
Documents and Records	378
Big Data	379

Synthesizing Results From Multiple Studies   381
    Narrative Review   381
    Systematic Review   381
    Meta-analysis   384
Key Points   386
Review and Apply   388
Study Further   388

Chapter 15 • The Analysis Process and Reporting Results   390

Learning Objectives   391
Overview   392
The Data Analysis Process   392
    Data Preparation   392
    Analysis File Preparation   393
        Data entry   393
        Data cleaning   393
        Names and labels   394
    Modification and Finalization   394
        Recoding and computing variables   394
        Reliability and validity   397
        Weighting   397
        Final frequencies   398
        Documentation   398
Overview of Quantitative Data Analysis   400
    Description   400
        Tables   401
        Percentages   402
        Central tendency   403
        Dispersion   403
    Contingency   404
    Correlation   404
    Regression   405
    Differences   405
    Hypothesis Testing   405
        Hypotheses   405
        Process   406
        Decision errors   408
    Validity and Substantive Significance   409
Overview of Qualitative Data Analysis   409
    Data Preparation   410
    Coding   410
    Themes and Conclusions   412
    Trustworthiness   413
        Credibility   413
        Transferability   413
        Dependability   413
        Confirmability   413
Reporting Research Results   414
    Abstract   415
    Introduction   416

- Background/Literature Review — 416
- Methods — 417
  - *Research design* — 417
  - *Subjects/participants* — 417
  - *Measurements/instrumentation* — 418
  - *Data collection* — 418
  - *Analysis* — 418
- Results/Findings — 418
- Discussion — 419
- References — 419
- Appendix — 419
- Other Components — 420
  - *Acknowledgements* — 420
  - *Funding support* — 420
  - *Human subjects protection* — 420
  - *Conflict of interest disclosure* — 420
- Authorship — 421
- Key Points — 422
- Review and Apply — 424
- Study Further — 425

Glossary — **427**

References — **443**

Index — **451**

• Preface •

In *Conducting Health Research: Principles, Process, and Methods*, I present an integrated and practical introduction to principles and strategies for planning, implementing, reporting, and assessing health research. My primary purpose is for this book to serve as a core textbook for graduate and advanced undergraduate health sciences students, particularly in public health, nursing, occupational therapy, physical therapy, disability studies, pharmacy, health education, health services management, medicine, and medical sociology. Also, it will serve as a useful reference for practicing health professionals.

As a developer and instructor of research methods courses for health sciences students, I have searched diligently for a text that presents the content as an integrated process and in a manner that is relevant to conducting health research. Unfortunately, I found I had to supplement texts that primarily presented overviews of methods and did not describe how to implement them. Also, most of the best texts were written for social science students. Consequently, I undertook writing *Conducting Health Research: Principles, Process, and Methods* to address the absence of the text I hoped to find.

It is essential for all health sciences students to understand the research process and how it is implemented. Although they did not anticipate a career conducting health research, many of my students have been surprised that one of their first postgraduation employment assignments involved research. Every one expressed appreciation for having been prepared to undertake and successfully complete those assignments. Accordingly, I have two major goals for this book, to prepare readers to

- participate in planning, implementing, and reporting health sciences research; and
- critically assess a study's strengths and limitations, to develop a trustworthy evidence-based practice and make informed policy decisions.

Moreover, this book provides a foundation for advanced study in research methods. I sincerely hope some readers will be inspired to do so.

I wrote *Conducting Health Research: Principles, Process, and Methods* from a teaching perspective, drawing on my extensive experience teaching research methods to health sciences students. I employ a balanced and integrated approach to understanding the research process, emphasizing how its various stages fit together and interact. I present each method with equal emphasis on its advantages and limitations, and I compare alternative methods and present guidelines for choosing among them. Rather than presenting the various methods and strategies as exclusive or competitive, I emphasize their complementarity. My goal is that readers will both understand how to select the most suitable method for a situation, and appreciate the value of employing multiple methods when appropriate and feasible.

Throughout, I present examples to illustrate applying principles and procedures to real health research problems. Where feasible, examples extend across methods so readers may follow familiar threads and appreciate how a problem may be approached in various ways. Also, I discuss practical aspects of planning and conducting research that too often are not addressed in textbooks, such as financial costs, time, staffing, and access to sites. Moreover, I describe how and why real-world situations often challenge researchers to be versatile in the face of unanticipated problems while preserving the integrity of their results.

Importantly, I focus on health research methods. Although this might appear self-evident from the title, I mention this because large portions of many methods textbooks are devoted to introductory statistics. Typically, my search for research methods texts yielded ones I describe as consisting mainly of a methods overview with a statistics primer appended to it. Data analysis certainly is an important component of the research process. I address analysis considerations as they relate to specifying the research question, research design, sampling strategy, measurement procedure, and data collection strategy. However, the main reason for reading a research methods book is to learn about research methods. Therefore, I used space that otherwise would be diverted to statistical techniques to address research methods more comprehensively and in greater depth than many competing research methods texts. Statistics can be covered more comprehensively and more effectively in a statistics textbook, of which there already are many excellent ones available. Moreover, I assume readers already have an understanding of basic statistical techniques, such as would be derived from completing an undergraduate-level course.

I structured the chapters to guide readers to an overall understanding of the nature and process of conducting and assessing health research. Nevertheless, I designed each chapter to be useful if read individually or in a different order, according to a reader's or an instructor's need or preference. Each chapter opens with an *Overview* that describes the main topic and its importance, followed by *Learning Objectives*. At the end of each major topic within a chapter, I guide the reader to *Check Your Understanding* about key concepts and strategies. At the end of each chapter, I provide a *Summary* of key points, present activities for readers to *Review and Apply* what they learned, and suggest readings to *Study Further*. A noteworthy aspect of the *Review and Apply* sections is that I guide readers through the process of planning a study about a health-related problem that interests them. In addition, throughout the book, I refer readers to online resources such as at the Centers for Disease Control and Prevention, regulations and training for conducting research with human subjects, sample size and power calculators, the Kahn Academy, questionnaire archives, and data archives.

To emphasize my focus on the research process as a whole, I did not divide this book into sections. However, as an overview, Chapters 1–3 may be viewed as presenting the foundations of the research process; Chapters 4–6 address research design; Chapter 7 addresses random sampling and assignment; Chapters 8–11 address measurement concepts and strategies; Chapters 12–14 address collecting and accessing data; and Chapter 15 describes the process of analyzing data and reporting results. A glossary of key terms is provided as well. The following is a brief summary of each chapter.

> *Chapter 1 The Nature and Process of Research.* Introduces the nature, logic, and stages of health research. Describes the key aspects of the scientific approach, the role of theory, the inference process, and the major determinants of research validity
>
> *Chapter 2 Conducting Ethically Responsible Research.* Describes research participants' rights and researchers' responsibilities to inform and protect research participants. Discusses the *Belmont Report*, the *Common Rule*, the institutional review board, the informed consent process, and privacy protection strategies.
>
> *Chapter 3 Variables and Relationships.* Describes what variables are and their various types, attributes of relationships, causal and noncausal relationships, and moderated and mediated relationships.
>
> *Chapter 4 Research Design Diagrams and Components.* Describes the basic components to consider when designing a study and the implications of decisions about those components for a study's validity. Explains how research design diagrams are developed and how they guide conducting a study.

Chapter 5 Research Design Validity. Distinguishes between observational and causal designs, describes internal validity threats and strategies, describes external validity threats and strategies, and presents guidelines for balancing internal and external validity.

Chapter 6 Research Designs. Presents observational, experimental, and quasi-experimental designs. Explains flaws in nonexperimental designs, and how to assess a design's strengths and weaknesses. Describes design variations that may enhance validity and efficiency.

Chapter 7 Random Sampling and Assignment. Presents reasons for selecting a sample and essential random sampling concepts. Describes advantages and disadvantages of nonprobability and probability samples, how to select random samples, and how to determine sample size by balancing statistical and logistical considerations. Describes strategies for assigning research participants to study conditions.

Chapter 8 The Measurement Process, Reliability, and Validity. Describes the measurement process from specifying constructs to operationalizing variables. Distinguishes between levels of measurement. Describes systematic and random error, and measurement reliability and validity. Presents reliability and validity assessment strategies.

Chapter 9 Developing a Measurement Instrument. Describes the instrument development process from specifying variables through field pretesting. Discusses advantages and disadvantages of using existing instruments. Describes how to develop single-item and multiple-item rating scales.

Chapter 10 Developing a Structured Questionnaire. Describes the advantages and disadvantages of a standardized measurement instrument, the cognitive response process, and satisficing theory. Describes the questionnaire development process, including cognitive interviewing and field pretesting. Discusses the relationship between questionnaire design and data collection mode. Presents guidelines for questionnaire format and structure.

Chapter 11 Writing Survey Questions. Describes advantages and disadvantages of closed and open question formats. Presents guidelines for question wording and structure. Presents guidelines for developing response choices.

Chapter 12 Survey Research Methods. Describes advantages and disadvantages of surveys. Describes survey data collection modes and compares them. Presents protocols for conducting a survey using each mode. Presents guidelines for conducting a survey interview.

Chapter 13 Qualitative Research Methods. Presents key characteristics of qualitative methods and their limitations. Describes how to conduct various types of qualitative interviews and observations. Describes qualitative sampling strategies and mixed methods designs.

Chapter 14 Secondary Analysis and Existing Data. Discusses advantages and disadvantages of conducting a secondary data analysis, and describes the secondary data analysis process. Discusses existing data sources and presents guidelines for assessing them. Describes strategies for synthesizing results from multiple studies.

Chapter 15 The Analysis Process and Reporting Results. Describes the process of preparing data for analysis, describes the analysis process, and presents overviews of quantitative and qualitative data analysis methods. Describes the major components of a research report.

Glossary. Presents definitions of key terms, which are highlighted by bold type the first time they appear in the text.

I extend my thanks to many who have influenced the preparation of this book. Some have done so indirectly, as they have been part of my career in conducting research and teaching research methods. In particular, Richard J. McKinlay introduced me to and nurtured my passion for the fascinating area of research methods. Robert Ferber modeled maintaining a healthy sense of humor and humility while addressing challenging methodological problems. Helen R. Grace and Paul S. Levy provided unparalleled support during the early stages of my career. I thank the many students whose insightful questions and comments contributed to honing my teaching skills. In addition, I am indebted to the many colleagues and predecessors whose contributions to the field of research methods are cited throughout the text.

Work on this book would have neither begun nor been completed without the continual encouragement, guidance, and support of Helen Salmon, SAGE Publications Senior Acquisitions Editor. An author could not ask for a more professional, competent, insightful, collegial, and supportive acquisitions editor. In addition, I am grateful for the excellent support and guidance of SAGE Publications staff, particularly Chelsea Neve, Associate Content Development Editor, and Megan O'Heffernan, Editorial Assistant, who coordinated bringing the manuscript to completion. I extend special thanks to Chelsea Neve for her contributions to pedagogical aspects of the text. Other SAGE staff who made noteworthy contributions to developing and producing this text are Eve Simon Oettinger, Nicole Wineman, and Bennie Clark Allen, Production Editor. In addition, the outstanding attention to detail and editing skills of copy editor Melinda Masson improved the overall readability of the text and consistency across chapters.

The following colleagues provided helpful comments on early chapter drafts: Anne Buffington, Michelle Choi Wu, Melissa A. Clark, Charles Hoehne, Timothy P. Johnson, Lisa M. Kuhns, Amy Lemke, April Y. Oh, and Meme Wang-Schweig. In addition, thoughtful suggestions and insights that helped to improve each chapter were provided by the following reviewers recruited by SAGE staff:

Michelle Renee Chyatte, University of Cincinnati

John R. Contreras, Westminster College

Cheryl G. Davis, Tuskegee University

Alexander Dawoody, Marywood University

Robert Duval, West Virginia University

Leslie J. Hinyard, Saint Louis University

Kerry-Anne Hogan, University of Ottawa

Russell S. Kirby, University of South Florida

Patrick M. Krueger, University of Colorado Denver

Robert G. LaChausse, California Baptist University

Richard S. Lockwood, University of Ottawa

Michael Ray, The College at Brockport

Janet Reid-Hector, Rutgers University

Amira Albert Roess, George Washington University

Jiunn-Jye Sheu, University of Toledo

Sheryl Strasser, Georgia State University

Katherine P. Theall, Tulane University

Elizabeth Walker, Emory University

My wife, Linda, donated her graphic design expertise to assist with searching for and selecting photographs. Above all, I express my love and thanks for her abiding love, grace, understanding, and support when so much of my time and attention were focused on developing and completing this project. Much of her is invested in this book. I thank her for sharing life with me.

• Companion Website •

The companion website for *Conducting Health Research* offers additional resources for both students and instructors.

Visit the companion website at: **study.sagepub.com/kviz**.

Password-protected **Instructor Resources** include:

- Editable, **chapter-specific PowerPoint® slides** that offer complete flexibility for creating course lectures
- **Chapter outlines** that summarize key concepts and can be used as in-class handouts for students or lecture notes
- **Full-text SAGE journal articles** carefully selected by the author to illustrate chapter concepts
- **Sample syllabi** that provide suggested models for structuring your course using the text
- **Figures and tables** from the book that are available for download

Open-access **Student Resources** include:

- **Full-text SAGE journal articles** carefully selected by the author to illustrate chapter concepts

• About the Author •

Frederick J. Kviz is Professor Emeritus, Community Health Sciences, at the University of Illinois at the Chicago School of Public Health. He completed his BA, MA, and PhD degrees in sociology at the University of Illinois at Chicago. In addition to *Conducting Health Research: Principles, Process, and Methods*, he authored (with Kathleen A. Knafl) *Statistics for Nurses: An Introductory Text*, which received an *American Journal of Nursing* Book of the Year Award. He has authored and coauthored 55 peer-reviewed publications, as well as many monographs, technical reports, and professional meeting presentations. Dr. Kviz has developed and taught a variety of courses and workshops on research methods and statistics for undergraduate and graduate health sciences students, and for academic and practicing health professionals. His teaching has been recognized by awards for excellence based on peer reviews and student recognition. Also, he was inducted as a faculty member in the Lambda Chapter of the Delta Omega Honor Society (the public health honor society). He is a former Project Coordinator and Assistant Director of the University of Illinois Survey Research Laboratory, and is an expert in survey research methods, research design, and measurement. He has served as a consultant to many public and private health-related agencies, including community-based organizations, health maintenance organizations, city and county health departments, and major medical centers. Dr. Kviz's research has focused on the influence of psychosocial and sociocultural factors on health promotion and illness prevention attitudes and behaviors, and health disparities. His research has involved employing most of the methods described in *Conducting Health Research: Principles, Process, and Methods*.

1

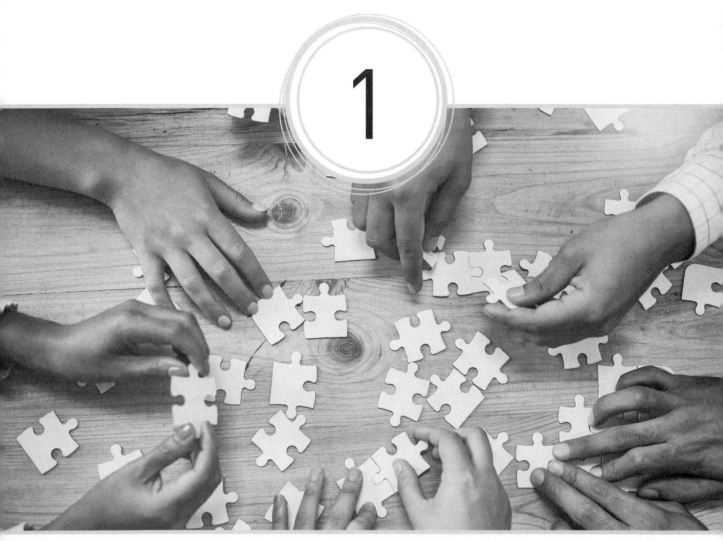

iStock.com/PeopleImages

The Nature and Process of Research

Chapter 1 • The Nature and Process of Research

Chapter Outline

Overview
Learning Objectives
The Nature of Research
    Research Objectives
    The Scientific Approach
    The Role of Theory
    Reasoning
    Inference
    Research Validity
The Research Process
    Problem Statement
    Research Question
    Conceptual Approach
    Research Design
    Subjects
    Data Collection
    Data Analysis
    Conclusions
    Next Study
    Pilot Study
Key Points

Learning Objectives

After studying Chapter 1, the reader should be able to:

- Describe the different types of research objectives and their purpose
- Identify the key aspects of the scientific approach and describe how they contribute to obtaining valid results
- Apply theory to guide planning a study and interpreting results
- Describe the inference process
- Describe the major determinants of research validity
- Identify the major stages in the research process and describe how they are interrelated
- Develop a research plan to address a specific research question

Overview

The ultimate goal of health research is to develop and enhance evidence-based policy and practice to promote health and prevent illness and injury. Pursuing that goal requires seeking answers to challenging questions about how complex factors, such as lifestyle, aging, social context, and the physical environment, may influence individual and population health. Moreover, health-related factors and health outcomes often vary substantially across individuals, populations, settings, conditions, and time. Health research seeks to describe, explain, and predict such variation. It does so by employing a systematic process comprising an integrated series of planning and activities to collect and analyze valid information.

The Nature of Research

Research Objectives

Each research study is focused on at least one specific objective determined by assessing the current state of scientific understanding of a problem and ascertaining how that understanding may be enhanced. Indeed, the first aspect of planning a research study is specifying the objective, which may range from an unstructured exploration of the fundamental aspects of an emerging problem to a highly structured evaluation of an intervention. As depicted in Box 1.1, the course of studying a particular problem generally entails a progressive series of studies with different objectives. When investigating a new problem about which little is known, initial studies commonly are **exploratory** and descriptive, with an objective to gain a basic understanding of the problem's nature and scope. The results of such studies might provide a foundation for developing and implementing an intervention strategy. If subsequent evaluations indicate an intervention is effective, further research might include developing a dissemination plan and proposing evidence-based policy and practice guidelines. Box 1.2 presents examples of research objectives for three different aspects of nutrition research.

> **Key Concept**
>
> *Studying a particular problem generally entails a progressive series of studies with different objectives.*

The Scientific Approach

Scientific research studies are guided by principles that distinguish them from the observations and conclusions people routinely make during the course of daily living. Deliberately and consistently applying those principles enhances the likelihood of deriving valid conclusions. Certainly, people making observations during the course of daily living also want to draw valid conclusions. However, those conclusions typically are not subjected

---

BOX 1.1: GENERAL PROGRESSION OF RESEARCH OBJECTIVES

- Exploration
- Description
- Intervention development
- Evaluation
- Dissemination

> **BOX 1.2: EXAMPLES OF RESEARCH OBJECTIVES**
>
> **Impact of Healthy Vending Machine Options in a Large Community Health Organization**
>
> Banner Health worked with its vending machine vendor to increase healthy vending options in 23 sites, including corporate, hospital, and other clinical settings, which provides [sic] vended food choices for employees and clients. We performed an evaluation of this organizational environmental change with the primary research question, "Did increasing the proportion of healthier 'right choice' (RC) options in vending machines at Banner Health corporate and patient-care sites decrease the amount of calories, fat, sugar, and sodium vended, while maintaining total sales revenue?"
>
> *Source:* Grivios-Shah et al. (2018, p. 1426).
>
> **Prevalence and Implementation Practices of School Salad Bars Across Grade Levels**
>
> The purpose of this article is to report on the prevalence of salad bars in Arizona schools by grade level (elementary, middle, high, and K-12). In addition, we will describe characteristics of school salad bars including type, format, and foods served on the salad bars by grade level.
>
> *Source:* Bruening, Adams, Ohri-Vachaspati, & Hurley (2018, p. 1376).
>
> **Physician Characteristics Associated With Sugar-Sweetened Beverage Counseling Practices**
>
> The objectives of this exploratory study were as follows:
>
> 1. To investigate what topics physicians discuss with patients who are overweight or have obesity when providing SSB-related counseling.
> 2. To examine the association between physicians' personal and medical practice characteristics, including physician personal SSB intake, and their SSB-related counseling practices for patients who are overweight or have obesity.
>
> *Source:* VanFrank, Park, Foltz, McGuire, & Harris (2018, p. 1366).

to the same scrutiny and standards as are applied to scientific research. Key components of the **scientific approach** are as follows:

- Objectivity
- Control
- Replication

Objectivity

To the extent possible, a research study should be conducted with **objectivity**, whereby researchers maintain an impartial posture, which sometimes is called *value neutrality*. The goal is to prevent **researcher bias** (also called "investigator bias" or "experimenter bias") whereby personal values might influence how researchers conduct a study and interpret its result. This threat to research validity especially is a serious concern in health research because it might lead to implementing an ineffective procedure or policy or even contribute to adverse health outcomes. It is not ethical to conduct a study or interpret its result deliberately in a biased manner. Nevertheless, researcher bias may be introduced inadvertently. Therefore, several strategies may be employed to guard against it.

Monitoring. Throughout the research process, it is important to monitor the research environment to identify potential sources of bias and employ appropriate countermeasures whenever feasible. There are two basic approaches to monitoring. One is **self-monitoring**, which involves routinely conducting self-reflective checks. Such checks are most effective when collaborating with colleagues who are committed to holding one another accountable. The other approach is **independent monitoring**, whereby by a third party (e.g., other researchers, practitioners, or community leaders) provide oversight for how a study is planned, conducted, and reported. This approach is more effective than self-monitoring because independent monitors have no vested interest in the research results. Such oversight may be exercised informally or semiformally, for example by sharing a research plan and progress reports in "brown bag seminar" presentations. Formal oversight typically involves convening an **advisory panel** of professional and/or lay experts that reviews plans and progress according to a predetermined protocol and schedule. Self-monitoring always should be employed. When feasible, the best practice is to employ both self- and independent monitoring.

Blinding. When evaluating an intervention, researcher bias might be introduced by favoring subjects in a **treatment group** that receives the intervention over ones in a **control group** that does not receive it. For example, as compared to control subjects, treatment subjects might be provided a more comfortable physical setting, or staff might communicate with them in a more supportive manner. Such actions may bias a study's result in favor of the treatment condition demonstrating a more positive outcome than the **control condition**. Consequently, a result might suggest an intervention is more effective than it actually is, or that it is effective when actually it is not.

Researcher bias may be prevented by employing a **researcher blind**, whereby researchers are not aware of which participants are assigned to which study condition/group. The underlying logic is that researchers and staff are likely to manage subjects and their data equitably if they do not know to which study condition subjects are assigned. Researcher **blinding** is implemented by engaging a third party to assign subjects to conditions using nondescript labels that do not disclose their assignment while a study is being conducted. The labels should be assigned using a random procedure to avoid a pattern, such as "Group A" always is treatment and "Group B" always is control. A **full blind** is applied at the time subjects are assigned to study groups, and the third party maintains custody of records regarding study condition assignments until all data are collected and analyzed. Thus, researchers may derive conclusions about differences in group outcomes while shielded from any potential influence associated with knowing to which conditions subjects were assigned.

Sometimes a full blind strategy is not possible. For example, if resources are not sufficient to employ independent health education staff, the researchers themselves might conduct educational sessions that are part of an intervention. Thus, they would know which subjects participate in those sessions. In such a situation, a **partial blind** might be applied, whereby the researchers are blinded to subject assignment during one or more parts of a study. For example, it might be feasible to apply a blind during data analysis by having a third party designate study conditions using nondescript labels that are disclosed only after data analysis is complete. Another example is data collection staff, such as interviewers, might be blinded regarding the condition to which subjects are assigned. That strategy might protect against potential **interviewer bias**, such as differences in probing or asking leading questions owing to expectations of obtaining certain types of responses from treatment versus control subjects.

In addition, validity may be enhanced by employing a **subject blind**, whereby the subjects are not told to which study condition they are assigned until after an intervention is implemented and outcome data are collected. The goal is to prevent study outcomes from being influenced by subjects reacting to their condition assignment. For instance, subjects who know they are assigned to receive a new intervention might expect to experience change, which might lead them to overreport positive outcomes and/or underreport negative outcomes. An example is that smoking cessation program participants might be reluctant to admit failure and not report occasions when they smoke cigarettes postintervention. Consequently, researchers might overestimate positive outcomes attributable to the smoking cessation program. On the other hand, control group subjects who are disappointed at not being assigned to receive an intervention might independently seek an alternative treatment outside the research context. If such compensatory behavior decreases control group smoking prevalence, the smoking cessation program's effectiveness might be underestimated. The term **single blind** applies to situations when only members of the research team or only subjects are blinded. In a **double blind** protocol, both researchers and subjects are blinded.

Empirical assessment. Scientific research results are derived from analyzing data collected through systematic empirical observation (Chapter 15). Furthermore, to the extent possible, analytic procedures should be employed that yield the same result regardless of who performs the analysis. The strongest support for the validity of data analysis is obtained when data are made available for independent verification of results by other researchers.

Full disclosure. **Full disclosure** includes reporting results, it is essential to disclose all aspects of how a study was designed and conducted so others may evaluate its validity and replicate it. When limitations of publication space or presentation time restrict the detail that may be reported, such as for a complex sampling design, a long section of a questionnaire, or a complex coding protocol, supplemental information should be provided on request or at a website. Full disclosure includes reporting all significant unanticipated problems encountered while conducting a study (e.g., recruiting subjects, gaining access to sites, staff turnover, and travel conditions), describing how they were addressed, and assessing their potential impact on a study's result.

Peer review. Most research studies undergo **peer review**, whereby independent researchers review a study proposal and/or reports of results. Typically, the peer review process begins when a research proposal is submitted to a funding agency. The proposal is reviewed by other researchers who evaluate features such as the significance of the research problem, innovative aspects of the research approach, the potential to produce important new information, the appropriateness of the study design and procedures, and the research team's capacity to conduct the study (based on training, experience, and resources). When a study is completed, the most rigorous reporting venues are publication in professional journals and presentations at professional meetings that require independent peer review prior to accepting a proposed manuscript or presentation. In most cases, the reviewers (called "referees," hence the term *refereed publication*) are blinded to the identity of the authors to prevent potential conflicts of interest and reviewer bias. Further, the readership or audience may raise questions about the research report and challenge the interpretation of a result.

Control

Control refers to managing the conditions under which a study is conducted and employing systematic protocols throughout the research process to enhance the comparability of results across individuals, groups, populations, settings, and time.

Conditions. Controlling conditions is a hallmark of **experimental research** (Chapter 6), whereby subjects are assigned to two or more **comparison groups**, such as treatment and control. Ensuring that all subjects experience the same conditions, except for intentional exposure to the treatment, enhances the validity of attributing an outcome difference to the treatment rather than to other differences in study conditions. If treatment exposure is the only substantial difference across groups, then treatment exposure is the most plausible explanation for different outcomes. Thus, alternative explanations may be ruled out.

Protocols. Employing systematic protocols reduces variation in activities such as recruiting subjects, exposing subjects to an experimental treatment, collecting data, and coding data in preparation for analysis. Such variation may influence the validity of a study's results. For example, suppose researchers studying stress related to conflict among coworkers give subjects the option to complete a self-administered questionnaire at the workplace or at home. The setting in which they complete the questionnaire might influence their responses. Those who complete it at the workplace, where they might discuss the questions with coworkers, might be inclined to enter responses that are more positive than those who complete the questionnaire in private at home.

Replication

In view of the various challenges to research validity, no study can be considered definitive. The body of scientific evidence about any problem derives validity from the collective results of multiple independent studies. As illustrated in Figure 1.1, when the preponderance of evidence from trustworthy studies converges on a particular answer to a research question, that answer is accepted as a functional understanding of the problem, pending convincing contradictory evidence. **Replication** refers to assessing whether consistent results are obtained from two or more studies using a design and procedures that are as similar as possible. While both the initial and replication studies may be conducted by the same researchers, the validity of replication results is enhanced if studies are conducted independently by different researchers, which controls for potential researcher bias that might enhance the similarity of results across studies.

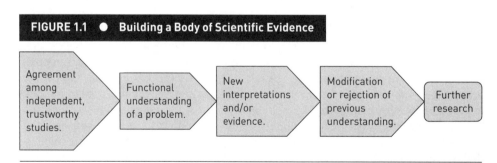

FIGURE 1.1 • Building a Body of Scientific Evidence

Sequential studies. Most often, replication studies are conducted sequentially. Exact replication across sequential studies is impossible because they are conducted in different time-related contexts. The more time that elapses between studies, the more likely their results will differ, for example owing to changes in social or political factors. Moreover, replication studies typically are conducted with different subjects and at different sites (e.g., different clinics, schools, or workplaces). Therefore, it is essential to take into account the potential that such factors might influence the comparability of results.

Simultaneous studies. A stronger replication approach is conducting simultaneous studies, as depicted in Figure 1.2. The most effective strategy for this approach is to divide an initial sample or pool of subjects randomly into **subsamples** of equal size so statistical power for analyzing results from the studies will be the same. Most often, it is not feasible to conduct simultaneous studies in the same setting owing to concern about contamination across studies. Instead, settings must be selected to be as similar as possible in terms of key characteristics that might be associated with the studies' results, such as high schools in the same geographic area with similar sociodemographic and academic profiles. Although replication across simultaneous studies may be conducted by the same research team, the best practice is for independent teams to conduct the replication studies. In comparison with sequential studies, an advantage of the simultaneous approach is it controls for potential differences in time-related contextual factors. However, an advantage of the sequential approach is it assesses the time invariance of results. Overall, the strongest replication evidence is derived when similar results are obtained from both approaches.

FIGURE 1.2 • Replication Across Simultaneous Studies

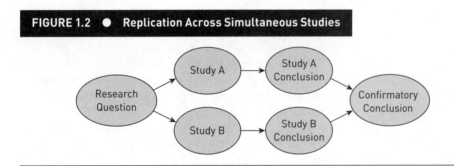

The Role of Theory

A **theory** is a conceptual model (sometimes called a **conceptual framework**) that identifies and defines key factors and describes relationships among them. Accordingly, it guides specifying the factors to measure and the factors to manipulate experimentally, planning data analysis, and interpreting results. Frequently used models of health behavior are the Health Belief Model (Rosenstock, Strecher, & Becker, 1988), the Theory of Planned Behavior (Ajzen, 1991), Social Cognitive Theory (Bandura, 2001), and the Social Ecological Model (McLeroy, Bibeau, Steckler, & Glanz, 1988). Although there are similarities among them, they differ in the factors and relationships they comprise.

> **Key Concept**
>
> *A theory is a conceptual model that identifies and defines key factors and describes relationships among them.*

Some models emphasize individual cognitive factors (e.g., Health Belief Model and Theory of Planned Behavior), while others emphasize social structural factors (e.g., Social Ecological Model). It is essential to be well acquainted with the various theoretical approaches that pertain to a particular problem in order to choose among them appropriately.

For example, suppose the Health Belief Model is chosen to guide developing and evaluating an intervention to increase the rate of mammography screening among a particular group of immigrant women. It would be posited that a woman is likely to obtain a mammogram if she perceives any of the following:

- She is susceptible to getting breast cancer (perceived susceptibility).
- Getting breast cancer will have a serious impact on her life situation (perceived seriousness/severity).
- Mammography is effective in detecting breast cancer early in its development (perceived benefits).
- She has access to obtain a mammogram (perceived barriers).
- She is capable of obtaining a mammogram (self-efficacy).

Therefore, each of those factors should be measured. Moreover, the intervention should be developed with the goal of influencing one or more of those factors in order to increase the likelihood that women who are exposed to it will get a mammogram.

Reasoning

Inductive reasoning

Inductive reasoning proceeds from empirical observations of specific instances to general conclusions. From an inductive perspective, the general research question may be stated as "What are the key factors that influence this problem, and how are they related?" Results from an inductive research approach may contribute to developing or modifying theories to guide further research, interventions, and policies. The term **grounded theory** refers to theory derived from interpreting empirical observations, rather than having been generated by speculation (Glaser & Strauss, 1967).

Most often, conducting research from an inductive perspective entails employing a fairly unstructured protocol to explore all aspects of a problem in a natural context. Such studies primarily collect **qualitative data** because there is insufficient understanding of the problem to guide collecting **quantitative data** (Chapter 13). For example, a study seeking to identify the key factors and relationships contributing to adolescent obesity might conduct unstructured individual interviews and/or focus groups with adolescents to explore their perceptions about various potential sources of influence on their food choices, such as peer pressure, body image, and the impact of obesity on health. Also, observations might be made of food choices and eating behavior in school lunchrooms.

Deductive reasoning

Deductive reasoning proceeds from general postulations derived from theory to specific predictions. From a deductive perspective, the general research question may be stated as "When certain factors are introduced or modified, do other factors that are expected to be related to them change in predictable ways?" A common application of deductive reasoning is evaluating an intervention or a policy. Conducting research from a deductive perspective typically entails employing a structured research protocol and collecting primarily quantitative data to test theory-based expectations (Chapter 15). Using a structured approach optimizes the validity of conclusions by controlling the data collection process and facilitating a standardized analysis. For example, the Theory of Planned Behavior might guide evaluating an intervention to prevent adolescent obesity by promoting healthy food choices in school lunchrooms. According to that theory, an effective intervention would be expected to promote positive attitudes toward eating healthy food to prevent obesity, promote a peer environment supportive of eating healthy food to prevent obesity, and enhance perceptions of behavioral control over food choices to prevent obesity.

A holistic perspective

The body of scientific evidence about any problem comprises contributions from both inductive and deductive perspectives. Moreover, a study may include aspects of both approaches, although typically one approach is emphasized. Figure 1.3 illustrates the general roles of inductive and deductive perspectives in research. Operating from the inductive perspective, observations are collected to explore a new problem or new aspects of an existing problem, which might lead to constructing a new or revised theory. Operating from the deductive perspective, observations are collected to test the validity of theory-based expectations about relationships or outcomes, which might lead to proposing policy/practice guidelines and directions for further research and/or theory development.

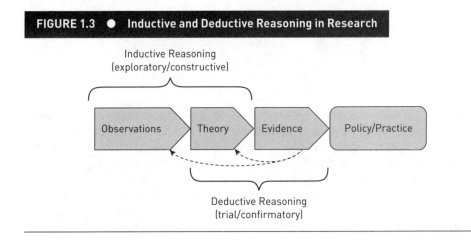

FIGURE 1.3 ● Inductive and Deductive Reasoning in Research

Inference

Most research studies do not include all members of a target population as subjects because doing so generally is prohibitively expensive, time-consuming, and logistically not feasible. For instance, it would not be reasonable to include all members of a population that includes hundreds of thousands or even millions of people, such as all high school students in a large city, all women age 50 or older in an urban county, or all adult cigarette smokers in the United States. Instead, most often research subjects are drawn in a sample, which is a subgroup selected to represent the target population (Chapter 7). Results from studying a sample are analyzed to draw inferences about what the results likely would have been had all members of the target population been studied. Figure 1.4 illustrates the **inference process** and introduces some key terms.

The set of entities targeted for a study is called a **population**. The individual entities in a population are called **elements**, which in most studies are individual people. However, other types of population elements may be studied, such as households, schools, and health clinics. Common notation uses capital Roman or Greek letters to designate population features. For example, N designates the number of population elements. Aggregate population characteristics are called **parameters**. For example, P_i (pronounced "P-sub-i") designates a population proportion with a particular characteristic (e.g., the proportion of middle school students participating in a school lunch program), and μ (Greek "mu") designates the population mean (i.e., arithmetic average) for a characteristic, such as the mean

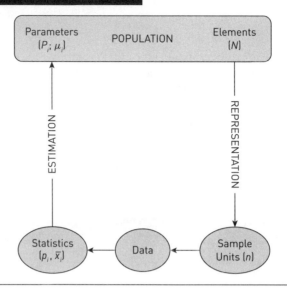

FIGURE 1.4 ● The Inference Process

number of fruit servings consumed per week by middle school lunch program participants. The subscript $_i$ indicates a proportion (P_i) or mean (μ_i) may be derived for more than one parameter. For example, for a population of middle school students, (P_1) might indicate the proportion participating in a school lunch program, (P_2) might indicate the proportion that is overweight, and (P_3) might indicate the proportion that is physically active.

Whenever possible, random sampling procedures (Chapter 7) generally are preferred for selecting a representative sample from a target population. The population elements to be included in a sample are called **sampling units**, which might be individual people, households, schools, or other entities, according to how the population elements are specified. While N designates the **population size**, n designates the **sample size**, the number of sampling units selected in a sample. Data are collected from or about the sampling units, and analyses are conducted to describe a sample's characteristics, called **statistics**, which are used to estimate corresponding population parameters.

The term *statistics* commonly is used to refer to analytical procedures, such as Student's *t* test (to assess differences between two means) (Chapter 15). However, technically those procedures are applied to data about sample characteristics (i.e., statistics), from which the generalized application of the term *statistics* to the analytical procedures is derived. According to common notation, lowercase Roman letters designate sample features. Accordingly, p_i designates the sample proportion with a particular characteristic and $\bar{x}_i$ (pronounced "x-bar sub-i") designates the sample mean for a characteristic. Thus, for example, the sample proportion of middle school students participating in a school lunch program (a statistic) would be used to estimate the proportion of middle school students participating in a school lunch program in the target population (a parameter).

For example, as shown in Table 1.1, if 40% of middle school students in a sample participate in a school lunch program, it would be estimated that approximately 40% of the population of middle school students participate in a school lunch program. Similarly, if the mean number of fruit servings consumed per middle school lunch program participant in a sample is 2.6 servings per week, then it would be estimated that the mean number of fruit servings consumed in the population of middle school students is approximately 2.6 servings per week. As described in Chapter 7, another aspect of making such inferences

TABLE 1.1 ● **Inferences From Sample Statistics to Population Parameter Estimates**

Variable	Sample Statistic	Inference Direction	Population Parameter Estimate[a]
Proportion of middle school students participating in a school lunch program	$p = .40$ (40%)	→	$\hat{p} = .40$ (40%)
Mean number of fruit servings consumed per week per middle school lunch program participant	$\bar{x}_i = 2.6$	→	$\hat{\mu} = 2.6$
Difference in mean number of fruit servings consumed per week by middle school lunch program participants (1) vs. nonparticipants (2)	$\bar{x}_1 - \bar{x}_2 = 0.7$	→	$\hat{\mu}_1 - \hat{\mu}_2 = 0.7$
Correlation between number of fruit servings consumed per week and body mass index (BMI) among middle school lunch program participants	$r = .35$	→	$\hat{r} = .35$

Note: The ^ symbol above a character representing a population parameter indicates the value is an estimate rather than the parameter's true value, which typically is not known when conducting a research study.

is computing confidence intervals for parameter estimates to account for variation in the random sampling process. Table 1.1 also illustrates that the inference process may be used to estimate a group difference and a correlation between variables.

Research Validity

In the research context, validity refers to the extent to which there is confidence in drawing conclusions based on research results. Validity is of the utmost importance in health research, where results may have a substantial impact on the health and well-being of many people. **Research validity** is a function of all aspects of how a study is designed, conducted, and analyzed. In general, the main factors that affect a study's validity are the following:

- Fit of the research design to the research problem
- Number and types of study groups
- Number and timing of observation points
- Number and types of subjects who participate
- Cooperation of subjects with a study protocol
- Setting(s) where a study is conducted
- Measurement instruments and procedures
- Analytical procedures

There is no definitive approach to assessing research validity. Thus, it is imperative to understand the research process and the factors that may influence validity.

Ultimately, a study's strengths are weighed against its weaknesses and limitations. All studies have weaknesses of some kind. Common examples are procedural variations (e.g., not implementing a data collection protocol consistently from one setting to another) and unavoidable, unanticipated problems (e.g., not being able to contact some subjects due to inclement weather). Moreover, virtually all studies have one or more limitations in the research plan. For example, instead of studying all schoolchildren in the United States, a study might be limited to those attending public schools and/or schools within a certain geographic area.

> **CHECK YOUR UNDERSTANDING 1.1**
>
> - List and briefly describe the major research objectives and their purpose.
> - Identify the key aspects of the scientific approach and describe how they contribute to obtaining valid results.
> - Describe the role of theory in planning a study and interpreting results.
> - Describe the two types of reasoning and their role in research.
> - Identify the inference process components and describe how they are related.
> - Describe the major determinants of research validity.

The Research Process

Figure 1.5 depicts the general process for planning and conducting a study. Research results often lead to specifying new research questions to be addressed in subsequent studies. Consequently, most studies are conducted in a context whereby they are preceded by other studies about the same or a related problem. Thus, the **research process** is a cyclical approach to building a valid body of scientific evidence about a particular problem.

> **Key Concept**
>
> A body of valid scientific evidence is developed by cycling through the research process.

Problem Statement

A study starts a **problem statement** identifying what is to be investigated. The more specifically the problem is stated, the better it provides guidance for the rest of the process. For example, Box 1.3 presents two statements about the same general problem. Statement A is an inadequate guide for planning a study because it does not specify the nature of the racial disparity in mammography screening rates or among which U.S. women the disparity is present. In contrast, statement B is more useful because it specifies three key aspects of the problem: (1) It focuses on women in a certain age group (50–74), (2) it identifies Asians as the main racial group of concern, and (3) it specifies the outcome criterion as the rate of self-reporting having a mammogram within the past two years.

Specifying a problem statement typically draws on a variety of sources. The process might begin with informal observation, such as noticing matters regarding health issues experienced professionally or personally, and reports in the news media (e.g., about an outbreak of gun violence). The most familiar source is a **literature review** to understand the current state of scientific understanding about a particular problem. A literature review might reveal important gaps or limitations in previous studies, such as populations that have not been represented adequately, or at all. Also, it might reveal contradictory results

FIGURE 1.5 ● The Research Process

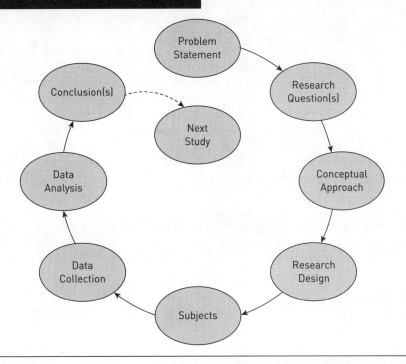

BOX 1.3: PROBLEM STATEMENTS

Problem Statement A

There is a racial disparity in mammography screening rates among women in the United States.

Problem Statement B

Among women aged 50–74 in the United States, Asian women have the lowest percentage who report having a mammogram within the past two years (Centers for Disease Control and Prevention, 2012).

that should be reconciled. Although most attention is given to publications in professional journals, it is important not to overlook presentations at professional conferences and reports from government and nonprofit agencies. Another valuable resource for specifying a research problem is consulting experts of various types. These include colleagues who are conducting research on the same or related issues, practicing health and social services professionals, and members of the prospective target population.

Research Question

The **research question** specifies the purpose and focus of a study. As such, it is the foundation for planning all the subsequent aspects of the research process. While typically there are multiple facets of virtually any problem, the research question specifies which

Key Concept

The research question is the foundation for all the subsequent aspects of the research process.

one(s) will be the focus for a particular study. Therefore, it is essential to state a research question clearly and specifically to guide developing and implementing a research plan.

Box 1.4 presents a research question corresponding to problem statement B from Box 1.3, specifying that a study will seek to identify the primary factors (rather than all factors) that account for the racial disparity in mammography screening. Also, it indicates the study will be exploratory in nature rather than one that will evaluate an intervention, for example. However, it does not specify the potential factors about which data should be collected. The next stage of the research process, specifying a conceptual approach, provides that guidance.

BOX 1.4: A RESEARCH QUESTION

What are the primary factors that account for Asian women aged 50–74 years in the United States having a lower percentage who report having a mammogram within the past two years than women of the same age in other racial groups in the United States?

Conceptual Approach

The **conceptual approach** specifies the key factors that will be studied and describes expected relationships among them. Thus, it guides identifying the variables to measure, developing a data collection plan, and developing a data analysis plan. Moreover, by specifying how key factors are expected to relate to one another, it guides interpreting a study's result, formulating conclusions, and proposing recommendations for policy, practice, and subsequent research.

A conceptual approach is derived by reviewing theories relevant to the research problem. Then, based on logic and previous research, the one that appears most appropriate for addressing the research question is selected. For example, to investigate a racial disparity in mammography screening among women in the United States, a theory would be considered that may be applied to understanding the process of engaging in health screening behavior, such as the Health Belief Model (Rosenstock et al., 1988) or the Theory of Planned Behavior (Ajzen, 1991). Although there are similarities among these theories, as summarized in Box 1.5, they differ in their key concepts and relationships. When conducting an exploratory study, it is wise to collect data about as many potentially key variables as is feasible to avoid overlooking them. Accordingly, a study to identify the primary factors that account for a racial disparity in mammography screening might collect data about the key factors specified by both the Health Belief Model and the Theory of Planned Behavior, and then assess which theory best fits the data.

Research Design

The **research design** specifies the pattern for how a study will be conducted. In general, a design comprises two main elements: the number and types of study groups and the number and timing of observation points. Research designs are discussed in detail in Chapters 4–6.

BOX 1.5: TWO CONCEPTUAL APPROACHES FOR ADDRESSING THE SAME RESEARCH PROBLEM AND RESEARCH QUESTION

Health Belief Model	Theory of Planned Behavior
Perceived susceptibility for getting breast cancer	Expectation about the outcome of getting a mammogram to detect breast cancer early
Perceived seriousness of getting breast cancer	Value of detecting breast cancer early
Perceived benefits of detecting breast cancer early	Perceptions of others' beliefs about getting a mammogram
Perceived barriers to obtaining a mammogram	Motivation to comply with others' beliefs
Self-efficacy to obtain a mammogram	Perceived control to perform the behavior of obtaining a mammogram

Subjects

The next stage in the research process involves specifying who will be the subjects and how they will be selected (Chapter 7). This stage involves specifying five key characteristics about subjects:

- Target population
- Units of study
- Inclusion/exclusion criteria
- Selection procedure
- Sample size

Target population

The **target population** is the set of entities (people or other elements) for which a study will seek to answer the research question. For example, to address the research question about a racial disparity in mammography screening, a study must include subjects who are Asian women in the United States aged 50–74. However, if only subjects with those characteristics were included, a study would not be able to identify effectively the primary factors that account for the racial discrepancy. That is because it would not be able to distinguish how Asian women differ from women in other racial groups in terms of the factors the conceptual approach posits might be related to mammography screening. Therefore, it would be essential also to include subjects who are women in the United States aged 50–74 but not Asian.

The most comprehensive approach would include women from all other racial groups, specifying the target population as all women in the United States aged 50–74. However, the more diverse the target population, the more challenging and expensive it likely will be to study. Greater diversity (i.e., variance) among the target population requires a larger sample size (Chapter 7). Also, it might require employing multiple strategies for selecting and recruiting subjects and collecting data. Finally, a more complex data analysis plan is necessary to assess differences across multiple groups. An alternative approach would be to focus on comparing only the two groups for which the disparity in mammography screening rates is highest: Asian and Black/African American women (Centers for Disease Control and Prevention, 2012). That approach would simplify the research plan, be more feasible to implement, and provide a more sensitive contrast. Accordingly, the target population would be specified as Asian and Black/African American women in the United States aged 50–74.

Units of study

The **units of study** are the entities in the target population about which a study will collect and analyze data. For instance, in a study about a racial disparity in mammography screening, the units of study likely will be individual women. However, the units of study also may be entities in which individuals are clustered, such as families, schools, workplaces, or health clinics. As will be discussed regarding cluster sampling design in Chapter 7, the most challenging situation is when the units of study are nested within other units. For example, a study of elementary school students might first select a sample of school districts, then schools within districts, then classes within schools, and finally individual students.

Inclusion/exclusion criteria

Every study must specify subject eligibility criteria. **Inclusion criteria** are characteristics target population members must meet to be eligible as subjects. **Exclusion criteria** are characteristics that disqualify target population members as subjects. Inclusion and exclusion criteria may be based on a variety of factors, including personal attributes (e.g., age, gender, race, health status, health history), behavior (e.g., use of certain services, alcohol consumption, tobacco use), and ability to participate (e.g., availability during the study time period, language proficiency, availability via a particular technological mode such as the internet). Typically, they include several factors in combination.

All target population members should be included unless there is a compelling reason for excluding them. Therefore, the rationale for invoking exclusion criteria must be considered carefully because they restrict the population to which results may be applied. Moreover, an important ethical concern (Chapter 2) is to avoid an inequitable exclusion of target population members. Generally, it is best to specify inclusion criteria first to ensure including as many target population members as possible and then specify exclusion criteria as appropriate. For example, to study a racial disparity in mammography screening among all women in the United States aged 50–74, inclusion criteria might be specified simply by reflecting the research problem and the research question: being women, residing in the United States, and being 50–74 years old.

Exclusion criteria should specify conditions other than those that do not meet the inclusion criteria and thus are redundant (e.g., not being a woman). A common reason for invoking an exclusion criterion is it would be inappropriate to include certain target population members. For example, to study a racial disparity in mammography screening, it would be reasonable to exclude women who already have been diagnosed with breast cancer. Also, in view of the research question's focus on having a mammogram within the past two years, it would be appropriate to exclude women who have not resided in the United States for at least two years.

Other exclusion criteria may be based on logistic factors, such as the data collection mode that will be employed. For instance, if data will be collected conducting in-person interviews, which are expensive and time-consuming, resource limitations might require excluding target population members who reside outside a prescribed geographic area to keep travel expenses and time manageable. Another common exclusion criterion is if subjects are not capable of participating in the study, such as not being sufficiently proficient in the language(s) that will be employed to collect data. Box 1.6 presents an example of inclusion and exclusion criteria for a study of a racial disparity in mammography screening among women in the United States aged 50–74. The criteria are based on the examples in the preceding paragraphs.

> **BOX 1.6: EXAMPLE OF INCLUSION AND EXCLUSION CRITERIA FOR A STUDY OF A RACIAL DISPARITY IN MAMMOGRAPHY SCREENING**
>
> | Inclusion Criteria | Exclusion Criteria |
> |---|---|
> | • Woman | • Diagnosed with breast cancer |
> | • U.S. resident | • U.S. resident for less than two years |
> | • Aged 50–74 | • Not proficient speaking English or Spanish |

Selection procedure

The main subject selection decision is whether to use a random or nonrandom procedure. In general, random selection provides more reliable target population inferences than nonrandom selection (Chapter 7). Nevertheless, there are situations where nonrandom selection not only is acceptable but might be preferred over random selection, such as when conducting exploratory research using primarily qualitative data collection methods (Chapter 13). Moreover, there are some situations where it is impossible, or nearly impossible, to select a sample randomly.

Sample size

Finally, the number of subjects to include must be specified. Specific strategies for determining sample size are discussed in Chapter 7. The main issue that must be addressed regarding sample size is determining the number of subjects sufficient to provide a trustworthy answer to the research question.

Data Collection

The **data collection** stage of the research process is particularly critical because it provides the information to answer the research question. Moreover, it typically involves the largest investment of resources and often is a point of no return. If serious problems are encountered after data collection is well under way, in most instances a study is not likely to have sufficient unexpended resources available to restart data collection with a revised protocol.

Key variables

It is essential to collect data about all the key variables specified by the research question and the conceptual approach. In addition, data should be collected about relevant background and contextual variables that might enhance understanding relationships among key variables. Care should be taken not to divert a study's focus and resources from the key variables at the expense of collecting data about variables that may be tangentially relevant to the research question.

Subjects

The data collection plan must be appropriate for the target population to secure constructive participation in a study. The first factor to consider is whether the intended subjects will be *able* to participate in the data collection process. For example, if a study will ask subjects to complete a questionnaire online (i.e., a web survey), target population members without internet access will not be able to participate. A second factor is whether the subjects will be *willing* to participate in the data collection process. For instance, some might decline an invitation to participate in a web survey if they do not think it is worth the investment of their time and effort.

Method

Many data collection methods (also referred to as "modes") are available. Taking resources into consideration, in general, a study should employ the data collection method that will provide the most valid and reliable measures (Chapter 8) of the key variables. The most substantial distinction among data collection methods is whether the type of data they typically collect is primarily qualitative or quantitative. No single method generally is best in all situations. Indeed, it is becoming increasingly common to employ mixed methods (Chapter 13), such as conducting focus groups in conjunction with a survey.

Data Analysis

Although data analysis is the last stage in the research process prior to drawing conclusions, it is vital to consider the analysis plan throughout the research process. Not attending to the analysis plan until data collection is complete introduces a serious risk of not being able to conduct the analysis that most effectively addresses the research question. Such a situation might occur owing to factors such as an avoidable deficiency in the research design, an unnecessary limitation in the subject selection plan, failing to collect data about a key variable, or not employing the most effective measurement strategy. It is too late to change such aspects of a study when data collection is complete.

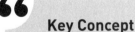

Key Concept

Consider the data analysis plan throughout the research process.

Before implementing a research plan, it is useful to review it in reverse order. Using that approach, first the data necessary to conduct an appropriate analysis is specified. Next, each preceding stage in the research process is reviewed to ensure the plan for that stage will lead to obtaining the necessary data. For instance, one may assess whether the data collection plan effectively will measure the key variables, the types of subjects are relevant for addressing the research question, and the research design is appropriate for conducting the planned analysis.

Conclusions

It might appear it is not possible to plan for the conclusions of a study until it is virtually complete. However, conclusions often may be anticipated based on theory and previous research. When planning a study, it is helpful to consider whether anticipated conclusions coincide with the problem statement and research question to ensure the research plan is focused appropriately. Also, consideration may be given to how a study's conclusions might guide planning a next study.

Next Study

After completing a study, consideration should be given to what might be the focus of a next study about the research problem and what subsequent research question(s) might be addressed. For example, when addressing the research question in Box 1.4, suppose results indicate social support is a primary factor for a disparity in mammography screening. In that case, the next research question might be "Are 50- to 74-year-old Asian women in the United States who participate in a program to enhance social support for obtaining a mammogram more likely to obtain a mammogram within the next two years?" Four questions generally are useful to ask when considering the focus of a next study:

- What was learned from the completed study that is trustworthy?
- What results from the completed study are questionable (e.g., do not fit the conceptual approach, appear counterintuitive, or contradict other results)?
- What aspects of the research problem merit further investigation?
- What new information would advance understanding the research problem?

Pilot Study

A **pilot study** is a small-scale, developmental study that may be conducted to assess the feasibility of and plan a larger-scale study. Box 1.7 presents four sets of common pilot study conditions and goals.

BOX 1.7: PILOT STUDY CONDITIONS AND GOALS

Conditions	Goals
Exploring a problem	Explore the nature and scope of an emergent problem
	Explore a new aspect of an existing problem
	Specify/refine research questions
Developing/refining an intervention	Assess potential effectiveness
	Develop/refine subject recruitment strategy
	Explore media alternatives
	Assess/refine delivery protocol
	Assess target population acceptance
	Assess feasibility of venues
Developing/refining a research method	Develop/refine subject selection strategy
	Develop/refine data collection protocol
	Develop/refine measurement instrument
	Develop/refine data processing/analysis strategy
Planning a large, complex study	Demonstrate potential significance
	Demonstrate feasibility
	Gain experience and demonstrate competence
	Specify administrative components

Plan and design

Sometimes a pilot study may be a complete study. Other times it may focus on developing and assessing one or more components of a research plan. Examples of such situations include assessing potential sites, negotiating access to and assessing the quality of records, estimating the number of eligible potential subjects in a target population, and developing a measurement instrument.

Subjects

When feasible, pilot study subjects should be selected from the future study target population. The best practice is *not* to include pilot study subjects also as subjects in the future study to avoid bias owing to participating in the pilot study. Sometimes the target population is small, such that selecting pilot study subjects from it would deplete the pool of subjects for a subsequent study. In that situation, pilot study subjects might be selected from another population, such as from another community with similar characteristics in the same city. The number of pilot study subjects typically ranges from about 30 to 100. However, more subjects may be included when planning a large, complex study, such as a nationwide interview survey.

Sites

In general, it is best to conduct a pilot study at the same site(s) that will be included in the future study. It is especially important for a pilot study to include sites with which there is little or no experience, or that might present a particular challenge. However, it is best not to include the same sites in a pilot study and in a future study if the pilot study might cause them to change in a way that is relevant to the research question. For example, conducting a pilot test of an intervention might change the way clinic staff subsequently interact with all patients of a certain type. Consequently, subjects assigned to a control condition for a future study might receive some or all aspects of an intervention that is being assessed. When feasible, that threat to validity may be avoided by conducting a pilot study at one or more alternative sites with similar characteristics (e.g., size, type, and location) as the future study site(s). If the future study will include multiple sites, an alternative strategy is to include only a representative sample of sites in the pilot study. When analyzing results from the main study, it should be assessed whether there are any systematic differences between pilot study sites and those that are included only in the main study. If such differences are detected, they should be taken into account when interpreting a study's result.

Data

The best practice is *not* to merge pilot study data with the future study data. When the number of future study subjects will be large, little is gained in analytic power by merging data from the typically small number of pilot study subjects with the future study data. Moreover, pilot study data and the future study data often may not be compatible for several reasons:

- A pilot study might not be a complete study.
- All aspects of a pilot study are not necessarily implemented in a manner identical with the future study plan.
- The time frame and conditions under which a pilot study is conducted will be different than for the future study.
- Based on the pilot study experience, the future study plan is likely to be revised.

Assessment

When assessing pilot study outcomes, it is common to seek answers to three questions:

- Is a future study worthwhile?
- How can a future study be conducted most effectively?
- How can a future study be conducted most efficiently?

First, the potential significance and return on investment for a future study should be assessed. In doing so, it is important to be mindful that owing to a smaller size a pilot study will not demonstrate outcomes at the same level of statistical significance as a larger study (Chapter 15). Second, potential factors that might threaten a future study's validity should be identified and strategies developed to address them in a future study. Examples are refining an intervention protocol and assessing alternative data collection strategies. Also, pilot study data may be used to estimate variance for key variables or the size of a treatment effect, which are important components for estimating sample size and statistical power for a future study (Chapter 7).

Third, a pilot study may provide valuable experience for refining logistic aspects that will affect the efficiency of a future, large-scale study, such as strategies for gaining access to sites, procedures for selecting and recruiting subjects, coordinating with external collaborators, and supervising data collection staff. Moreover, pilot study data provide a foundation for developing or refining an analysis plan, such as devising a coding scheme for administrative records, identifying potential confounding variables, planning subgroup analyses, or developing a preliminary multiple regression model. Finally, a valuable pilot study outcome is it provides an experiential foundation for refining budget and time schedule estimates.

CHECK YOUR UNDERSTANDING 1.2

- List and briefly describe the stages of the research process.
- Describe how the research process stages are interrelated.
- Describe the general characteristics and purposes for conducting a pilot study.

Key Points

The Nature of Research

Research Objectives

The course of studying a particular problem generally entails a progressive series of studies with different objectives.

The Scientific Approach

Research seeks to derive valid conclusions by following certain principles throughout the research process: objectivity, control, and replication.

The Role of Theory

A theory is a conceptual model that identifies and defines key factors and describes relationships among them.

Reasoning

Inductive reasoning proceeds from empirical observations of specific instances to general conclusions.
Deductive reasoning proceeds from general theoretical postulations to specific predictions about a particular problem.

Inference

Most often, a study focuses on a sample selected from a target population. A sample's characteristics (statistics) are analyzed to draw inferences about the population's characteristics (parameters).

Research Validity

Research validity is the extent to which there is confidence in drawing conclusions based on research results. It is a function of all aspects of how a study is designed, conducted, analyzed, and reported.

The Research Process

The research process is a cyclical approach to building a valid body of scientific evidence about a particular problem. It comprises the following major stages:

- Problem statement
- Research question
- Conceptual approach
- Research design
- Subjects
- Data collection
- Data analysis
- Conclusions
- Next study
- Pilot study (optional)

Review and Apply

Identify a health-related problem that interests you or choose one from U.S. Department of Health and Human Services, *Healthy People 2020 Leading Health Indicators: Progress Update*, available at https://www.healthypeople.gov/2020/leading-health-indicators/Healthy-People-2020-Leading-Health-Indicators%3A-Progress-Update.

1. Write a problem statement.
2. Conduct a brief search of the research literature about the problem and describe why it is important.
3. Choose a theory you consider appropriate to guide research about the problem, identify its key factors, and describe how they are related.

4. Write a research question to address the problem.

5. If you were to plan a study to address your research question:

   a. What key variables would you measure?
   b. How many and what types of study groups would your research design include?
   c. Would you collect data at one observation point or more than one?
   d. What would be the target population and the units of study?
   e. What inclusion and exclusion criteria would you specify?
   f. Would you collect qualitative, quantitative, or both kinds of data?
   g. Without getting into technical statistical aspects, what general type of analysis would be appropriate to answer your research question?
   h. Review your research plan in reverse order, beginning at the data analysis stage. Did you make any changes in your research plan? If so, why?

6. How might your research plan benefit from conducting a pilot study? Be specific in identifying aspects of your research plan that you might assess in a pilot study.

Study Further

Fink, A. G. (2014). *Conducting research literature reviews: From the internet to paper* (4th ed.). Thousand Oaks, CA: Sage.

Glanz, K., Rimer, B. K., & Viswanath, K. (2015). Theory, research, and practice in health behavior. In K. Glanz, B. K. Rimer, & K. Viswanath (Eds.), *Health behavior: Theory, research, and practice* (5th ed., pp. 23–42). San Francisco, CA: Jossey-Bass.

Rychetnik, L., & Frommer, M. A. (2002). *A schema for evaluating evidence on public health interventions* (version 4). Melbourne, Australia: National Public Health Partnership. Retrieved from http://www.health.vic.gov.au/archive/archive2014/nphp/publications/phpractice/schemaV4.pdf

U.S. Department of Health and Human Services. (2018, last updated March 8). *Definitions of criteria and considerations for research project grant (RPG/X01/R01/R03/R21/R33/R34) critiques*. Retrieved from https://grants.nih.gov/grants/peer/critiques/rpg_D.htm

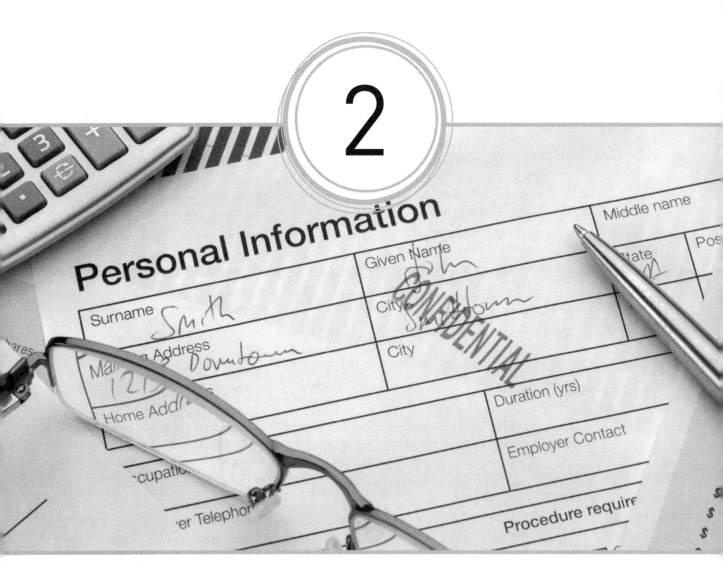

2

Conducting Ethically Responsible Research

Chapter Outline

Overview
Learning Objectives
Ethical Principles of Research With Human Subjects
    Respect for Persons
    Beneficence
    Justice
Federal Regulations and the IRB
    The Common Rule
    Institutional Review Board (IRB)
    Training
    Informed Consent
    Proposed Changes in Federal Regulations
Privacy Protection
    Privacy
    Anonymity
    Uses of Identifiers
    Maintaining Confidentiality
Key Points

Learning Objectives

After studying Chapter 2, the reader should be able to:

- Identify and apply the three ethical principles of human subjects research
- Identify and describe the three types of potential research harms
- Assess relative risks and benefits of human subjects research
- Differentiate the three types of institutional review board (IRB) review
- Identify the key elements that should be included in an IRB protocol
- Comply with requirements for training in protecting human subjects
- Summarize the basic elements and process of informed consent
- Implement procedures to protect the privacy of research information

Overview

A critical aspect of the validity of research involving human subjects in health-related research is individuals' trust and willingness to participate. Human subjects must always be treated with respect and protected from potential participation-associated risks to the extent feasible. Most importantly, prior to participating, they must be informed about what participation entails and any associated potential risks or benefits. Research involving human subjects must comply with well-defined principles and a diligent oversight process.

Ethical Principles of Research With Human Subjects

Subsequent to the termination of the Tuskegee syphilis study (Box 2.1), in 1974 the National Research Act (PL 93-348) created the National Commission for the Protection of Human Subjects of Biomedical and Behavioral Research. The commission was charged to identify basic ethical principles for conducting biomedical and behavioral **research** involving **human subjects**, and to develop guidelines for ensuring that research is conducted accordingly. In the ***Belmont Report*** (1979), the Commission delineated three principles that provide the current ethical framework for conducting research with human subjects:

> **Key Concept**
>
> *The* Belmont Report *delineated three principles that guide ethical practice for conducting human subjects research.*

- **Respect for persons:** Individuals should be treated as autonomous agents, and persons with diminished autonomy should be protected.
- **Beneficence:** Possible benefits should be maximized, and possible harms should be minimized.
- **Justice:** The burdens and benefits of participating in research should be distributed fairly.

BOX 2.1: SUMMARY OF THE TUSKEGEE STUDY

Current standards for ethical treatment of human research subjects were established in response to several widely publicized cases of abuse. One of the most infamous of these was the Tuskegee Study of Untreated Syphilis in the Negro Male, conducted by the U.S. Public Health Service between 1932 and 1972 to study the natural progression of untreated syphilis.

Subjects were 600 African American men in rural Alabama who were told they were being treated for "bad blood," a vague colloquial term for various ailments, and enticed by incentives including free medical examinations, meals on examination days, and a burial stipend. They were not informed about the true purpose and nature of the study, or about the risks associated with participation. Among the participants, 399 who contracted syphilis prior to or during the study were not told they had the disease, and they were neither provided treatment nor informed about available treatment (although by 1947 penicillin had become the standard treatment for syphilis, it was withheld as a part of the study).

Owing to press exposure in 1972, the study was terminated, 40 years after it began and 25 years after an effective treatment for syphilis became available. By that time, many of the infected subjects had died from the disease directly or from related health problems. Also, many family members and others had become infected with syphilis through contact with the infected men.

Respect for Persons
Self-determination

Individuals have a right to decide whether to participate in research. Participation should be *voluntary* and based on adequate information about what research participation involves. The primary procedure for implementing this principle is the process of **informed consent**, which is discussed later in this chapter. Individuals who are not capable of appropriately exercising self-determination, such as children and cognitively impaired adults, should be protected from undue influence to participate in research.

Human subjects should not be recruited through explicit or implied coercion. For example, participation should not be required by an agent of authority, such as a workplace supervisor, school principal, or clinic administrator. Also, care should be taken that individuals who choose not to participate in research do not reasonably perceive that their choice might result in negative consequences. For instance, deciding not to participate in research should not diminish workers' expectations of opportunities for career advancement, students' expectations of opportunities to participate in special activities, or patients' expectations of their ability to access quality health care as needed. A related concern is that incentives (e.g., money, gifts, or services) offered to induce individuals to participate in research sometimes might influence them to consent to an activity in which they otherwise would not engage. In particular, this issue arises when the value of an incentive is disproportionately large relative to the participation burden, and when subjects are financially or otherwise disadvantaged.

Vulnerable populations

Special protections should be provided for individuals who are vulnerable to manipulation owing to reasons such as diminished cognitive capacity, a power differential, or a lack of resources. Such conditions may be related to characteristics of individuals or situations, and they may be temporary or permanent. Part C.3 of the *Belmont Report* (1979) defines individuals in a **vulnerable population** as those such as racial minorities, the economically disadvantaged, the very sick, and the institutionalized, who may be manipulated owing to being readily available in a research setting, their dependent status, and/or their diminished capacity to freely consent. Department of Health and Human Services (DHHS) regulations governing protection of human subjects in research (45 CFR part 46) specify that special protections should be provided for the following vulnerable groups of subjects:

- Pregnant women (subpart B)
- Prisoners (subpart C)
- Children (subpart D)

In addition, researchers and institutions may designate other groups as vulnerable, such as students or employees of the institution conducting research. The particular special protections that should be implemented for vulnerable groups depend on the nature and degree of their vulnerability and the nature of the research. Examples of such protections are subjects' advocates, monitoring by external agents, limiting the scope of a research protocol, and renewing consent at specified stages of a study.

Beneficence

There are two aspects to the **beneficence** principle. First, it specifies that any *possible benefits* should be *maximized*. It does not require that human subjects necessarily should derive any benefits from participating in research. Second, it specifies that any *possible risks* should be *minimized*. It does not require that human subjects' participation in research should be risk free. In some situations, human subjects might not derive any benefit from participating in research, and it might not be possible to conduct a study in a manner such that there is no risk to human subjects. The beneficence principle requires assessing the possible benefits against the possible risks for human subjects.

Benefits

There are two types of possible research benefits: benefits to subjects and benefits to others. **Subjects** might derive *direct benefits* such as learning about warning signs for heart disease, being helped to stop a risky health behavior (e.g., smoking cigarettes), or being aided to adopt a health-promotive behavior (e.g., regular physical activity). Incentives to induce subjects to participate in research, or compensation for travel or other expenses related to their participation, should not be considered as benefits of participating in a study. Subjects might derive *indirect benefits*, such as ones that might be realized from providing information that contributes to improving conditions in their community (e.g., developing strategies for reducing street violence or improving access to health services). Typically, it is impossible to guarantee subjects will realize any benefits because the purpose of research is to identify and assess *potentially* effective strategies to address existing problems. Also, while it is not feasible to identify all possible benefits in advance of conducting a study, all reasonable possible benefits should be identified.

Participating in research might benefit other people by contributing to a body of generalizable knowledge about a problem. For example, research about knowledge, attitudes, and behaviors of subjects diagnosed as HIV-positive might lead to developing strategies to prevent others from being infected. Obviously, such research will not benefit the research subjects who already are infected. Nevertheless, such contributions should be considered when assessing the possible benefits of conducting a study.

Risks

Research should be planned and conducted to minimize possible risks to human subjects. Federal regulations (45 CFR part 46.102.h.1) define **minimal risk** as follows:

> The probability and magnitude of harm or discomfort anticipated in the research are not greater in and of themselves than those ordinarily encountered in daily life or during the performance of routine physical or psychological examinations or tests.

It often is not possible to conduct research risk free or even to identify all possible risks in advance. For instance, among the reasons for evaluating an innovative intervention is to identify possible negative outcomes associated with it.

Assessing risks

Any risk beyond minimal risk that reasonably may be anticipated should be assessed as to whether a study's potential benefits justify exposing subjects to it. For each risk, the assessment should consider the probability it actually will cause harm or discomfort, the number of subjects who might incur harm or discomfort, and the nature of the possible harm or discomfort (severity, duration, and treatability). Consideration should be given to whether a risk might be minimized or avoided, for example by employing an alternative research strategy or incorporating safeguards, such as monitoring by external agents.

Justice

Inclusion

All target population members should be eligible for being included in a research study unless there is a justifiable reason for excluding them, such as a scientifically valid purpose or to protect a vulnerable population from unwarranted risks. For example, when conducting research about a racial disparity in mammography screening among women, it would be appropriate to exclude men as subjects. However, excluding a major racial group from such a study without compelling justification would violate the **justice** principle.

Treatment

Subjects should be treated equitably while participating in a research study. Whenever possible, experimental research subjects should be given equal opportunity to be assigned to treatment and control conditions. Unless there is a justifiable reason, no subgroup should be given preference for receiving a potentially beneficial treatment, nor should any subgroup be systematically denied an opportunity to receive a treatment. Random assignment (Chapter 7) is the most effective strategy for equitably assigning subjects to study conditions. Also, the distribution of participation incentives and reimbursements for participation-related expenses should be equitable, in terms of both the opportunity to receive them and their value.

> ### CHECK YOUR UNDERSTANDING 2.1
>
> - Identify and briefly describe the three ethical principles for conducting research with human subjects delineated in the *Belmont Report* (1979).
> - Write a definition of *minimal risk* in your own words and compare it with its specification by federal regulations in 45 CFR part 46.102.h.1.

Federal Regulations and the IRB

The Common Rule

DHHS regulations (45 CFR part 46, subpart A), known as the **Common Rule**, are based largely on the *Belmont Report*. The Common Rule specifies basic protections for human subjects in biomedical and behavioral research that is

- sponsored by a federal agency;
- conducted by investigators at institutions that receive federal funding, regardless of whether a particular study is supported by federal funding;
- conducted within or outside the United States (if either of the first two conditions applies); or
- conducted by investigators employed by institutions that require compliance with the federal policy, regardless of funding sources.

The Common Rule applies to research conducted by virtually all academic institutions and agencies affiliated with them. It outlines basic requirements for reviewing and criteria for approving protocols for research with human subjects. Individual institutions where research is conducted have discretion in establishing policies and procedures for implementing the Common Rule, with oversight by the U.S. Office for Human Research Protections (OHRP) (research involving drugs is monitored by the U.S. Food and Drug Administration, or FDA).

The Common Rule specifies the following definitions of research and human subjects, which are keys

> **Key Concept**
>
> *The Common Rule specifies basic protections for human subjects.*

to determining whether an activity is subject to regulations about research with human subjects:

- *Research* (45 CFR part 46.102.d): "A systematic investigation, including research development, testing and evaluation, designed to develop or contribute to generalizable knowledge."
- *Human subject* (45 CFR part 46.102.f): "A living individual about whom an investigator (whether professional or student) conducting research obtains (1) Data through intervention or interaction with the individual, or (2) Identifiable private information."

In most situations, the key factor in the research definition is the phrase "designed to develop or contribute to generalizable knowledge." For example, suppose college administrative staff collect and analyze data about students' demographic characteristics and academic performance. If the sole purpose is to conduct an internal assessment of administrative policies about matters such as recruiting and grading, the activity would not meet the Common Rule definition of research. However, if instead of, or in addition to, an internal assessment the results will be reported through publication in a professional journal or a presentation at a professional association meeting, the activity would be defined as research.

The human subject definition excludes deceased individuals. However, in some situations, collecting data about deceased individuals might present a risk to living individuals, who should be protected from possible harm. For example, psychological harm might result from discussing conditions surrounding the death of a family member. In such a situation, the Common Rule regulations for conducting research with human subjects (i.e., surviving family members) would apply.

Institutional Review Board (IRB)

Purpose and composition

Each institution where research is conducted that is subject to the Common Rule is required to have an **institutional review board (IRB)** that operates in accordance with guidelines and oversight from the OHRP. An IRB is responsible for reviewing and approving all protocols for research with human subjects before the research may be initiated. It also is responsible for continuing review of approved research while it is being conducted to ensure compliance with federal regulations and the institution's policies. IRB members are drawn primarily from within the institution, although at least one member must be unaffiliated. IRB membership should be diverse in terms of individual backgrounds (e.g., race, gender, and culture), professional disciplines, and experience with the types of research activities commonly conducted at the institution.

> **Key Concept**
>
> An IRB reviews all human subjects research protocols and continues to review approved research.

IRB protocol

Prior to initiating any research that involves human subjects, a protocol must be submitted for review and approval by the institution's IRB. The protocol must include sufficient information for an IRB to assess possible risks to human subjects and possible benefits of conducting the research in accordance with the *Belmont Report* principles, the Common

Rule, and the institution's policies. After a protocol is approved, the IRB must review and approve any changes to the research protocol that might affect human subjects.

An IRB protocol typically is a separate document from a research proposal. It should include a description of the research plan and copies of all materials pertaining to human subjects. Particular attention should be given to specifying the target population, inclusion and exclusion criteria, subject selection procedures, number of subjects, informed consent procedure, participation incentives, reimbursement for participation costs, procedures for monitoring subject safety, and procedures for assessing and addressing possible harms. Box 2.2 lists key elements that commonly should be included in an IRB protocol. Subject recruiting materials include items such as email solicitations, hardcopy handouts, posters, and oral scripts. Data collection instruments include items such as questionnaires, interview guides, and focus group moderator guides. Data collection materials include items such as photographs, drawings, and videos that will be shown to subjects.

BOX 2.2: KEY ELEMENTS OF AN IRB PROTOCOL

Research Plan	Materials
• Objectives and significance	• Recruiting materials
• Research design	• Informed consent documents
• Subjects	• Data collection instruments
• Data collection plan	• Data collection materials
• Data management plan	

IRB review

There are three types of IRB review: exempt, expedited, and convened, summarized in Box 2.3. The IRB, not the researcher, decides the type of review that is appropriate for a study. A protocol must be submitted for the IRB to decide whether a study is exempt. Moreover, qualifying for exempt review does not relieve a researcher of responsibility for adhering to the *Belmont Report* principles and other ethical guidelines. Exempt and

BOX 2.3: TYPES OF IRB REVIEW

Feature	Exempt	Expedited	Convened
Conditions	No more than minimal risk and meet at least one exempt category listed in 45 CFR part 46.101.b	No more than minimal risk or minor change(s) in an approved protocol	More than minimal risk and/or a vulnerable population
Review	IRB staff and/or at least one designated IRB member	IRB chairperson and/or one or more designated IRB members	Entire IRB convened in session

expedited review policies may vary by institution. The following are examples of research that is likely to qualify for each review type:

- **Exempt:** focus groups with adults about attempting to stop smoking
- **Expedited:** adding questions to a previously approved questionnaire for a survey about college students' study habits
- **Convened:** interviews about safe-sex practices with men who have sex with men

Research with human subjects may not be initiated until an IRB issues a written notice of approval. Also, a funding agency may require written notice of IRB approval before issuing an award. A research protocol may be disapproved only by a convened IRB review. If a protocol is not approved by an expedited or exempt review, it is referred for a convened review. Prior to issuing an approval, an IRB may require additional information to be submitted, or it might require specific modifications to be made to a protocol.

It is important to allot time to prepare an IRB protocol and for an IRB to review it. Also, time should be allotted for responding to any IRB requests for additional information or required modifications. Typically, IRB review proceeds most efficiently by consulting with IRB staff in advance of preparing and submitting a protocol. Such consultation is helpful in identifying aspects such as the type of review to anticipate and the protocol submission deadline, and addressing in advance issues about which an IRB might be concerned.

While conducting a research study, a researcher must notify the IRB promptly about any problems involving human subjects. Examples are subjects experiencing unanticipated risks or harms, or a violation of the approved protocol by research staff. Also, IRB approval is required in advance of implementing any changes in a protocol. Typically, that may be done by submitting an amendment to the approved IRB protocol, which the IRB must approve before the revisions may be implemented.

Training

The National Institutes of Health (NIH) requires education on the protection of human research subjects for all key personnel involved in proposed research before funds are awarded (https://grants.nih.gov/grants/guide/notice-files/not-od-00-039.html; accessed October 25, 2018). Moreover, an IRB typically requires certification of completing training before a research protocol may be submitted for review, including one that might qualify for an exempt review. **Key personnel** are individuals involved in the design or conduct of human subjects research. This includes ones who are not compensated from an award supporting the research, and collaborators who are not employed by or otherwise affiliated with the institution at which the research is conducted. The **principal investigator** is the lead researcher and is responsible for ensuring that all key personnel receive adequate training and supervision to ensure compliance with all human subjects policies.

The NIH does not require any specific educational program(s). Training programs are the responsibility of IRBs, which may develop programs or designate ones available from third parties. Some IRBs subscribe to the online courses offered by the Collaborative Institutional Training Initiative (CITI) (https://about.citiprogram.org/en/homepage/; accessed August 1, 2018). In addition to initial training, IRBs may require continuing education training to ensure researchers and staff stay up-to-date on human subjects policies and best practices.

Informed Consent

Process

As required by the principle of **respect for persons**, individuals have a right to decide whether to participate in research. There are two aspects of informed consent. First, subjects must have a clear and complete understanding (i.e., be informed) about what their participation in research will entail. Second, subjects must be competent to give voluntary consent to participate in research. Informed consent is a process that begins when initial contact is made with a subject and ends when the subject completes his or her participation. Subjects should be provided a sufficient opportunity to understand what participation will involve and to consider whether to participate. This includes reviewing any documents, asking questions, and consulting with others, as appropriate.

The consent process and documents should be presented in clear language using terms that are in common use. Technical terms or professional jargon should not be used unless absolutely necessary. They should be defined when they are used. Also, the consent process should use language in which subjects are proficient. As appropriate, scripts and documents should be translated, and the person obtaining consent should be proficient in the subjects' preferred language. Accommodations should be made for subjects who are illiterate or have a seeing, speaking, hearing, or writing disability. Informed consent may not include any exculpatory language, oral or written, whereby subjects waive or appear to waive their legal rights or release or appear to release researchers, staff, institutions, or funding agencies from liability for negligence.

Individuals who are not competent adults are not legally capable of giving consent independently. However, they may be included in research by obtaining consent on their behalf from a legally authorized representative (e.g., parent, guardian, spouse, or other agent). In such situations, *assent* to participate should be obtained from individuals who are not capable of providing informed consent. The Common Rule (45 CFR part 46, subpart D 402.b) defines assent by children as "a child's affirmative agreement to participate in research. Mere failure to object should not, absent affirmative agreement, be construed as assent." For individuals with a chronic cognitive impairment or whose cognitive capacity is fluctuating (e.g., owing to illness or intoxication), screening procedures should be employed to assess their competence to consent. If participation will involve an extended period of time, as in longitudinal research, subjects' competency should be reassessed at specified points. As stated in part B.1 of the *Belmont Report* (1979):

> The extent of protection afforded should depend upon the risk of harm and the likelihood of benefit. The judgment that any individual lacks autonomy should be periodically reevaluated and will vary in different situations.

Elements

Box 2.4 presents eight basic elements the Common Rule (45 CFR part 46.116.a) requires informed consent to include.

An IRB may require additional informed consent elements to enhance subjects' understanding of research and voluntary decision making. Some elements may be required as an IRB's general policy. Other elements might be required as an IRB deems appropriate in view of subjects' risks as participants in a particular study. Box 2.5 lists additional informed consent elements that IRBs commonly may require. It is strongly recommended to include those elements even if an IRB does not require them.

Assessment

After subjects consent to participate, the person obtaining consent should assess their understanding of their consent. In general, this includes understanding the research

BOX 2.4: BASIC ELEMENTS OF INFORMED CONSENT PER THE COMMON RULE

1. A statement that the study involves research, an explanation of the purposes of the research and the expected duration of the subject's participation, a description of the procedures to be followed, and identification of any procedures which are experimental.
2. A description of any reasonably foreseeable risks or discomforts to the subject.
3. A description of any benefits to the subject or to others which may reasonably be expected from the research.
4. A disclosure of appropriate alternative procedures or courses of treatment, if any, that might be advantageous to the subject.
5. A statement describing the extent, if any, to which confidentiality of records identifying the subject will be maintained.
6. For research involving more than minimal risk, an explanation as to whether any compensation and an explanation as to whether any medical treatments are available if injury occurs and, if so, what they consist of, or where further information may be obtained.
7. An explanation of whom to contact for answers to pertinent questions about the research and research subjects' rights, and whom to contact in the event of a research-related injury to the subject.
8. A statement that participation is voluntary, refusal to participate will involve no penalty or loss of benefits to which the subject otherwise is entitled, and the subject may discontinue participation at any time without penalty or loss of benefits to which the subject is otherwise entitled.

BOX 2.5: POTENTIAL ADDITIONAL ELEMENTS OF INFORMED CONSENT

- Who is conducting the research: principal investigator and institution.
- Agency that is funding the research.
- How and why subjects were selected.
- Approximate number of subjects involved in the research.
- Incentives and/or reimbursements, if any, for participating; the conditions to receive them; the process by which subjects will receive them.
- Circumstances under which the subject's participation may be terminated by the principal investigator.
- Disclosure of any conflicts of interest by the investigator(s) and/or institution.

purpose, what participation will involve, and implications of giving consent. In most situations, this may be done by briefly interviewing the subject and/or legally authorized representative, as appropriate. Depending on factors such as a study's complexity, the nature of risks, and the nature of the population, an IRB might specify questions to be posed to subjects. Box 2.6 presents examples of consent assessment questions.

> **BOX 2.6: EXAMPLES OF QUESTIONS TO ASSESS INFORMED CONSENT**
>
> - What is the purpose of this research study?
> - Why are you being asked to participate in this study?
> - Do you have to take part in this study, or is it OK to say "no"?
> - What will you do as a participant in this research study?
> - Once you start participating, can you drop out if you don't want to continue?
> - Tell me what the main risks are to you of being in this study.
> - What are the potential benefits of this study to you or others?
> - How will your privacy and confidentiality be protected?
> - How much will you be paid for participating in this study?
> - What questions do you have about participating in this study?
> - Considering everything we've discussed about this study, are you willing to take part in it?

Documentation

The preferred procedure for documenting informed consent is obtaining written consent, whereby a subject or legally authorized representative signs a form approved by an IRB (45 CFR part 46.117.a).

Written consent. The IRB specifies guidelines for preparing a written consent form and typically will require using a template that may be downloaded from a website. As appropriate, the person obtaining consent may read the consent form aloud instead of, or in addition to, the subject reading it him- or herself. The consent form is signed and dated by the subject, or legally authorized representative, and the person obtaining consent. Depending on the nature of the study and population, an IRB might also require a signature from a witness, such as a subjects' advocate. The signed consent form is retained for the study files, and a copy is given to the subject and anyone else who signs it.

Box 2.7 presents an example of a consent form that was used to conduct focus groups with Korean American men about cigarette smoking and health. The English version shown in the box was translated into the Korean language for use in the study. The person who obtained informed consent was fluent in English and Korean.

Waivers and alterations. An IRB may waive obtaining written documentation of consent from some or all subjects under either of two conditions (45 CFR part 46.117.c):

1. The only record linking the subject and the research would be the consent document, and the principal risk would be potential harm resulting from a breach of confidentiality.

2. The research presents no more than minimal risk of harm to subjects and involves no procedures for which written consent is normally required outside of the research context.

An example of the first condition is conducting interviews with subjects who might have committed a crime and be at risk of prosecution. An example of the second condition is

BOX 2.7: INFORMED CONSENT FORM EXAMPLE

University of Illinois at Chicago
Consent for Participation in Research
"Smoking and Health Focus Groups" (KA)

Why am I being asked?

You are being asked to participate in a research study about smoking and health because you volunteered to participate in it and you meet the study's eligibility requirements, which are that you must be either a current or former cigarette smoker, age 45 to 74, your background is Korean, and you are a fluent speaker of Korean. A total of about 130 persons are being asked to participate in this research study.

Read this consent form carefully and ask any questions you may have before you agree to participate in this research. Your participation in this research is voluntary. Your decision whether or not to participate will not affect your current or future relations with the University or any community service agency where you might have found out about this research.

What is the purpose of this research?

The purpose of this research is to learn what current and former cigarette smokers think about how smoking is related to their health.

What procedures are involved?

If you agree to participate in this research, we will ask you to do three things:

1. Background Questionnaire. Complete a brief questionnaire that will take about 10 minutes to provide information about your background and smoking history.
2. Group Discussion. Participate in a group discussion that will take about 1½ hours to talk with about 10 other persons like you about how you think smoking cigarettes is related to your health.
3. Follow-up Questionnaire. Complete a brief questionnaire that will take about 5 minutes to provide any final comments you might have about the group discussion.

The total time for your participation in this research will be about 2 hours.

What are the potential risks and discomforts?

Talking about your experiences and beliefs about how smoking may affect your health might cause you to be worried about becoming ill.

Are there benefits to taking part in this research?

Helping the researchers to understand how current and former smokers think about smoking and health can help them to develop more effective programs to help people like you to quit smoking. Although there are no direct benefits to you from participating in this research, participating in the group discussion might help you to understand better your beliefs about how smoking may affect your health.

What about privacy and confidentiality?

Although the other participants in the group discussion will be asked not to tell other people what you say, the researchers cannot guarantee that this will not happen. The only other people who will know that you are a participant in this research are members of the research team. Reports of the results of this research will not include any information that would reveal your identity. No information about you will be disclosed to others without your written permission. The questionnaire that you complete will not contain any information that will identify you. Information about your name, telephone number, and address will be stored in locked file cabinets and in computer files that are protected by a password. These files can be accessed only by authorized members of the research team.

The group discussion will be recorded on audio tape to help keep track of what is discussed. The researchers will listen to the tape and the tape also will be transcribed onto paper to help the researchers to review the discussion. The transcription of the tape will not include any identifying information about you, such as your name. If there is a time when you do not feel comfortable about this, the tape recording will be stopped. When the research is finished, your questionnaire and the tape will be destroyed.

Will I be reimbursed for any of my expenses or paid for my participation in this research?

You will be paid $ 50 in cash for your participation.

Whom should I contact if I have questions later?

This research study is directed by Dr. Frederick J. Kviz, a professor in the School of Public Health at the University of Illinois at Chicago. You may contact Dr. Kviz at (312) 996–4889.

What are my rights as a research subject?

If you have any questions about your rights as a research subject, you may call the UIC Office for Protection of Research Subjects at (312) 996–1711. You will be given a copy of this form for your information and to keep for your records.

Remember

Your participation in this research is voluntary. Your decision whether or not to participate will not affect your current or future relations with the University. If you decide to participate, you are free to withdraw at any time without affecting that relationship.

Signature of Subject or Legally Authorized Representative

I have read (or someone has read to me) the above information. I have been given an opportunity to ask questions and my questions have been answered to my satisfaction. I agree to participate in this research. I have been given a copy of this form.

_____   _____
Signature of Subject   Date

_____
Printed Name of Subject

_____   _____
Signature of Person Obtaining Consent   Date (must be same as above)

_____
Printed Name of Person Obtaining Consent

conducting an internet survey that does not include any questions about **sensitive topics**. If written consent is waived, a researcher still should implement other aspects of the informed consent process. When feasible, an IRB may require that subjects are provided a written description of the research that is similar to a written consent form, but that subjects are not asked to sign.

In some situations, an IRB may approve a consent procedure that does not include or alters some or all of the informed consent elements, or may waive the requirements to obtain informed consent. To do so, the Common Rule (45 CFR part 46.116.d) requires the following:

1. The research involves no more than minimal risk to the subjects;
2. The waiver or alteration will not adversely affect the rights and welfare of the subjects;
3. The research could not practically be carried out without the waiver or alteration; and
4. Whenever appropriate, the subjects will be provided with additional pertinent information after participation.

An example of an informed consent alteration is conducting a telephone interview survey that does not include any questions about sensitive topics, and an interviewer script presents a brief overview of the study prior to initiating an interview.

Some research cannot be conducted when subjects are provided information about its purpose in advance if that is likely to result in them not participating in a natural manner. In such situations, valid research cannot be conducted without an element of deception. An alteration of the informed consent process must be approved by an IRB before deception may be employed. A deception should not involve more than minimal risk. When their participation is complete, subjects should be debriefed about the nature of the deception and the reason why it was necessary.

Proposed Changes in Federal Regulations

The U.S. DHHS and 15 other federal departments and agencies proposed revisions to the Common Rule "to modernize, strengthen, and make more effective the Federal Policy for the Protection of Human Subjects that was promulgated as a Common Rule in 1991 . . . better protect human subjects involved in research, while facilitating valuable research and reducing burden, delay, and ambiguity for investigators . . . [and] simplify, and enhance the current system of oversight." On January 2, 2019 the National Institutes of Health (NIH) announced the revised Common Rule will be effective as of January 21, 2019. Further information is available at https://grants.nih.gov/grants/guide/notice-files/NOT-OD-19-050.html; accessed January 3, 2019.

CHECK YOUR UNDERSTANDING 2.2

- According to the Common Rule, what is the definition of each of the following?
    - Research
    - A human subject
- Describe the purpose of an institutional review board (IRB).
- Describe the informed consent process and its main elements.

Privacy Protection

Privacy

Privacy is the concept that free individuals have a right to control others' access to them and to information about them. The Common Rule (45 CFR part 46.102.f) defines **private information** as

> information about behavior that occurs in a context in which an individual can reasonably expect that no observation or recording is taking place, and information which has been provided for specific purposes by an individual and which the individual can reasonably expect will not be made public (for example, a medical record).

In general, publicly available information is not considered private. Examples are observations of behavior in public places (e.g., recording the amount of time women and men spend viewing a museum display about fetal development) and extracting information from public records (e.g., marriage licenses issued by a county during a certain time period). Technical distinctions aside, what constitutes an *invasion of privacy* may differ across individuals and settings. Researchers should be sensitive to such differences and treat human subjects with courtesy and respect in all situations. For example, suppose a researcher plans to make on-the-scene video recordings of family members grieving over gun violence victims. A question may be raised about whether recording such intimate behavior is insensitive, and it might be argued that although it is observed in public places (e.g., streets, playgrounds, and parks), it should be respected as private.

Research sometimes involves collecting private information from or about human subjects. The concept that individuals have a *right to privacy* does not prohibit approaching subjects to solicit their participation in a study, or to request consent to access private information (e.g., medical or school records) about them. Researchers should treat subjects with respect and implement measures to protect their privacy. Collecting private information might present a risk of harm to subjects, particularly when the information is about a sensitive topic, such as substance abuse, sexual behavior, or illegal activities. When appropriate, the Common Rule (45 CFR part 46.111.a.7) requires that an IRB ensures that a protocol includes "adequate provisions to protect the privacy of subjects and to maintain the confidentiality of data." The **Privacy Rule** of the Health Insurance Portability and Accountability Act of 1996 (HIPAA) and the Family Educational Rights and Privacy Act of 1974 (FERPA) established federal policies for protecting the privacy of individually identifiable information for research that requires access to medical and school administrative records.

In addition to complying with regulations, implementing measures to protect subjects' privacy might enhance data quality, especially when a study involves collecting information about a sensitive topic. Privacy protections reduce subjects' concerns about how their information might affect them outside the research context. Subsequently, they may be more likely to participate in research, and provide more complete and accurate information.

Anonymity

When feasible, **anonymity** is the most effective means for protecting subjects' privacy. Under anonymity, it is not possible even for research staff to associate individual subjects with any information obtained from or about them either directly by name or indirectly through an **identifier** that may be linked to them. Examples of identifiers are a subject's address, telephone number, email address, Social Security number, medical record code, employee identification number, and student identification number.

Not recording identifiers

A strategy for providing subjects anonymity is not maintaining a record of identifiers. It applies when subjects are identifiable prior to collecting data, such as a sample selected from a list or roster of the target population. For example, a sample might be selected from a list of patients who received services from a certain source of health care during a particular time period. In addition to patients' names, the list is likely to include identifiers such as medical record codes, addresses, telephone numbers, and email addresses. Anonymity may be provided by not assigning subject identification codes to data collection instruments. For example, to provide anonymity in a standard mail questionnaire survey, no identifiers would appear on questionnaires or return envelopes. Thus, it would not be possible for anyone, including research staff, to associate information on a completed instrument with an individual subject. Also, the absence of identification codes effectively assures subjects that the information they provide is anonymous. However, for data processing purposes, such as verifying data entry accuracy by comparing electronic data records to raw questionnaire data, study-specific identification codes may be assigned randomly to completed data collection instruments when they are logged in for data processing.

Not collecting identifiers

Not collecting identifying information about subjects may be employed when they are not identifiable prior to collecting data. For example, when selecting subjects by convenience sampling (Chapter 13), such as recruiting individuals who attend a community health fair, it is not possible in advance to know their identities. Anonymity may be maintained simply by not collecting identifiers from them.

De-identification

De-identifying data may be employed when conducting a *secondary data analysis* (Chapter 14), where existing data collected by a third party are analyzed. The data might have been collected for research purposes (e.g., a health behavior survey) or administrative purposes (e.g., health clinic records). When such data include identifiers, anonymity may be provided by arranging for the data proprietor to remove identifiers, a procedure called **de-identification**, before delivering a copy of the data for secondary analysis.

Uses of Identifiers

In many situations, anonymity is not feasible because individual subject identifiers are essential to or substantially enhance conducting a study. The following sections describe common uses of identifiers during the data collection process and after data collection is complete.

Prenotification

Providing information about a study in advance may encourage subjects to participate. This strategy enables subjects to review the information in their own time, discuss the research with others, verify a study's legitimacy, and pose questions about it. As appropriate, prenotification may be done by standard mail, email, or telephone. Prenotification often is employed prior to contacting subjects to participate in a survey (Chapter 12). However, it also may be used in advance of implementing other data collection procedures, such as conducting unstructured interviews. Box 2.8 presents a list of elements commonly included in prenotification. Although most prenotification elements also are included in informed consent, prenotification should be presented as a brief and cordial invitation to participate in research.

BOX 2.8: PRENOTIFICATION ELEMENTS

- The purpose and importance of the research.
- How subjects were selected.
- What participation will involve.
- Incentives and/or reimbursements, if any, for participating.
- Assurance of confidentiality.
- Who is conducting the study and how to obtain further information (e.g., telephone number, email address, project website).
- When and how subjects will be contacted to participate.

Scheduling

Identifiers may be required to contact subjects to schedule their participation in research. For example, the time and place for focus group sessions must be arranged in advance. Also, for studies that employ an experimental design, it might be necessary to schedule when subjects will attend training sessions or support groups.

Follow-up

Identifiers often are used to make follow-up contacts with subjects in a survey (Chapter 12), as well as with other data collection modes. Three types of follow-up contacts commonly are employed in a survey. First, they may be used to remind subjects about a study and encourage their participation. For example, when conducting a mail or web survey, a follow-up letter or email message may be sent to subjects shortly after they receive a questionnaire by mail or are provided a link to one online. The second type of follow-up is to make additional attempts to gain subjects' participation if the initial attempt is not successful. The third type of follow-up may be employed in a telephone or in-person interview survey with subjects who have been contacted but break off an interview before it is complete (e.g., because of a lack of time) or refuse to participate at all. As appropriate, such subjects might be contacted later during the data collection period in an attempt to obtain their responses to questions following the point of a break-off, or to convert an initial refusal to an interview. Strategies for these types of follow-up attempts are discussed further in Chapter 12.

Data collection evaluation

When conducting large numbers of interviews, as is common for many telephone and in-person surveys, typically interviews are conducted by a staff of several interviewers. A common practice in such situations is to evaluate interviewers' performance to ensure they are complying with instructions and employing strategies to obtain data that are as accurate and complete as possible. In most situations, it is sufficient to randomly select a portion (e.g., 10%–15%) of each interviewer's completed cases throughout the data collection period. An interviewer supervisor contacts the subjects, usually by telephone, to confirm the interview was conducted and to ask subjects whether they were treated appropriately (Chapter 12). A similar procedure may be employed in studies where data are extracted from records and transferred to coding forms. For example, a supervisor may randomly select a portion of each coder's completed cases for comparison against the original records.

Missing data recovery

Data quality is a function of two factors, completeness and accuracy. In survey research, **item nonresponse** is a condition where subjects respond to most but not all questions (items) in a questionnaire. Item nonresponse might occur owing to several reasons: subjects being distracted when completing a self-administered questionnaire; subjects or interviewers not following instructions; subjects choosing not to answer certain questions; or subjects being unable to provide the information requested. Instances of missing data also might occur with other data collection modes, such as extracting data from records. For example, data items might be missing in some records, or errors might occur when transferring data from records to an analysis file. To enhance data quality, attempts should be made to recover missing data. When feasible, subjects might be contacted to request the missing information. Another strategy is linking to other data sets that contain subject identifiers and the missing data. If data appear to have been lost during transfer to an analysis file, the primary source should be accessed to recover them.

Data verification/clarification

Situations may arise where there is a need to contact subjects to verify or clarify information that has been collected from or about them. Logical inconsistencies might be detected; for example, a subject reports there are no children living in her household when responding to one survey question, but responds to a later question by reporting that two children living in her household are enrolled in high school. Other times, information may appear implausible. For example, assuming data are collected in the year 2016, if a subject's year of birth is recorded incorrectly as 1831 instead of 1931, the subject's age would be computed as 185 instead of 85. Rather than assume the error was only in one particular digit and make an administrative correction, it is best to verify the year by contacting the subject or checking a data record, as appropriate. In other situations, clarification may be sought regarding matters such as illegible handwriting by subjects or staff, illogical statements, slang terms, or unclear abbreviations.

Payments

Identifiers are required to distribute and record payment of participation incentives and/or reimbursements.

Linking data sets

Subject identifiers are essential when a research plan includes linking data from two or more sources. An example is linking subjects' responses to survey questions with medical record data. Identifiers also are necessary to link baseline and outcome data for subjects in pretest–posttest experimental and quasi-experimental designs (Chapter 6).

Tracking

Subject identifiers are essential for studies that employ longitudinal designs, whereby data are collected from or about subjects at multiple time points (Chapter 6). In addition to linking data over time, identifiers facilitate tracking subjects whose contact information changes during the course of a study, making it possible to contact them at the next data collection point(s).

Sharing results

Identifiers enable distributing a summary of research results by mail or email, or notifying subjects when and where they may view results online. Also, subjects may be notified about the time and place where they might attend a presentation of research results at a public community forum.

Maintaining Confidentiality

When identifiers are used, subjects' privacy should be protected by treating their participation in research confidentially. Maintaining **confidentiality** applies to two aspects of research participation: not disclosing that a subject participated in a study, and not disclosing any information collected from or about him or her.

Subject identification codes

Subject-specific identifiers (names, addresses, telephone numbers, medical record codes, etc.) that might allow others to link subjects to their participation in research or their data never should be entered on data collection instruments or in data analysis files. Standard practice for linking subject identifiers and contact information to their data is to assign **study-specific codes** that may be linked to subjects by research staff only. This protects subjects' identities from being detected while data are being collected or entered into an analysis file, and if data documents should be accessed by an unauthorized person.

Subjects' identification codes should not be composites of their personal information that might be decoded by others, such as a subject's digital birth date or the last four digits of his or her telephone number. A simple and common method to generate subject identification codes is to randomly assign numbers from 1 to n (the number of subjects). For example, if a study includes 200 subjects, they may be assigned numbers from 1 to 200, or 001 to 200. Code numbers also may be designed to include other study-specific information. For instance, when conducting an experiment, assignment to treatment and control conditions might be designated by the leading numerals 1 and 2, respectively. Accordingly, if a study assigns 100 subjects to a treatment condition and 100 to a control condition, treatment subjects may be assigned codes 1001 to 1100, and control subjects may be assigned 2001 to 2100. The leading numerals designating condition assignment facilitate data collection and data processing. In a blinded study, such a coding scheme should not be disclosed to subjects and/or staff, as appropriate.

Security

Subjects' identification codes, contact information, and other identifiers should be recorded in a log that is stored separate from data collection instruments and analysis files. Access to the log should be restricted to staff who need it to conduct the research, and they should access it for that purpose only. Physical documents containing data and/or identifiers (e.g., questionnaires, focus group transcripts, or unstructured interview notes) should be stored in locked cabinets in locked rooms, with restricted access. Electronic files should be password-protected using strong password construction, and password access should be restricted. When identifiers and data must be transferred electronically, files should be encrypted and transferred over a secure network. When they are no longer needed for collecting or analyzing data, all hard-copy and electronic documents and files containing subject identifiers should be properly disposed of. Research institutions often have specific policies about storing, archiving, and disposing of such research material.

Nondisclosure

Nondisclosure means research staff should not share information that might disclose subjects' identities outside the research context, such as showing completed data collection instruments or discussing any specific subject's data. Even when instruments or data files do not contain subject-specific identifiers, it is important to protect against potential **deductive disclosure**, whereby others who are familiar with subjects might be able to identify them from their data. For example, subjects might be identified based on a unique combination of characteristics, such as date and place of birth, schools attended, and employment history. Whenever feasible, research results should be reported in a summary format, such as the percentage of subjects who regularly engage in physical activity for exercise.

When feasible, staff should not be assigned to collect data from or about subjects with whom they might be familiar, such as interviewing neighbors. If such conditions are not avoidable, the importance of maintaining confidentiality should be emphasized. Also, staff should not share with others any observational information they obtain while interacting with subjects that is not part of the data collection plan. For example, they should not share information about a subject's personal appearance, hygiene, or behavior, or the contents or upkeep of his or her dwelling. Such observations obtained without a subject's expectation or consent that they would be shared with others should be treated as private.

To the extent possible, appropriate measures should be taken to protect subjects from **inadvertent disclosure**, whereby individuals who are not members of the research staff become privy to a subject's data. For example, interviews should be conducted in settings where they cannot be overheard. When feasible, subjects should be protected from **disclosure by association**, which might result from being observed participating in research by others who are familiar with them. This is particularly a concern when being identified as a participant in research that others know addresses a certain topic may disclose private information about subjects. For example, if subjects are seen entering a site where a substance abuse treatment program is being evaluated, others might conclude they are substance abusers.

Subjects should not be identified when reporting results in writing or orally (Chapter 15). When it is necessary to report results on an individual basis, pseudonyms should be employed. For example, when reporting results from unstructured interviews or focus groups, quotes from subjects often are presented to illustrate their thought process, manner of expression, and passion about a topic. Pseudonyms may be designated simply as Subject A, Subject B, and so on. Essential basic subject characteristics, such as sex, may be indicated as Female Subject A, and so on. However, caution must be exercised not to include so many individual characteristics that unique combinations might enable others to identify a subject, for example "a 35-year-old mother of twin girls age 12, who is employed part-time at the community library and resides near the intersection of Main and West Streets."

Collect necessary information only

The potential for a breach of confidentiality increases with the number of identifiers that must be protected. Thus, confidentiality protection may be enhanced by collecting and maintaining the minimum number of subject identifiers necessary for conducting a study. Similarly, the risk of subject harm increases with the amount of information collected about them. Therefore, data should be collected only if necessary to address a study's research question. Other data should not be collected out of curiosity or with the notion that it might come in handy in some unspecified way in the future. For example, collecting extensive demographic background information might enable others who are familiar with a subject to identify him or her without access to direct identifiers. In particular, information about a sensitive topic should be collected only if it is essential and only at the level of detail necessary.

Limitations of confidentiality

Statements to subjects about protecting their privacy by maintaining confidentiality should clearly acknowledge certain limitations, as appropriate. The first limitation is that confidentiality is not the same as anonymity, and despite measures to maintain confidentiality, it may be possible for subjects to be identified and linked to their data. Second, a researcher ethically or legally might be compelled to report certain information to appropriate authorities, whether it is discovered through data collection or observations while interacting with subjects. In general, the confidential relationship between a researcher and subjects is not legally protected. A researcher may be compelled by subpoena to disclose a subject's identity and his or her data. Such conditions should be included in the informed consent form when it is anticipated that they might arise owing to the research topic, setting, or study population.

> **Key Concept**
>
> *Confidentiality is not the same as anonymity.*

Certificate of Confidentiality

When potential harm to subjects from disclosure is severe, such as a risk of criminal prosecution or civil action, an application should be submitted to obtain a **Certificate of Confidentiality (CoC)**, which may be issued by the NIH and other federal agencies, including the Centers for Disease Control and Prevention and the FDA. A CoC protects identifiable research information from forced disclosure, with the intention of enhancing a researcher's ability to collect information subjects would be reluctant to provide otherwise. Accordingly, a researcher may refuse to disclose identifying information about subjects in any civil, criminal, administrative, legislative, or other proceeding, whether at the federal, state, or local level. However, a researcher may *voluntarily* disclose information in compliance with ethical principles or laws. Such intentions should be specified in the informed consent form and process. When protected by a CoC, a researcher still should implement all appropriate methods for protecting against a breach of confidentiality.

A CoC is issued automatically to NIH-funded researchers through their award if they will collect or use identifiable sensitive information. Federal research funding is not a prerequisite for obtaining a CoC. One may be requested for any biomedical, behavioral, or other type of research involving sensitive information about identifiable subjects. Generally, information is sensitive if it might be damaging to an individual's financial standing, employability, or reputation within the community or might lead to social stigmatization or discrimination. Examples of sensitive information are sexual attitudes, preferences, or practices; use of alcohol, drugs, or other addictive substances; illegal conduct; and mental health status. Further information is available at the NIH CoC Kiosk (https://humansubjects.nih.gov/coc/index; accessed October 25, 2018).

> **CHECK YOUR UNDERSTANDING 2.3**
>
> - What are the three anonymity strategies discussed in this chapter?
> - Identify and describe at least five of the ten uses of identifiers discussed in this chapter.
> - Identify and describe at least four of the six strategies for maintaining confidentiality discussed in this chapter.

Key Points

Ethical Principles of Research With Human Subjects

The Belmont Report (1979) delineated three ethical principles for research with human subjects:

- Respect for persons
    - Individuals should be treated as autonomous agents.
    - Persons with diminished autonomy should be protected.
- Beneficence
    - Possible benefits should be maximized.
    - Possible harms should be minimized.
    - Whenever possible, research should involve no more than minimal risk.
- Justice
    - Inclusion: All target population members should be included unless there is a justifiable reason for excluding them.
    - Treatment: Subjects should be treated equitably.

Federal Regulations

Department of Health and Human Services regulations (45 CFR part 46, subpart A), known as the Common Rule, specify basic protections for human subjects in biomedical and behavioral research.

The Common Rule applies to research conducted by virtually all academic institutions and agencies affiliated with them.

Institutional Review Board (IRB)

The Common Rule requires each institution to have an IRB that does the following:

- Reviews all protocols for research with human subjects before it may be initiated
- Conducts continuing review of approved research

There are three types of IRB review:

- Exempt
- Expedited
- Convened

Training

The National Institutes of Health requires human subjects training for all key personnel involved in proposed research before funds are awarded.

IRBs typically require human subjects training before a research protocol may be submitted for review.

Informed Consent

Informed consent requires that subjects do the following:

- Have a clear and complete understanding about their participation in research
- Are competent to consent voluntarily

Written consent is the preferred documentation of informed consent.

Under certain conditions, an IRB may waive written consent or approve an altered informed consent process.

Privacy Protection

Collecting private information may present a risk of harm to subjects, particularly when the information is about a sensitive topic.

Anonymity is the most effective means for protecting subjects' privacy.

When individual subject identifiers are essential to or substantially enhance a study, subjects' privacy should be protected by maintaining confidentiality.

Review and Apply

1. Review the research plan you developed in the Review and Apply section of Chapter 1.
    a. Identify the possible benefits of your project, if any, to subjects and/or to others.
    b. How might the possible benefits of your project be enhanced?
    c. Identify the types of potential harms to subjects in your project. If they involve more than minimal risk, present a justification for them.
    d. How might the possible harms in your project be reduced?
    e. Describe the informed consent procedure you would implement for your project.
    f. What procedures would you employ to protect subjects' privacy?
    g. Which type of IRB review do you think would be appropriate for your project? Why?
    h. Obtain the appropriate IRB protocol form and prepare a draft of it.
2. Check if your institution has an IRB. If it does, visit the IRB website. Otherwise, visit the IRB website at another institution. Explore the information and resources at the site. In particular, examine the policies, training requirements, and forms.
3. If you have not already done so, complete the human subjects training available from an IRB. This might be provided in-person and/or online.

Study Further

Anderson, E. E. (2015). Ethical considerations in collecting health survey data. In T. P. Johnson (Ed.), *Handbook of health survey methods* (pp. 487–511). Hoboken, NJ: John Wiley & Sons.

National Research Act (NRA) (P.L. 93-348). (1974). Retrieved from https://history.nih.gov/research/downloads/PL93-348.pdf.

U.S. Department of Health and Human Services. (n.d.). Office for Human Research Protections (OHRP). Retrieved from http://www.hhs.gov/ohrp/index.html

World Health Organization (WHO). (2018). *Ethical standards and procedures for research with human beings*. Retrieved from http://www.who.int/ethics/research/en/

3

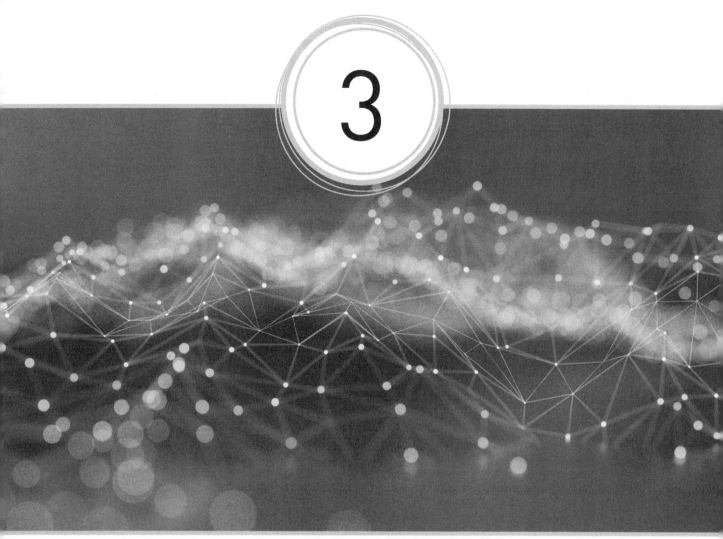

iStock.com/gremlin

Variables and Relationships

Chapter Outline

Overview
Learning Objectives
Types of Variables
    Levels of Measurement
    Discrete Variables
    Continuous Variables
Attributes of Relationships
    Contingency
    Direction
    Strength
Causal Concepts
    Independent and Dependent Variables
    Path Diagrams
    Necessary and Sufficient Conditions
    Noncausal Relationships
    Inferring Causality
    Multiple Causes and Multiple Effects
    Reciprocal Causality
    Mediated Causal Relationships
    Multiple Mediator Models
    Moderated Causal Relationships
    Mediation and Moderation Combined
    Complex Causal Models
Key Points

Learning Objectives

After studying Chapter 3, the reader should be able to:

- Distinguish between different types of variables
- Distinguish between different types of relationships among variables
- Classify variables as independent and dependent
- Draw and interpret a path diagram model of relationships between variables
- Identify causal and noncausal relationships
- Identify and assess mediated and moderated relationships

Overview

The general goal of research is to describe, explain, and predict patterns of variation across empirical observations. A **variable** is an attribute of an observation unit (individual, group, place, event, etc.) whose quality and/or quantity may be different (vary) from one observation to another. Variables may differ in their nature, the ways they may be measured, and how their measurements may be analyzed. Some variables may vary only across observation units, but not within the same unit across time (e.g., each individual has one birthplace).

Other variables may vary across units (e.g., ages of clinic patients) and/or within the same unit across time (e.g., an individual's age changes over time). In addition, variables may be related to one another in different ways. Some relationships may be causal, while others may be noncausal. Moreover, a relationship between two variables may be influenced by one or more other variables.

Types of Variables

Levels of Measurement

The way variables are measured influences the procedures that may be applied when analyzing research results. Measured variables are classified in a series of levels (nominal, ordinal, interval/ratio; see Chapter 8), according to the nature and amount of information a measurement captures. Sometimes the **level of measurement** is intrinsic to a variable's nature. For example, only two categories may be applied to classify a person as living or deceased, which is a measurement at the **nominal level**. However, for most variables, the **measurement level** is a function of the measurement procedure that is employed. For instance, a woman's height may be measured at the **ordinal level**, in terms relative to the height of other women (e.g., shorter than average, about average, or taller than average), or at the **interval/ratio level**, in terms of standard units, such as inches or centimeters.

Key Concept

Measured variables are classified in a series of levels, according to the nature and amount of information a measurement captures.

When a qualitative data collection method is employed (Chapter 13), the level of measurement is nominal, whereby observations are made in terms of the kind (quality) of a variable's attributes. For example, a study might record the type of store where individuals purchased groceries most recently, or the main reason they chose to purchase groceries at that store. When a quantitative data collection method is employed, measurements distinguish between observations in terms of the amount (quantity) of attributes (Chapter 8). For example, a study might record the number of times during the past 30 days individuals purchased fresh produce at a particular store, or their rating on a 5-point scale of the quality of fresh produce usually available at that store.

Discrete Variables

A **discrete variable** may be measured only in terms of particular units. Not all values across the measurement range from minimum to maximum are possible for a discrete variable. An example of a discrete variable is a count, which may be measured only in terms of whole units. For instance, it is not possible to observe that a woman made 2.37 prenatal clinic visits during her most recent pregnancy. Nevertheless, when analyzing aggregate data for a group of pregnant women, it is possible to compute the average (mean) number of prenatal clinic visits per woman in other than whole units, such as 2.37 visits (Chapter 15).

Continuous Variables

A **continuous variable** may be measured in terms of an infinite number of possible values because observations may occur at any point across the measurement range. For example, when measuring a person's height, the measurement scale may be demarcated in terms of feet, inches, half-inches, quarter-inches, and so forth, theoretically without limit.

However, in practice, continuous variable measurements are limited by the precision of the measurement instrument, such as the increments in which a ruler is marked off. Moreover, for simplicity of interpretation and presentation, measurements of a continuous variable may be grouped into intervals or ordinal categories. For example, American College of Cardiology guidelines (www.acc.org/latest-in-cardiology/articles/2017/11/08/11/47/mon-5pm-bp-guideline-aha-2017; accessed August 20, 2018) group blood pressure reading into the following ordinal categories:

- Normal: less than 120/80 mm Hg
- Elevated: systolic between 120 and 129 *and* diastolic less than 80
- Stage 1: systolic between 130 and 139 *or* diastolic between 80 and 89
- Stage 2: systolic at least 140 *or* diastolic at least 90 mm Hg
- Hypertensive crisis: systolic over 180 and/or diastolic over 120

CHECK YOUR UNDERSTANDING 3.1

- Provide examples of at least two discrete variables.
- Provide examples of at least two continuous variables.

Attributes of Relationships

Measurements of individual variables are useful for describing the status of a target population in terms of characteristics such as the mean (average) age and percent who smoke cigarettes. Studying relationships among variables provides an understanding of complex phenomena, such as factors that may contribute to disparities in use of breast cancer screening services by women of different races/ethnicities. Relationships are complex because they involve more than one variable. Additionally, they may occur in a wide variety of social, cultural, political, and physical contexts comprising many other variables that must be taken into account.

Contingency

A **contingency analysis** assesses whether an observation in a particular category of one variable is *contingent* on the category in which that observation occurs for another variable. Typically, that is done by casting data into a **contingency table** (also called a "cross-classification table") that simultaneously classifies observations in categories of two or more variables, to assess whether observations in categories of one variable are contingent on the categories in another variable. The most information is communicated by a contingency table when both the number and percentage of cases in each cell are presented. For example, Table 3.1 displays the contingency between cigarette smoking status and alcohol use disorder among a group of 220 men, based on data available from the National Institute on Alcohol Abuse and Alcoholism at https://pubs.niaaa.nih.gov/publications/AA71/AA71.htm (accessed August 20, 2018). Most of the men (45%) are either never or former smokers and have no alcohol use disorder. The second most prevalent condition is that 24% both are current smokers and have an alcohol use disorder. However, the table does not enable drawing a conclusion about whether smoking is a *cause* of alcohol use disorder, or that the presence of an alcohol use disorder is a *cause* of smoking status.

TABLE 3.1 • Cigarette Smoking Status and Alcohol Use Disorder Among Men

Smoking Status	Alcohol Use Disorder		Total ($N = 220$)
	No	Yes	
Never/former smoker	45% ($N = 99$)	15% ($N = 33$)	60% ($N = 132$)
Current smoker	16% ($N = 36$)	24% ($N = 52$)	40% ($N = 88$)
Total	61% ($N = 135$)	39% ($N = 85$)	100% ($N = 220$)

Direction

Another attribute of a relationship is its **direction**, which refers to whether one variable changes in a predictable direction when another variable changes in a certain direction. In a **positive relationship**, both variables change in the same direction. That is, as values for variable X increase, values for variable Y also increase, and vice versa. In a **negative relationship**, variables change in opposite directions: As values for variable X increase, values for variable Y decrease, and vice versa. The terms *positive* and *negative* do not impart any interpretation of the quality of a relationship, such that a positive relationship is desirable and a negative relationship is undesirable. Such value-based interpretations depend on the context. For example, a negative relationship between regular physical activity and heart disease risk is a desirable condition because it indicates that regularly engaging in physical activity is correlated with a lower heart disease risk. Thus, it is important not to confuse the direction of a relationship with how it might be valued from a practice or policy perspective.

Table 3.2 illustrates how the direction of a relationship is determined at the most basic level, for two dichotomous variables. In this situation, direction is assessed in terms of whether the presence or absence of one variable's attribute is correlated with the presence or absence of another variable's attribute. In a positive relationship, attributes of the two variables are the same: Both are present or absent. In a negative relationship, attributes of the two variables are opposite: One is present; the other is absent. Using Table 3.2 as a model, Table 3.1 depicts a *positive* relationship because the predominant pattern is for both smoking and alcohol use disorder to be either absent or present. A related example of a negative relationship is if completing a smoking cessation intervention is correlated with not smoking at the end of the intervention. That is, when completing the intervention is present, smoking is absent. Analysis of contingency tables is discussed in further detail in Chapter 15.

For variables that are measured at the ordinal, interval, or ratio levels (Chapter 8), a pattern of change may be observed over a range of values, which provides a more precise description of a relationship than whether the presence or absence of one variable's attribute is correlated with that of another variable's attribute. Figure 3.1 depicts directional patterns of relationships for two variables, X and Y. The patterns of data plots shown in the bottom panel of the figure generally may be described as **linear relationships** because the trends of the data tend to describe straight lines.

Not all relationships are linear. Some relationships change over the range of one or both variables. For example, a **nonlinear relationship** might be found between age and the average number of days per week on which adults engage in physical activity. As depicted

TABLE 3.2 ● Direction of Relationship for Dichotomous Variables

Variable A	Variable B	
	Absent	Present
Absent	Positive	Negative
Present	Negative	Positive

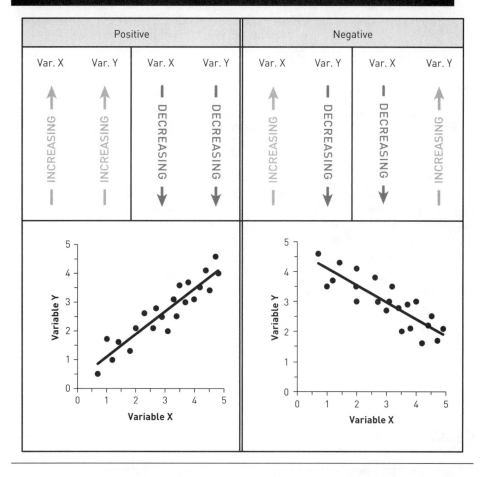

FIGURE 3.1 ● Relationship Directions for Ordinal-, Interval-, and Ratio-Level Measurements

in Figure 3.2, physical activity is high among young adults, declines among middle-aged adults, and then is low among older adults. Another example of a nonlinear relationship in Figure 3.2 is a reversed *J*-shaped relationship between self-rated health status and the number of physician visits individuals report making during the past 12 months. Perhaps in response to a high level of need, the number of physician visits is high among individuals whose health status is low. The number of physician visits decreases as health status increases, up to a certain point. Thereafter, the number of physician visits is somewhat higher among individuals with the highest health status, which might be attributable to accessing health care that increases their health status rating.

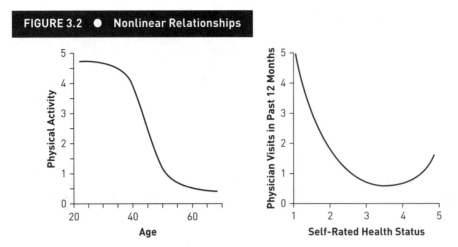

FIGURE 3.2 • Nonlinear Relationships

Strength

The **strength of a relationship** refers to how reliably the amount of change in one variable may be predicted when another variable changes by a certain amount. The most common method for measuring relationship strength is computing a **correlation coefficient** (e.g., Spearman's rho and Pearson's r). A correlation coefficient's value ranges from 0 (no relationship) to 1.00 (a perfect relationship); a coefficient's sign (+/−) indicates a relationship's direction. For example, the correlation coefficient (Pearson's r) for the positive relationship displayed in the graph in Figure 3.1 is .93, indicating a very strong relationship, which also may be discerned by the compact distribution of the data points along the trend line. The correlation coefficient for the negative relationship in the figure, for which the data points are more widely distributed, is −.85, indicating a slightly less strong relationship than for the positive one. Analysis of correlations is discussed in further detail in Chapter 15.

CHECK YOUR UNDERSTANDING 3.2

- Identify and briefly describe the three aspects of a relationship between variables.

Causal Concepts

The goal in assessing potential **causal relationships** is to identify which variables account for changes in other variables, the process through which change happens, and the conditions under which change occurs.

Independent and Dependent Variables

As depicted in Figure 3.3, a basic causal relationship consists of two variables, a **cause** and an **effect**, with the direction of influence in the relationship proceeding from the cause to the effect. A cause is a factor that, when it is present or changed, produces the presence or a change in the value of another factor, called its effect. For example, a cause might be a health education program, and its effect might be change in a particular health behavior. The cause is called the **independent variable**, indicating that its values change independently of any change in the effect. The effect is called the **dependent variable**, indicating that its values are dependent to some degree (an effect may have more than one cause) on values of an independent variable.

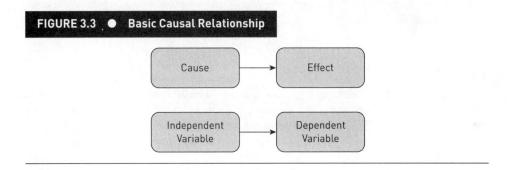

FIGURE 3.3 • Basic Causal Relationship

Path Diagrams

Figure 3.4 illustrates how the direction of a relationship is indicated in a **path diagram**, which indicates the pathways through which variables influence other variables. A **straight, single-headed arrow** linking variables indicates a **path** from a cause (independent variable) to an effect (dependent variable). A "+" or "−" symbol alongside a path arrow indicates whether the relationship is positive or negative, respectively. In addition, the strength of a relationship may be indicated by placing a correlation coefficient (or another appropriate statistic) alongside a path arrow. For instance, as shown in Figure 3.4, a positive relationship, such as between social support and mammography screening, might be indicated by placing the correlation coefficient .48 alongside the path arrow (by convention, a positive correlation is implied by the absence of a symbol). A negative relationship, such as between participating in a smoking cessation program and quitting smoking, might be indicated by placing the correlation coefficient −.32 alongside that path arrow. As will be discussed further in the next section, **temporal precedence** of the independent variable (i.e., it must change before the dependent variable changes) is an essential condition of a causal relationship. Accordingly, in Figure 3.4, with time progressing left to right per convention, independent and dependent variables are aligned horizontally, from left to right, respectively.

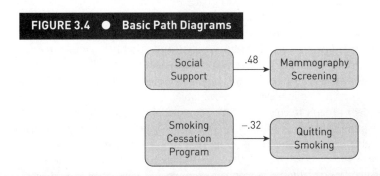

FIGURE 3.4 • Basic Path Diagrams

Exogenous variables

An **exogenous variable** is one whose value is determined by factors *externally*, outside the context of a causal model. Thus, a causal model does not account for changes in it.

Path arrows do not point toward exogenous variables; path arrows point *only from* exogenous variables.

Endogenous variables

An **endogenous variable** is one whose value is determined *internally*, within the context of a causal model, that is, by other variables in the model. Thus, path arrows point *toward* endogenous variables.

Necessary and Sufficient Conditions

Change in an independent variable is a **necessary condition** for causality if a dependent variable changes *only* if the independent variable changes. Conversely, the dependent variable does not change if the independent variable does not change. However, this does not mean the dependent variable always changes whenever the independent variable changes. There might be one or more other causes of the dependent variable that must change as well. As illustrated in Figure 3.5, it is necessary that both variables X and Z change to cause a change in variable Y. However, neither independent variable alone is sufficient to cause variable Y to change.

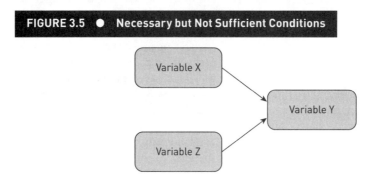

FIGURE 3.5 • Necessary but Not Sufficient Conditions

Most often, a dependent variable is influenced by multiple causes that operate in combination and/or through a process, such that change in a particular independent variable alone is not sufficient to cause a dependent variable to change. For example, drinking alcohol is necessary for alcohol dependency to occur. However, drinking one drink, one time, is not sufficient to cause alcohol dependency, which develops after consuming larger amounts of alcohol, more frequently and over a longer time period. Moreover, alcohol dependency also is influenced by genetic, attitudinal, social, and other behavioral factors.

Change in an independent variable is a **sufficient condition** for causality if a dependent variable changes whenever the independent variable changes. Although a sufficient condition *always* produces a change in a dependent variable, it might not be necessary for that particular independent variable to change. A dependent variable might change owing to change in one or more other variables as well. As illustrated in Figure 3.6, it is sufficient that *either* variable X or variable Z changes to cause a change in variable Y. However, it is not necessary that either independent variable changes to cause variable Y to change. Variable Y will change whenever variable X or variable Z changes. For example, if it rains, then the sidewalk will get wet, but the sidewalk might get wet from a lawn sprinkler, whether or not it rains.

In practice, virtually no independent variable is a necessary and sufficient cause, whereby it is both required to produce an effect (necessary cause) and able by itself to produce an effect (sufficient cause). Health research typically entails studying complex systems of **component causes** (Rothman, 1976), whereby sufficient causal conditions

FIGURE 3.6 ● Sufficient/Not Necessary Condition

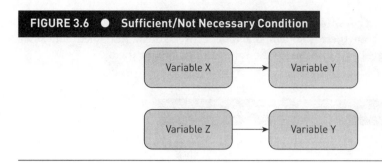

may comprise various combinations of independent variables in different contexts. For example, simply being exposed to someone who has the flu is not sufficient for another person to contract the disease. The flu virus must be transmitted to the other person, and that person's immune system must be susceptible to it. A more complex example is the Health Belief Model (Rosenstock, Strecher, & Becker, 1988), which specifies several independent variables (perceived susceptibility, perceived seriousness, perceived benefits, perceived barriers, cues to action, and self-efficacy) that may function as components of sufficient conditions for performing a health promotion behavior.

> **Key Concept**
>
> Health research entails studying complex systems of component causes that may comprise various combinations of independent variables.

CHECK YOUR UNDERSTANDING 3.3

- Describe the difference between an independent and a dependent variable.
- Describe the difference between a necessary and a sufficient condition for causality.

Noncausal Relationships

Risk factor

Some independent variables are neither necessary nor sufficient causes of certain outcomes. For example, obesity is not a necessary cause of heart disease because some people who are not obese may develop heart disease. Also, obesity is not a sufficient cause of heart disease because not every obese person develops heart disease. Thus, while obesity increases the probability for a person to develop heart disease, it is neither necessary nor sufficient to cause heart disease. Epidemiologists use the term **risk factor** to indicate a variable that increases the probability of incurring a particular adverse health outcome. Accordingly, obesity is a risk factor for heart disease. Moreover, many risk factors are not specific to a particular health problem. For example, obesity also is a risk factor for stroke and type 2 diabetes as well as other health problems.

Common cause

The top panel of Figure 3.7 depicts a noncausal relationship between two variables, A and B, which are correlated because both are dependent variables of the same independent variable. This is called a **common cause** condition. Variables A and B are aligned vertically in the diagram to indicate there is no temporal order between them. Also, their noncausal relationship is indicated by a **two-headed curved arrow** linking them.

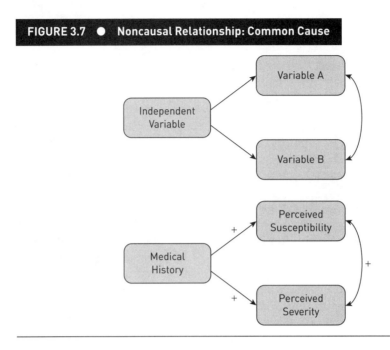

FIGURE 3.7 ● Noncausal Relationship: Common Cause

Key Concept

Correlation implies a potential causal relationship; it does not ensure causality.

For example, drawing on the Health Belief Model (Rosenstock et al., 1988) and as depicted in the bottom panel of Figure 3.7, a person's perceived susceptibility for a disease (e.g., cancer) and perceived severity of that disease are correlated. However, they both are dependent variables of a common cause, medical history. For instance, if a person's medical history includes cancer, he or she is more likely to perceive being susceptible to cancer and also is likely to perceive cancer as a serious health threat.

Although a correlation between two variables implies a *potential* causal relationship, that alone does not ensure causality (see the section on inferring causality). As illustrated in Figure 3.7, variables may be correlated but not be in a causal relationship. Therefore, when variables are found to be correlated, it is essential to assess whether the correlation might indicate causality or the influence of a common cause. That assessment should comprise two components. The first of these is to consider whether the correlation conforms to logic and a trusted theory, such as the relationship between perceived susceptibility and perceived severity as specified in the Health Belief Model. The second component is an empirical analysis, in which other variables that might account for a noncausal correlation are taken into consideration.

Spurious relationship

A **spurious relationship** (*spurious* means false or not authentic) is a noncausal relationship that may appear to be causal but is explained by the influence of a third variable. It is important to assess whether an apparent causal relationship actually is spurious to avoid misinterpreting a research result. As depicted in Figure 3.8, in a spurious relationship, a purported independent variable X is correlated with a purported dependent variable Y, but their relationship is not causal. Instead, they are related owing to both being dependent variables that are influenced by a common cause, variable Z.

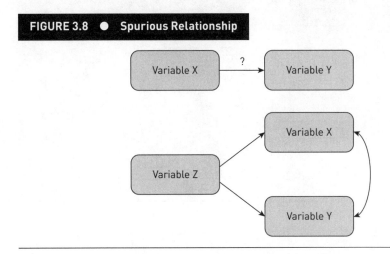

FIGURE 3.8 • Spurious Relationship

The third variable that accounts for a spurious relationship is called an **extraneous variable** because it is external to the initial two-variable relationship. When an extraneous variable explains a spurious relationship, social scientists refer to it as an **explanatory variable**. Epidemiologists refer to the extraneous variable as a **confounder variable**, to indicate that not taking its influence into account might lead to misinterpreting a non-causal relationship as causal. For an extraneous variable to account for a spurious relationship (i.e., to be an explanatory or a confounder variable), it must be

- correlated with the purported independent variable (risk factor/exposure),
- correlated with the purported dependent variable (outcome/disease/injury), and
- not in the causal pathway between the purported independent and dependent variables (i.e., extraneous).

For example, suppose women who regularly get a mammogram, as recommended by their physician, are found to be more likely than women who do not regularly get a mammogram to be diagnosed with stage I breast cancer. It might be concluded that regular mammography screening causes stage I breast cancer and therefore physicians should not recommend that women should regularly get a mammogram. However, that interpretation and recommendation contradicts logic and trusted theory. As shown in Figure 3.9, that conclusion would be false. Regularly getting a mammogram and a stage I breast cancer diagnosis are correlated because they both are influenced by medical history, specifically whether a woman has a family history of breast cancer, which is a breast cancer risk factor. Women with a family history of breast cancer are more likely than others to get a mammogram regularly. Also, regular mammography screening increases the chance of detecting a cancerous tumor at an early stage (i.e., stage I).

Women who do not have a family history of breast cancer are less likely than those with a family history of breast cancer to get a mammogram regularly. Therefore, if they are diagnosed with breast cancer, it is more likely to be at a later stage. As seen in the bottom panel of Figure 3.9, medical history, the extraneous variable, meets the three conditions

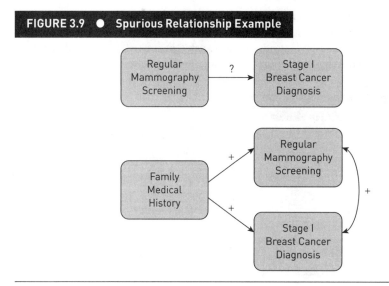

FIGURE 3.9 • Spurious Relationship Example

for being considered an explanatory or a confounder variable. It is correlated with the purported independent variable (regular mammography screening), it is correlated with the purported dependent variable (stage I breast cancer diagnosis), and it is not in the causal pathway between the purported independent and dependent variables (i.e., extraneous).

Ecological fallacy

When participants are studied in aggregates (e.g., students in schools, or residents in communities) instead of as individuals, the results must be interpreted at the same aggregate level. Interpreting aggregate-level results at the individual level may result in committing a logical error called the **ecological fallacy**, which is erroneously attributing causality at the individual level based on aggregate-level evidence (Robinson, 1950). The ecological fallacy functions in a manner similar to a spurious relationship in the sense that an error in attributing causality results from failing to take into consideration the influence of extraneous factors.

For example, suppose a positive correlation is found between the number of flu vaccinations and the number of new flu cases in a city. It might be concluded that receiving the flu vaccine caused an increase in new flu cases, and therefore people should be advised not to get vaccinated against the flu. However, as shown in Figure 3.10, that would be an erroneous causal attribution. Population flu vaccination rates and the incidence of flu cases are correlated because they both are influenced by the time of year. In particular, during flu season, both the number of people who get vaccinated and the number of flu cases increase. However, those patterns occur at the aggregate level, for the population of the city. It is not reliable to conclude that the individuals who are vaccinated also are those who get the flu. Indeed, it is most likely that most of the new flu cases occur among individuals who do not get vaccinated.

CHECK YOUR UNDERSTANDING 3.4

- Present an example of a spurious relationship.
- Present an example of an ecological fallacy.

FIGURE 3.10 ● Ecological Fallacy

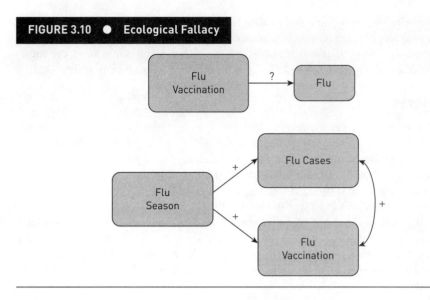

Inferring Causality

In most situations, it is not possible to observe directly one variable causing another variable. For example, it is not possible to actually see individuals' medical history causing them to perceive they are susceptible to a particular disease. Instead, logic, theory, and a process of systematic testing must be employed to *infer* causal relationships. Although several formulations have been proposed (Bollen, 1989; Hill, 1965; Rothman, 1976; Shadish, Cook, & Campbell, 2002; Susser, 1973), in general, there are five conditions for inferring a causal relationship:

- **Covariation:** A pattern of concordant change occurs in terms of amount and direction (essential).

- **Temporal precedence:** Change in the independent variable precedes change in the dependent variable (essential).

- **Alternative explanations:** Plausible noncausal alternative explanations for a relationship are ruled out (essential).

- **Mechanism/Process:** A relationship is explainable by a plausible causal mechanism or process.

- **Consistency:** A relationship is observed independently across various conditions.

Covariation, temporal precedence, and ruling out alternative explanations are essential conditions. However, none of the five conditions alone is sufficient evidence of a causal relationship. Confidence for inferring a causal relationship is derived from the overall strength of evidence for all of the conditions. The more conditions that are met, and the more convincingly they are met, the more confidence there is for inferring a causal relationship.

Covariation

Covariation is essential for inferring causality. Under this condition, the joint distribution of observations for two variables displays a pattern of concordant change in terms of amount and direction (see Figures 3.1 and 3.2). In general, covariation indicates there is a correlation between two variables. In data analysis (Chapter 15), a correlation may be assessed by a variety of measures, such as computing the covariance, a measure of association, a regression coefficient, or a correlation coefficient. However it is measured, the stronger the correlation, the more confidence there is for inferring a causal relationship.

Temporal precedence

For a relationship to be causal, change in the cause (independent variable) must precede change in the effect (dependent variable) (see Figure 3.3). In some situations, temporal precedence may be based on logic. For example, it is logical to posit that unsafe working conditions cause work-related injuries (rather than work-related injuries cause unsafe working conditions), or that cigarette smoking is a cause of lung cancer (rather than being diagnosed with lung cancer is a cause of cigarette smoking). However, in most situations, the strongest evidence for temporal precedence is obtained by employing a longitudinal design, especially one that includes a pretest–posttest structure (Chapter 6). The more an independent variable may be controlled to manipulate when and by how much it changes, the more reliably subsequent change in the dependent variable may be attributed to change in the independent variable (Chapter 5).

Some researchers (e.g., Holland, 1986) contend that assessments of causality should be restricted to independent variables that are subject to **manipulation**. The rationale for that approach is research should focus on developing knowledge that leads to intervention strategies (e.g., a health education curriculum) that influence dependent variables by manipulating independent variables. However, as Bollen (1989) has argued, manipulation is not an essential condition for causality. Moreover, if causal research were confined only to independent variables that may be manipulated, it would not address important effects of many variables that are not subject to manipulation. For example, there might be no research about racial/ethnic disparities in access to health care and health outcomes, or the public health impacts of natural disasters, because an individual's race/ethnicity and the occurrence of natural disasters cannot be manipulated.

Alternative explanations

Confidence for inferring a causal relationship is enhanced when plausible alternative explanations for a correlation may be ruled out. Alternative explanations are derived from logic and theory, which also may be employed to rule them out. However, empirical evidence is most effective for ruling out plausible alternative explanations. Empirical strategies include employing a research design that controls variation in potential alternative explanatory variables (Chapters 5 and 6), assessing threats to internal validity (Chapter 5), and measuring potential alternative explanatory variables to test for their influence when analyzing results.

Mechanism/process

A causal relationship should be explainable by a plausible mechanism or process through which the independent variable is posited to affect the dependent variable. Such explanations are derived from theoretical models and logical reasoning. For example, suppose a positive correlation is found between women's ratings of social support from family and friends, and their intention to get a mammogram. Confidence in postulating this correlation as a causal relationship, in which social support is the independent variable, is increased if a plausible process can be described whereby social support might influence health screening behavior. For instance, according to the Health Belief Model (Rosenstock et al., 1988), it might be hypothesized that social support reinforces perceived benefits of screening and reduces perceived barriers to getting a mammogram. Thus, increasing social support would be expected to increase the likelihood that a woman will get a mammogram.

Specifying a plausible causal mechanism or process is one of the most challenging conditions for inferring causality. Although it is easiest to think in terms of only two variables, independent and dependent, causal relationships are not so simple. Virtually always, they involve influence from other variables. For example, consider a situation where there is an increase in knowledge about warning signs for heart disease among African American men at the conclusion of a multifaceted, community-wide educational campaign. A knowledge increase might be caused solely by the campaign, or by the campaign in combination with other variables, such as medical history. Also, consideration should be given to whether a knowledge increase is attributable to the campaign as a whole, to only one component of it, or to some combination of its components.

Consistency

Confidence for inferring a causal relationship is enhanced by corroborating empirical evidence from multiple independent studies. As discussed regarding replication in Chapter 1, the validity of knowledge about a problem increases with the cumulation of supportive evidence from studies conducted by different researchers, at different times, with different populations, in different settings, and using different methodology.

Guidelines for inferring causality

The following series of questions provides a guide for assessing whether there is a causal relationship between two variables.

- Does the direction of correlation between the independent and dependent variables make sense and comply with theory?
- How strong is the correlation between the independent and dependent variables?
- What is the theoretical, logical, and empirical support for temporal precedence of the independent variable?
- What plausible alternative explanations might account for the correlation between the independent and dependent variables, and can they be ruled out?
- Through what mechanism or process might the independent variable affect the dependent variable?
- Is corroborating evidence available from independent studies conducted at different times, with different populations, in different settings, and using different methodology?

> **CHECK YOUR UNDERSTANDING 3.5**
>
> - Identify and briefly describe the three *essential* conditions for inferring causality.

Multiple Causes and Multiple Effects

Multiple independent variables, individually or in combination, may be causes of a particular dependent variable. For example, there are multiple risk factors for heart disease, including cigarette smoking, obesity, diabetes, stress, and family history. Theories such as the Health Belief Model posit that multiple factors may influence health promotion

Key Concept

Health research typically involves studying complex constellations of multiple causes and effects.

behaviors. Moreover, an independent variable may be a cause for multiple dependent variables. For example, cigarette smoking may cause several cancers, heart disease, stroke, emphysema, and chronic obstructive pulmonary disease (COPD). Similarly, obesity may cause heart disease, stroke, and type 2 diabetes as well as other health problems. Thus, health research typically involves studying complex constellations of multiple causes and multiple effects. An illustration of such a situation is presented in Figure 3.11, where two independent variables (cigarette smoking and obesity) influence two dependent variables in common (heart disease and stroke). In addition, they each separately influence two other dependent variables (cigarette smoking affects lung cancer, and obesity affects diabetes).

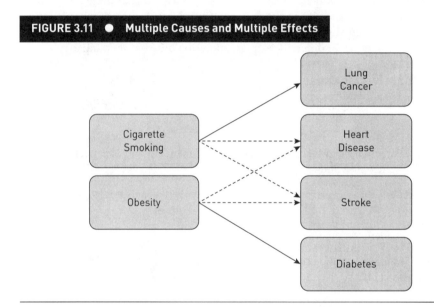

FIGURE 3.11 • Multiple Causes and Multiple Effects

Reciprocal Causality

Sometimes it is difficult or impossible to discern which of two variables changes first. There are two conditions that contribute to this dilemma. One is when two variables both change quickly, such that the temporal sequence is very short. This situation is complicated further by the second condition, which is when it is plausible that either variable may be a cause of the other one. Thus, two variables may appear to affect and be caused by each other virtually simultaneously. This type of relationship is referred to here as **reciprocal causality**, although sometimes other terminology is used, such as a feedback relationship, simultaneous causality, mutual causality, and reverse causality. As depicted two ways in Figure 3.12, reciprocal causality refers to a relationship in which two variables are both independent and dependent variables of each other.

For example, as illustrated in Figure 3.13, on one hand, it is plausible that health beliefs influence a person's health behavior. On the other hand, it also is plausible that a person's health behavior influences his or her health beliefs. For instance, people who believe they will not experience adverse health effects from cigarette smoking might smoke cigarettes (beliefs cause behavior). Also, people who smoke cigarettes and do not

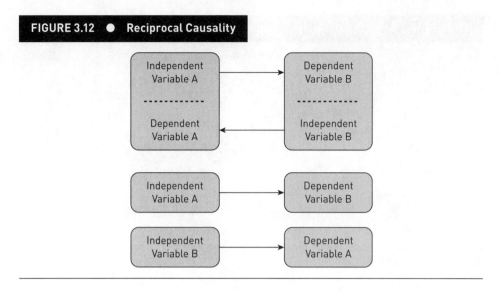

FIGURE 3.12 ● **Reciprocal Causality**

experience any apparent smoking-related health problems might believe their health is not at risk from smoking cigarettes; therefore, they continue to smoke, and so on (behavior causes beliefs).

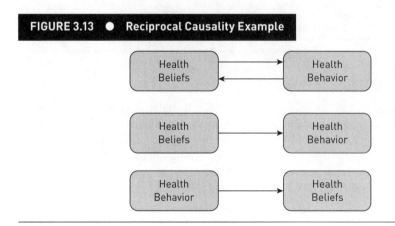

FIGURE 3.13 ● **Reciprocal Causality Example**

An alternative way to represent a reciprocal causal relationship that often is employed in a path diagram is to align variables vertically to indicate that a temporal order between them is indistinguishable. As illustrated in Figure 3.14, access to health care is a common cause of clinic visits and health status. Clinic visits and health status are represented as having a reciprocal causal relationship, such that clinic visits affect health status and vice versa. That is, in general, poor health status tends to increase the number of clinic visits, and more health care utilization tends to have a positive effect on health status.

Reciprocal causal relationships typically are more complicated than as depicted in Figures 3.13 and 3.14 because by nature they extend over long time periods during which there may be multiple cause–effect iterations. As illustrated in Figure 3.15, health beliefs influence both health behavior and subsequent health beliefs. Similarly, health behavior influences both health beliefs and subsequent health behavior. The most effective strategy

FIGURE 3.14 ● **Path Diagram of a Reciprocal Causal Relationship**

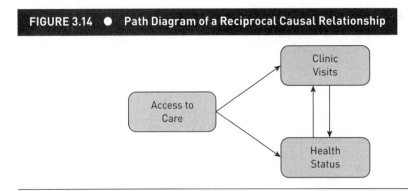

for studying the dynamics of a reciprocal causal relationship is employing a **longitudinal design** (Chapter 6), whereby observations are collected from the same individuals at multiple successive time points.

FIGURE 3.15 ● **Longitudinal Reciprocal Causality Example**

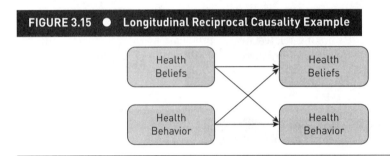

Mediated Causal Relationships

In virtually all causal relationships, the independent variable does not have a simple **direct effect** on the dependent variable. Instead, to some extent, the independent variable typically has an **indirect effect** by acting through at least one other variable, called a **mediator variable** (sometimes also called an intervening variable). A **mediated relationship** is one where an independent variable influences a dependent variable through its effect on a mediator variable.

Basic mediation model

Figure 3.16 depicts the basic mediation model, whereby the independent variable influences the dependent variable through its influence on the mediator variable, which then affects the dependent variable. The diagram in the lower panel of the figure illustrates that the mediator variable plays two roles by virtue of its position in the causal pathway between the independent and dependent variables. First, it is an intermediate dependent variable that is influenced by the primary independent variable. Subsequently, it functions as an intermediate independent variable that influences the ultimate dependent variable.

A situation where mediation commonly occurs is when research is conducted to evaluate a health behavior intervention. As illustrated in Figure 3.17, a health behavior intervention program functions through a process whereby program components affect **intermediate outcomes** such as changes in knowledge, attitudes, and social support, which then affect health behavior. For example, a program to encourage married women to obtain regular mammography screening might focus on increasing knowledge about obtaining a

FIGURE 3.16 ● Basic Mediation Model

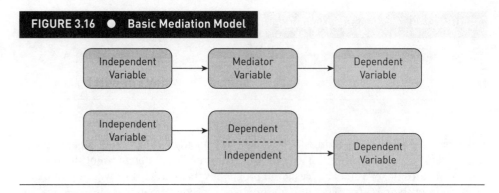

mammogram, perceived susceptibility to breast cancer, and spousal support for obtaining a mammogram, with the expectation that those variables will affect health behavior. If the program is effective, the mammography screening rate should increase among women who participate in it.

FIGURE 3.17 ● Mediated Intervention Program

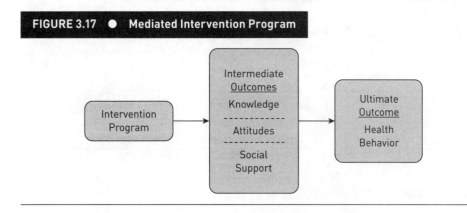

In the preceding example, all of the effects of the independent variable (the intervention program) on the mediator variables are positive, causing each mediator to increase. Moreover, each mediator has a positive effect on the dependent variable (mammography screening). However, mediated causal relationships are not necessarily positive. As illustrated in Figure 3.18, an intervention to encourage women to obtain a mammogram might focus on decreasing barriers to obtaining a mammogram, such as providing free mammograms. In this example, although it is intended that the intervention program will have a positive outcome effect on mammography screening, its intended effect on the mediator variable is negative (although reducing barriers is a "positive" outcome). In addition, barriers have a negative effect on screening: The fewer the barriers, the more likely a woman is to get a mammogram. Nevertheless, the program's effect on mammography screening is positive because by reducing barriers the program makes it more likely a woman will get a mammogram.

The overall direction and size of an effect in a path diagram, as displayed in Figure 3.18, is determined by multiplying the effects of variables in the same causal pathway. Thus, the product of two negative effects yields a positive effect overall. For example, suppose the correlation between the program and barriers is −.52 and the correlation between barriers and screening is −.45. The effect of the program on screening would be .23, computed as −.52 × −.45.

Figure 3.19 presents another perspective on a health behavior intervention program and mediation. In this example, the program's short-term goal is to cause a change in health

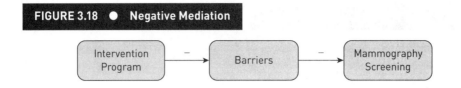

FIGURE 3.18 ● Negative Mediation

behavior as a **proximal outcome** that mediates the program's long-term goal to improve health status (e.g., prevent illness) as a **distal outcome**. The intended short-term effect (proximal outcome) of a smoking cessation program is that participants will stop smoking by the end of the program. The ultimate program goal (distal outcome) is to reduce the incidence of smoking-related disease, such as lung cancer. Thus, stopping smoking mediates the program's effect on lung cancer incidence.

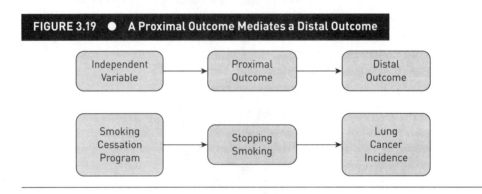

FIGURE 3.19 ● A Proximal Outcome Mediates a Distal Outcome

Complete mediation

Figure 3.20 depicts a **completely mediated** causal relationship, in which all of the independent variable's effect on the dependent variable is expressed through a mediator variable. In this condition, the independent variable has only an indirect effect on the dependent variable, through the mediator.

Partial mediation

Figure 3.21 depicts a **partially mediated** causal relationship, in which the independent variable's effect on the dependent variable comprises two components. One component is an indirect effect through the mediator variable, along paths a and b. However, not all of its effect is expressed through the mediator variable. It also has a direct effect through path c. The independent variable's **total effect** on the dependent variable is computed as the sum of its indirect effect and direct effects. Accordingly, as shown in Figure 3.21, the total effect is a × b (indirect effect) + c (direct effect).

Suppose as in the prior example of an intervention program to encourage mammography screening (Figure 3.18) the correlation between the program and barriers is −.52 and the correlation between barriers and screening is −.45. As shown in Figure 3.22, the indirect effect of the program on screening would be .23. In addition, suppose the correlation between the program and screening is .26, which is the program's direct effect. Adding the indirect and direct effects, the program's total effect on screening is .49.

FIGURE 3.20 ● Complete Mediation

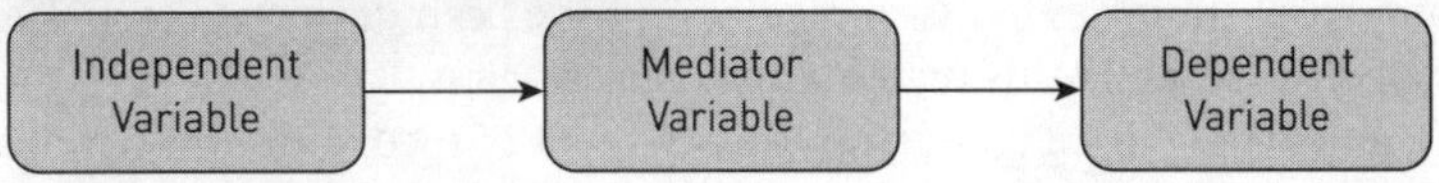

Independent Variable → Mediator Variable → Dependent Variable

FIGURE 3.21 ● Partial Mediation

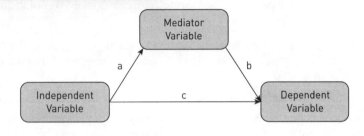

Indirect Effect = a × b
Direct Effect = c
Total Effect = Indirect Effect + Direct Effect = (a × b) + c

FIGURE 3.22 ● Indirect, Direct, and Total Effects

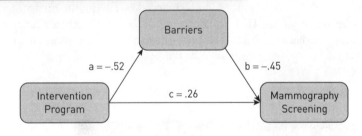

Indirect Effect = −.52 × −.45 = .23
Direct Effect = .26
Total Effect = Indirect Effect + Direct Effect = .23 + .26 = .49

Analyzing mediated causal relationships

When planning a study, it is essential to identify plausible potential mediator variables to ensure measuring them and being able to analyze their effects. Potential mediator variables are identified by drawing on theory, logic, and results from previous studies. There are three essential conditions for a variable to be a mediator of a causal relationship. A variable mediates a causal relationship if

- it is affected by the independent variable,
- it has an effect on the dependent variable, and
- the independent variable's effect on the dependent variable is reduced (or eliminated in the case of complete mediation) when the mediator's effect on the dependent variable is taken into account.

Baron and Kenny (1986) specified a strategy for assessing whether a variable mediates a causal relationship by conducting a series of three regression analyses. Since then, more advanced analytical strategies to assess mediation have been developed (e.g., Hayes, 2009) that are beyond the scope of this presentation. Nevertheless, Baron and Kenny's strategy is used widely, and it provides a conservative assessment of mediation in the sense that it is less likely than other strategies to conclude incorrectly that a causal relationship is mediated (see type I error in Chapter 15). Baron and Kenny's three-step strategy is as follows:

1. The independent variable affects the mediator variable when the mediator is regressed on the independent variable (the dependent variable is not included in the regression model).

2. The independent variable affects the dependent variable when the dependent variable is regressed on the independent variable (the mediator is not included in the regression model).

3. The mediator variable affects the dependent variable, and the independent variable's effect on the dependent variable is reduced (or eliminated in the case of complete mediation) when the dependent variable is regressed on both the independent and mediator variables.

The first two steps assess whether the independent variable affects both the mediator variable and the dependent variable, as illustrated in the top panel of Figure 3.23. If those conditions are not supported, a mediated causal relationship is not possible, and there is no need to proceed to the third step. The logic for the third step is as follows. If a causal relationship is mediated, then the independent variable's direct effect on the dependent variable when assessed in isolation should be reduced by adding the mediator variable to the step-two regression model. That would happen because the mediator variable accounts for some (partial mediation) or all (complete mediation) of the independent variable's isolated direct effect. This pattern is seen in the bottom panel of Figure 3.23, where the

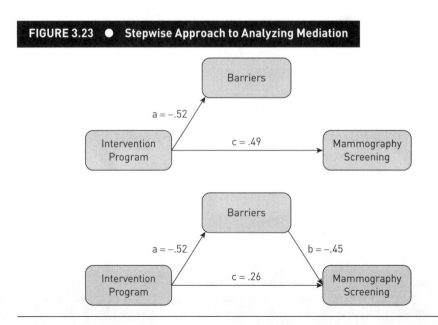

FIGURE 3.23 ● Stepwise Approach to Analyzing Mediation

independent variable's direct effect is reduced from .49 to .26 when the mediator's effect on the dependent variable is taken into account. If adding a presumptive mediator variable does not diminish the direct effect, then it does not mediate the causal relationship.

Multiple Mediator Models

Simultaneous/parallel multiple mediator model

Most causal relationships involve more than one mediator variable. For example, as shown in Figure 3.24, drawing on the Health Belief Model, in addition to reducing barriers, a mammography screening intervention program simultaneously may increase perceptions of susceptibility to breast cancer, the seriousness of breast cancer, and the benefits of mammography screening. For this simultaneous or parallel multiple mediator model, the total effect of the intervention program is the sum of its four indirect effects through the mediator variables plus its direct effect on mammography screening.

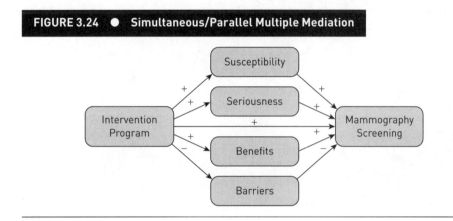

FIGURE 3.24 ● Simultaneous/Parallel Multiple Mediation

Sequential/serial multiple mediator model

Multiple mediator variables also may operate sequentially or serially, whereby a mediator variable affects one or more mediator variables in succession. Figure 3.25 depicts a sequential/serial multiple mediator model in which an intervention program's effect on mammography screening is mediated by increasing social support, which reduces barriers; by reducing barriers, the likelihood of obtaining a mammogram is increased. For this model, the intervention program's indirect effect is the product of its effect on social support, the effect of social support on barriers, and the effect of barriers on mammography screening.

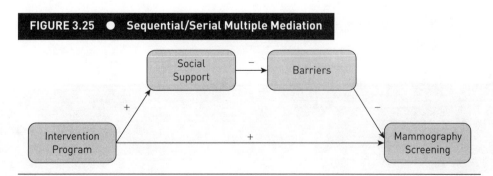

FIGURE 3.25 ● Sequential/Serial Multiple Mediation

Mixed multiple mediator model

Figure 3.26 depicts a mixed multiple mediator model, in which both simultaneous/parallel and sequential/serial mediation occur. In addition to a program's effect on mammography screening being mediated sequentially/serially through social support and barriers, Figure 3.26 includes a second mediation path, whereby the program simultaneously has a direct effect on barriers in addition to its indirect effect on barriers through social support. Thus, in this model, the program has two indirect effects on mammography screening: a path mediated by social support and barriers, and a path mediated by barriers only. For example, the program might reduce barriers indirectly by increasing social support, which then reduces a woman's reluctance to obtain a mammogram owing to fear of finding a problem. In addition, the program might reduce barriers directly by increasing a woman's access to mammography screening services.

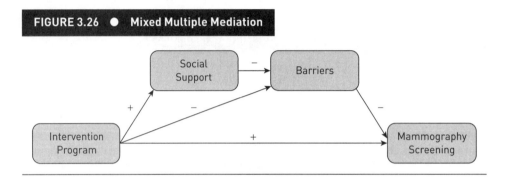

FIGURE 3.26 • Mixed Multiple Mediation

Multiple independent variable mediation

One variable may mediate the effects of multiple independent variables as illustrated in Figure 3.27, which is based on the Theory of Planned Behavior (Ajzen, 1991). According to that theory, behavioral intention mediates the effects on behavior from three independent variables: attitude toward the behavior, subjective norm, and perceived control. Thus, there are three indirect effects: a × d, b × d, and c × d.

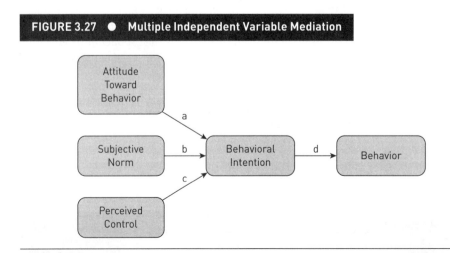

FIGURE 3.27 • Multiple Independent Variable Mediation

Moderated Causal Relationships

A **moderated causal relationship** occurs within a context where other variables, such as individual characteristics, family or household characteristics, and aspects of the social and physical environment, might influence it. A **moderator variable** modifies the strength and/or direction of the independent variable's effect on the dependent variable. For example, health risks may vary across individuals or populations, and delivery of an intervention program may vary across staff or settings. It is important to assess the influence of moderators to specify for whom, when, and/or under what conditions a particular causal relationship is observed.

Basic moderation model

Figure 3.28 depicts the basic moderation model. Unlike previous diagrams, the path arrow for the moderator variable's effect does not point to another variable. Instead, it points to the path from the independent variable to the dependent variable, indicating the moderator variable *interacts* with the independent variable to influence its effect on the dependent variable. Although a moderator variable may also have a direct effect on the dependent variable, it is not an essential condition for a moderated causal relationship (Baron & Kenny, 1986). In the basic moderation model, the independent variable's total effect on the dependent variable is the sum of its direct effect and its **interaction effect** with the moderator variable.

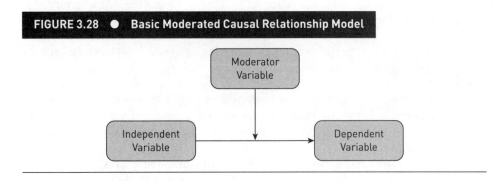

FIGURE 3.28 • Basic Moderated Causal Relationship Model

For example, as illustrated in Figure 3.29, women participating in an intervention program to promote mammography screening might have different outcomes depending on their medical history, which might moderate the causal relationship between the intervention program and screening. Accordingly, a higher postintervention mammography screening rate might be found among women with a family history of breast cancer than

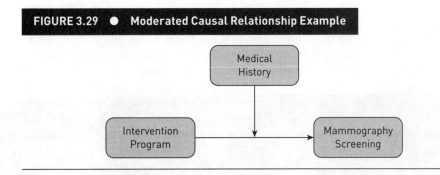

FIGURE 3.29 • Moderated Causal Relationship Example

among women without a family history of breast cancer. This example illustrates how a moderator variable may influence the strength of a causal relationship. That is, the intervention program's effect will be stronger among women with a family history of breast cancer than among women without that characteristic.

A moderator variable also may influence the direction of a causal relationship. For example, in general, a negative relationship is likely to be found between health status and use of health care services. Owing to a greater need, people in poor health status are likely to seek health care services more often than those in good health status. Thus, the lower their health status, the higher will be their use of services, such as the number of health clinic visits per year. However, age might moderate the relationship between health status and use of health care services. For instance, a negative relationship might hold among younger people, who generally are in good health and tend to seek health care services mainly in response to experiencing a health problem. Thus, for them, poorer health status is correlated with increased health care services use. However, among older people, a positive relationship might be found, such that older people might be likely to use health care services when their health status is good to maintain their health through regular check-ups and preventive screening. Thus, for them, a higher health status is correlated with increased health care services use.

Analyzing moderated causal relationships

When planning a study, it is essential to identify plausible potential moderator variables to ensure measuring them and being able to analyze their effects. As with mediator variables, potential moderator variables are identified by drawing on theory, logic, and results from previous studies. No variables are exclusively or standard moderator variables. However, in general, among the most often identified moderator variables at the individual level are age, gender, education, occupation, race/ethnicity, and health history. At the household/family level, income, insurance coverage, marital status, number of children, and type of housing often are potential moderator variables. At the setting or organizational level, potential moderator variables often are public versus private ownership (e.g., schools or hospitals), location (e.g., urban or rural), and size (e.g., number of hospital beds or number of employees).

A moderated causal relationship may be assessed by examining whether there is an interaction effect between the independent variable and the proposed moderator variable (Baron & Kenny, 1986). Depending on the level of measurement for the independent, moderator, and dependent variables, moderation may be assessed by employing various strategies, including analysis of variance (ANOVA), regression, contingency analysis, and more advanced methods (Hayes, 2009).

Table 3.3 presents a contingency analysis for moderation of an intervention program to encourage women to obtain regular mammography screening (also see Figure 3.29). If medical history moderates the program's effect, then Table 3.3 should display a difference in outcomes depending on the value of the moderator variable (medical history). Such a difference would indicate an interaction between medical history and the program, moderating the causal relationship between the program and mammography screening. In particular, based on the Health Belief Model, the more women perceive they are susceptible to breast cancer, the more likely they will be to get a mammogram. Accordingly, since a family history of breast cancer is a breast cancer risk factor, the proportion of women who receive a mammogram within 18 months postintervention would be expected to be higher among those with a family history of breast cancer than among women without a family history of breast cancer.

Of 130 women who participated in the program, 60% ($N = 78$) got a mammogram within 18 months. However, the outcome differed depending on a woman's medical history. While

TABLE 3.3 ● Mammography Screening by Medical History Among Intervention Program Participants

Medical History	Mammogram Within 18 Months		Total ($N = 130$)
	No	Yes	
No breast cancer	63% ($N = 38$)	37% ($N = 22$)	100% ($N = 60$)
Breast cancer	20% ($N = 14$)	80% ($N = 56$)	100% ($N = 70$)

37% of women without a family history of breast cancer got a mammogram within 18 months, more than twice as many, 80%, of those with a family history of breast cancer got a mammogram. Therefore, medical history moderated the program's effect. As this example demonstrates, if moderation is not taken into account, an erroneous conclusion might be drawn about a causal relationship's strength and/or direction. For instance, based on the overall outcome that 60% of the women got a mammogram within 18 months, it might be recommended that the program worked fairly well for women in general. However, after taking moderation into account, it might be recommended that different versions of the program should be tailored according to a woman's medical history.

Multiple moderator models

Most causal relationships involve more than one moderator variable. For example, in Figure 3.30, medical history, age, and marital status moderate the intervention program's effect on mammography screening.

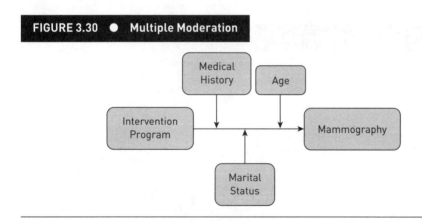

FIGURE 3.30 ● Multiple Moderation

Mediation and Moderation Combined
Mediated moderation

The top panel of Figure 3.31 presents the basic mediated-moderation model, where the independent variable's effect is moderated and then mediated. This is illustrated in the bottom panel, where response to the intervention program is moderated by medical history; then the moderated effect is mediated by perceived susceptibility.

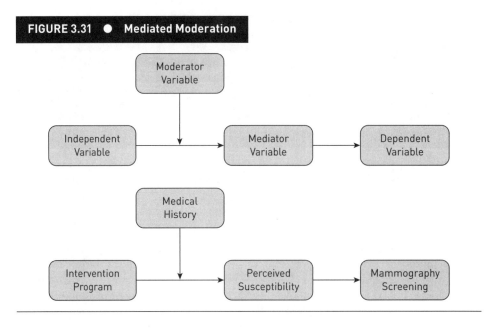

FIGURE 3.31 ● Mediated Moderation

Moderated mediation

The top panel of Figure 3.32 presents the basic moderated-mediation model, where the independent variable's effect is mediated and then moderated. This is illustrated in the bottom panel, where response to the intervention program is mediated by perceived susceptibility; then the mediated effect is moderated by medical history.

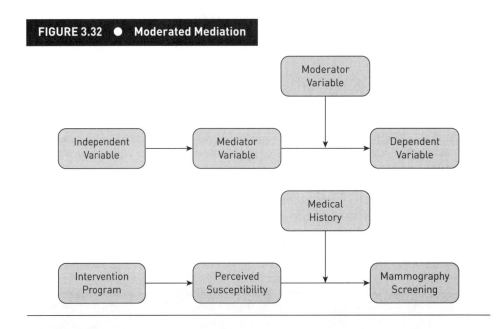

FIGURE 3.32 ● Moderated Mediation

Does the sequence matter?

For both mediated moderation and moderated mediation, the independent variable's total effect is the *product* of its **moderated effect** and its **mediated effect**. The mediated-moderation and moderated-mediation models presented in Figures 3.31 and 3.32 are mathematically equivalent:

moderated effect × mediated effect = mediated effect × moderated effect.

Thus, from a mathematical perspective, the order in which mediation and moderation occur is irrelevant (Muller, Judd, & Yzerbyt, 2005). However, their order does indicate conceptual and practical differences in the causal conditions and process. In the examples, the mediated-moderation model posits that women *participate* in the intervention differently depending on their medical history. For example, their medical history might influence their attentiveness and compliance with the intervention. The moderated-mediation model posits that women participate in the intervention similarly but they *respond* to it differently depending on their medical history. Box 3.1 presents an example of a study that assessed both mediation and moderation.

Complex Causal Models

Virtually all causal relationships involve multiple mediators and moderators. For example, as shown in Figure 3.33, researchers might posit a causal model that includes both mediated moderation and moderated mediation, whereby

- the intervention program has a direct effect on mammography screening;
- the intervention program has an indirect effect on mammography screening that is mediated by perceived susceptibility;
- the intervention program has an indirect effect on mammography screening that is mediated by social support, which is mediated by barriers;
- the intervention program's effect on perceived susceptibility is moderated by medical history;
- perceived susceptibility's effect on mammography screening is moderated by age; and
- social support's effect on barriers is moderated by marital status.

The role of any particular variable in a causal relationship depends on the context. For example, in a study about causes of heart disease, hypertension might be an independent variable, but it might be a dependent variable in a study about the health effects of smoking cigarettes. In another study, it might be a mediator of the effect of smoking cigarettes on heart disease, or it might be a moderator of how participants respond to a health education program about preventing heart disease.

Virtually always, it is possible to identify additional moderators and mediators that might be included in a causal model. A model easily can become unwieldy by attempting to account for every conceivable influence on every variable, and every variable's effect on other variables. In general, compared to a needlessly complex model, a model that is focused on key variables is a more effective guide for conducting research and optimizes translating research results into evidence-based practice.

FIGURE 3.33 ● **A Complex Causal Model**

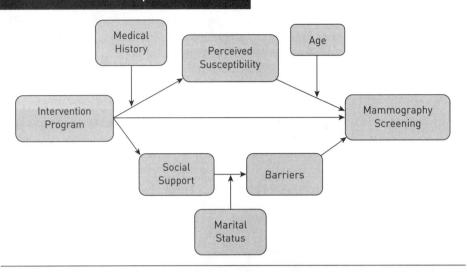

BOX 3.1: EXAMPLE OF ASSESSING MEDIATION AND MODERATION

UNPACKING THE EFFECT OF PARENTAL MONITORING ON EARLY ADOLESCENT PROBLEM BEHAVIOR: MEDIATION BY PARENTAL KNOWLEDGE AND MODERATION BY PARENT–YOUTH WARMTH

Lippold, Greenberg, Graham, and Feinberg (2014) analyzed effects of three components of parental monitoring on two adolescent problem behaviors, taking into account mediation by parental knowledge and moderation by the affective quality of the parent–youth relationship. An adapted version of their conceptual model is as follows:

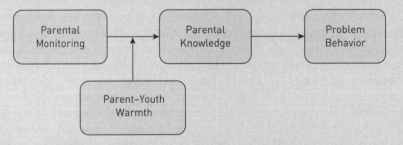

They collected data from the same students and their mothers selected randomly from 28 rural communities and small towns in Iowa and Pennsylvania at three points: fall of Grade 6, spring of Grade 6, and spring of Grade 8.

They found parental knowledge mediated the effect of two components of parental monitoring (parental actions and youth disclosure) on both problem behaviors (delinquency and substance use). The third independent variable, parental supervision, had no effect on problem behaviors. The effect of parental actions on substance use was partially mediated by parental knowledge. Parental knowledge completely mediated all other effects on delinquency and substance use.

Parent–youth warmth moderated the relationship between parental actions and parental knowledge (mediated moderation), such that it was stronger among families with higher levels of parent–youth warmth than families with lower levels. There were no other moderation effects.

Lippold et al. (2014) concluded: "Active parent monitoring efforts and youth disclosure are important components of the monitoring process and both are protective against youth delinquency and substance use. . . . However, interventions that target active parent monitoring efforts may be most effective if they concurrently provide parents with strategies to improve the emotional quality of the parent–youth relationship" (p. 1819).

Source: Lippold et al. (2014). Reproduced with permission from SAGE.

CHECK YOUR UNDERSTANDING 3.6

- Describe a mediated relationship and present an example of one.
- Describe a moderated relationship and present an example of one.

Key Points

Types of Variables

A variable is an attribute of an observation unit whose quality or quantity may change (vary) from one observation to another.

- Measured variables are classified in a series of levels of measurement (nominal, ordinal, and interval/ratio) according to the nature and amount of information a measurement captures.
- A discrete variable is measurable only in terms of particular units.
- A continuous variable is measurable in terms of an infinite number of possible values.

Attributes of Relationships

- Contingency: Occurrence of an observation in a particular category of one variable is contingent on the category in which that observation occurs for another variable.
- Direction: Values for one variable change in a predictable way when values for another variable change.
  - Positive relationship: Variables change in the same direction.
  - Negative relationship: Variables change in opposite directions.
- Strength: Indicates how reliably the amount of change in one variable may be predicted given the amount of change in another variable.

Causal Concepts

Causal relationships account for change in other variables, the process through which change happens, and the conditions under which change occurs.

- Independent variable: An independent variable causes change in a dependent variable.
- Dependent variable: Values depend on an independent variable's values.

- Necessary condition: A dependent variable changes only if the independent variable changes.
- Sufficient condition: A dependent variable changes whenever the independent variable changes.

Noncausal Relationships

- A risk factor is an independent variable that is neither a necessary nor a sufficient cause.
- Variables may be correlated because they are dependent on a common cause.
- A spurious relationship is explained by the influence of a third variable, which may be called an extraneous variable, an explanatory variable, or a confounder.
- An ecological fallacy occurs when causality is erroneously attributed at the individual level based on aggregate-level evidence.

Conditions for Inferring Causality

- Covariation
- Temporal precedence
- Ruling out alternative explanations
- A causal mechanism/process
- Consistency

Types of Causal Relationships

- Multiple causes and effects.
- Reciprocal: Two variables are both independent and dependent variables of each other.
- Mediated: An independent variable affects a dependent variable through its effect on a mediator variable.
- Moderated: A moderator variable modifies the strength and/or direction of the independent variable's effect on the dependent variable.

Review and Apply

1. Review the research plan you developed in the "Review and Apply" section of Chapter 1. If you did not do that activity previously, either do it now or identify a health-related problem that interests you. Write a problem statement and a research question, and choose a theory you consider appropriate to guide research about the problem.

    a. List the key variables you would measure to address your research question, placing them in the following categories:

    (1) Independent variable (limit to one variable)

    (2) Dependent variable (limit to one variable)

    (3) Key moderator variables (limit to no more than three)

    (4) Key mediator variables (limit to no more than five)

    b. Using the theory you selected as a guide, draw a causal model using path diagram methods to describe how you posit the variables are related. Label each path with a letter and a + or − sign to indicate the direction of each relationship.

    c. Choose one of the moderator variables in your causal model and describe how you would assess whether it truly is a moderator.

d. Choose one of the mediator variables in your causal model and describe how you would assess whether it truly is a mediator.

2. Suppose a positive correlation is found between sales of coffee and sales of alcoholic beverages in a particular community. For each of the following possible conclusions, state whether you think it is appropriate and explain why.

   a. Drinking coffee causes alcohol use (e.g., to counter the stimulating effect of caffeine).
   b. Alcohol use causes people to drink coffee (e.g., to get sober).
   c. There is another explanation for finding a positive correlation in this situation.

3. Compute the following effects for relationships in Figure 3.34.

   a. The intervention program's indirect effect on mammography screening that is mediated by perceived susceptibility
   b. The intervention program's indirect effect on barriers that is mediated by social support
   c. The intervention program's indirect effect on mammography screening that is mediated by social support and barriers
   d. The intervention program's total effect on mammography screening

4. Based on your analysis of Figure 3.34, if you were able to implement only one component of the intervention program, would you chose to implement the component that affects perceived susceptibility or the one that affects social support and barriers? Explain why.

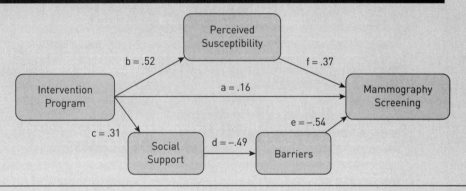

FIGURE 3.34 • A Complex Causal Model for a Mammography Screening Program

Study Further

Kahn Academy. (n.d.). *Correlation and causality*. Retrieved from https://www.khanacademy.org/math/statistics-probability/designing-studies/modal/v/correlation-and-causality

Shadish, W. R., Cook, T. D., & Campbell, D. T. (2002). *Experimental and quasi-experimental designs for generalized causal inference*. Boston, MA: Houghton Mifflin.

Trochim, W. M. (2006). *The research methods knowledge base* (2nd ed.). Retrieved from http://www.socialresearchmethods.net/kb/

4

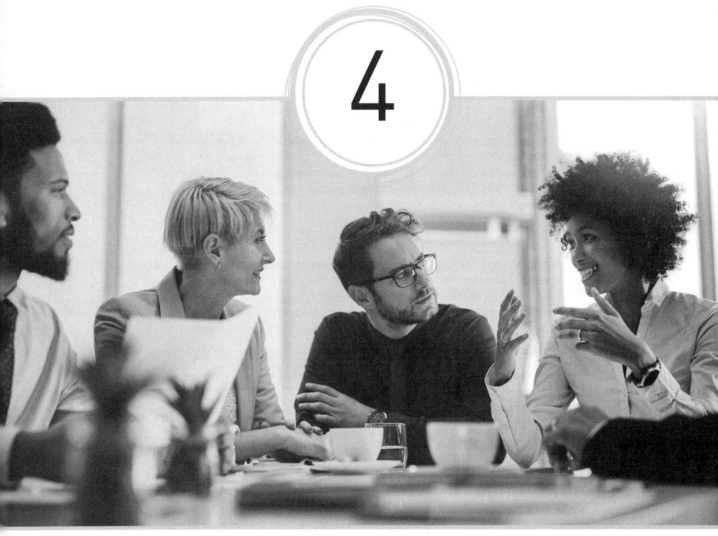

iStock.com/PeopleImages

Research Design Diagrams and Components

Chapter Outline

Overview
Learning Objectives
Research Design Diagrams
Research Design Components
    Time Frame
    Groups
    Conditions
    Observation Points
Key Points

Learning Objectives

After studying Chapter 4, the reader should be able to:

- Identify the four basic components in a research design diagram
- Draw and interpret a research design diagram
- Appropriately employ one-group and multiple-group designs
- Apply the control group model to simulate the counterfactual model
- Address ethical considerations related to control group conditions
- Apply strategies for specifying the timing of observation points

Overview

A research design is the pattern for how a study is conducted. As described in Chapter 1, the research question is the primary guide for specifying a research design. Chapter 5 presents several of the most often used basic designs. However, many variations of those designs, as well as other design formulations, may be employed. It often happens that while the research design for a particular study is similar to a "basic" one, it includes one or more alterations to accommodate a study's unique purpose and context. Selecting, modifying, or developing an appropriate research design requires understanding the principles of how design components function, interact, and influence the validity of results.

Research Design Diagrams

A **research design diagram** is a graphic device for developing a design, assessing potential threats to validity, implementing a research plan, and guiding analyzing and interpreting results. There are four basic components in a research design diagram:

- *Time*—the sequence in which other components will be implemented
- *Groups*—one or more groups of participants

- *Conditions*—the context in which participants will be observed
- *Observations*—measurements of variables at predesignated time points

It is essential to understand the principles that guide specifying and combining these components in a research design.

Although there is some variation among researchers regarding preferred symbols and format, Box 4.1 depicts the basic structure of a research design diagram. It shows the prototypical experimental research design, called the **pretest–posttest control group design**, which also commonly is called a **randomized controlled trial (RCT)**. The application, logic, advantages, and disadvantages of that design are discussed in detail in Chapter 5. Briefly, the design comprises two groups of participants who are randomly assigned (R) to different study conditions. The **treatment** group is exposed to an experimental treatment (X), while the control group is not exposed to the treatment. Observations (O) are made for both groups at two time points: pretest (prior to treatment implementation) and posttest (after treatment completion).

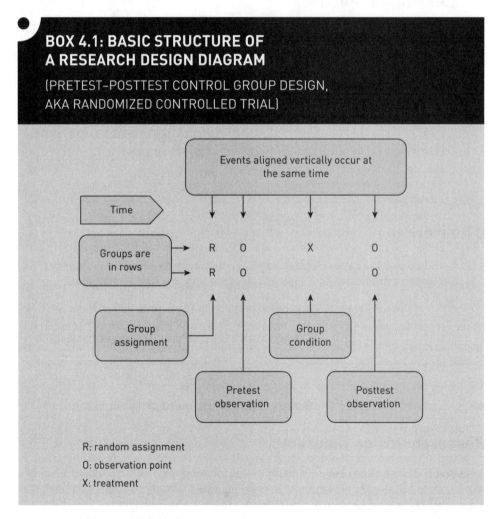

BOX 4.1: BASIC STRUCTURE OF A RESEARCH DESIGN DIAGRAM
(PRETEST–POSTTEST CONTROL GROUP DESIGN, AKA RANDOMIZED CONTROLLED TRIAL)

R: random assignment
O: observation point
X: treatment

Time progresses from left to right: Components to the right of others occur later; components aligned vertically occur simultaneously. The horizontal space between components does not necessarily indicate the length of time between components. Time points may be labeled, such as is shown in Box 4.2.

BOX 4.2: DIAGRAM WITH TIME LABELS

	February	March	April
R	O	X	O
R	O		O

Groups are arranged in rows, one row per group. Typically, groups are not labeled (e.g., "treatment" and "control") if they are readily identifiable from the group condition component of a diagram. However, for a design that is complex or unusual, it is helpful to insert group labels. The R in Boxes 4.1 and 4.2 indicates that **random assignment**, also sometimes indicated by RA, such as a lottery drawing, will be used to determine to which study conditions the groups will be assigned. Random assignment is the most effective strategy for creating comparable groups (Chapter 7). By convention, group assignment typically is indicated at the start of each row. However, that does not necessarily indicate that random assignment is done before the first observation point. The discussion of random assignment in Chapter 7 explains why it is most effective to conduct group assignment *after* the first observation point, whenever possible. Instead of cluttering a diagram with details, it is best to present them in narrative text accompanying a diagram.

When a design includes two or more groups/conditions, the rows often are referred to as "arms." For example, the design in Box 4.2 comprises two common conditions or arms: treatment and control. The *X* represents a treatment, such as an education program, social support, or a drug therapy. It appears in the row for the treatment group, which typically, but not necessarily, is presented in the top row. The absence of a condition symbol for the second group, the control group, indicates it is a **no-treatment control condition** that will be exposed neither to the experimental treatment nor to an alternative treatment. If the control condition will receive a treatment, such as standard care, then that condition should be indicated by an appropriate symbol, such as SC.

A research design diagram includes one or more observations (O) when variables will be measured. The number and timing of observations vary according to a study's purpose and context. When a design includes one or more treatment conditions, the terminology for identifying observation points indicates whether they occur before (pretest) or after (posttest) a treatment is implemented. The pretest–posttest terminology derives from research for which observations are made by administering "tests," such as to assess knowledge or ability. However, in current usage, those terms have evolved to a generic reference to observations taken before or after treatment implementation regardless of the measurement method. For example, they may refer to interviews about attitudes or behavior.

CHECK YOUR UNDERSTANDING 4.1

- Identify and briefly describe the four basic components in a research design diagram.

Research Design Components

The following sections describe further the features of the four research design components, including principles to guide modifying them according to a study's purpose and context.

Time Frame

There are two aspects of time in a research design. The first and perhaps most obvious one is the **timing** of when group assignment, observations, and group conditions will be implemented. That aspect of time will be addressed separately relative to each of the other design components in the following sections. This section addresses the second time aspect, which is the **time frame** in which a research design is implemented. The focus is on the period that typically starts with selecting and recruiting participants, and ends when all observations are completed. It does not refer to the entire study performance period, which includes activities such as hiring and training staff, purchasing supplies and equipment, processing and analyzing data, and reporting results. Strategies for indicating a design's time frame are including it in a diagram's title and/or inserting date labels above events as depicted in Box 4.2.

Accessibility

Access to research participants and/or sites may vary by the time of year when a study is conducted. For example, at certain times, some individuals are more likely to be away on vacation. Schools, teachers, and students are more accessible when schools are in session. In some situations, it might not be feasible to conduct a study at all during certain times of year, such as observing water safety at beaches in northern states during winter when beaches are closed. Moreover, even when individuals or sites are accessible, there are times when they might be less likely to cooperate, such as during a busy holiday season or near the end of a school term. For similar reasons, research staff responsible for collecting data and/or implementing a treatment also might not be available at certain times of year.

Seasonally inclement weather may restrict travel by participants (e.g., for a focus group at a central location) and/or research staff (e.g., to conduct face-to-face interviews at participants' homes). When planning to conduct a study in a location where weather conditions might be a hindrance at certain times of the year, the time schedule should be adjusted as appropriate. An alternative strategy is to consider other approaches for achieving a study's purpose. For example, travel may be avoided by conducting telephone interviews instead of face-to-face interviews. Another option is to consider a location where weather conditions are not likely to be a factor.

Observations

The nature and quality of data collected at observation points may vary by the time of year. For example, some variables are sensitive to seasonal fluctuations, such as type, frequency, and intensity of outdoor physical activity; access to fresh produce; traditional holiday food choices; and exposure to certain health problems, such as influenza. Thus, data about physical activity, dietary patterns, and health status might vary according to the time of year when they are collected. In most situations, the best strategy to address such potential issues is to schedule observation points to avoid them. Although in some situations data might be collected retrospectively through self-reports (e.g., interviews or questionnaires), their validity might be impaired owing to recall errors. In general, the less significant the events and the longer the time period over which individuals are asked to recall them, the less complete and accurate their reports tend to be (Bradburn, Sudman, & Wansink, 2004).

Treatment implementation

Whenever feasible, the time of year when a treatment is implemented should be planned to avoid coinciding with other potential influences on the dependent variable. Specifically, a threat to the validity of conclusions about the effectiveness of an experimental treatment, called a **history effect**, may be incurred (Chapter 5). The threat derives from the potential that a time-related extraneous variable (Chapter 3) either is the cause of a change in the dependent variable instead of the treatment, or is confounded with the treatment's effect. For example, throughout the year, there are many months, weeks, and days that are designated for observance of certain health issues (see National Health Information Center, 2018). If the timing of a treatment evaluation coincides with the observance period for the health issue the treatment is intended to address, the evaluation results might be influenced by the observance period instead of or in addition to the treatment. For instance, if a study implements a program to promote breast cancer screening during October, which is National Breast Cancer Awareness Month, the response to the program might be confounded with access to information and services associated with that month's special observance. Other examples are potential changes in physical activity in response to New Year's resolutions, or deviations from usual dietary practices during holiday feast/fasting periods. The best strategy to address such history threats is to schedule treatment implementation to avoid them.

In addition to addressing such predictable potential sources of extraneous influence, it is important to be alert for special conditions that might influence a study's results. For example, response to a program promoting mammography screening might be confounded by media reports that a widely respected celebrity recently has been diagnosed with breast cancer. Thus, when conducting such a study, it is essential to monitor the environment to detect potential extraneous influences. If such an event occurs, it is important to assess whether participants were exposed to it and how it influenced them. The event's occurrence and potential influence on a study's validity must be included in any report of results. Finally, if the potential influence of an extraneous event is deemed to be so strong as to have a devastating impact on a study's validity, then the best course of action is to suspend the study until it may be resumed in an appropriate context.

CHECK YOUR UNDERSTANDING 4.2

- Identify and describe ways that a study's time frame may influence the validity of its conclusions.

Groups

The following sections focus on the number of groups and their composition. Procedures for selecting individuals and assigning them to study conditions are presented in Chapter 7.

Number

The number of groups included in a research design may range from one to two or more. It is determined by the study purpose and the research question.

One group. As described further in Chapter 5, some research designs focus on a single group. The most simple and one of the most common designs is the **cross-sectional design**, which collects data from or about one group at one observation point. For example, a cross-sectional design might be employed for a community health needs assessment (see Centers for Disease Control and Prevention, 2016; and Community Commons, 2016) to develop a profile of community residents and their environment. The observation point might include measuring variables such as demographic characteristics, health status, health knowledge and beliefs, health behaviors, access to and satisfaction with health care services, access to healthy food sources, and so forth. Such information might be used to guide developing or modifying programs or policies to address health disparities.

Other one-group designs, generally referred to as **repeated-measures designs**, include two or more observation points. As will be discussed in a following section, such designs are not effective for assessing a treatment's effect because they do not include a control group. However, they are effective for assessing change/stability within a group under prevailing conditions during a certain time period, or for monitoring a group's status at specific time intervals (Chapter 6). For example, Box 4.3 depicts a basic **panel design**, whereby one group of individuals (the **panel**) is measured at multiple observation points (three points are presented for illustrative purposes). An example of a study using a panel design is the ongoing National Longitudinal Study of Adolescent to Adult Health (Add Health) that was initiated with a nationally representative sample of more than 20,000 adolescents in Grades 7–12 in the United States in 1994–1995. The goal is to examine the influence of social contexts (families, friends, peers, schools, neighborhoods, and communities) on health and risk behaviors over the course of adolescence and early adulthood (www.cpc.unc.edu/projects/addhealth/design; accessed August 24, 2018).

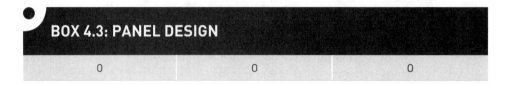

BOX 4.3: PANEL DESIGN

O   O   O

Multiple groups. Research designs include two or more groups to make comparisons across

- similar groups under different conditions, or
- different groups under similar conditions.

Comparisons of *similar groups under different conditions* are used to assess causality and the size of the effect of an independent variable on a dependent variable. For example, the pretest–posttest control group design comprises two groups: a treatment group that will be exposed to an experimental treatment (X) and a control group that will not be exposed to the treatment. The analysis will assess whether there is any difference between groups that may be attributed to being exposed to the treatment (i.e., a "treatment effect"). A design may include more than two groups. For example, the pretest–posttest control group design might be expanded by adding a third group that would receive standard care. Another application of multiple groups is to compare *different groups under similar conditions*, where the goal is to assess factors that account for a particular group difference. For instance, a study might seek to assess the cause of a disparity in the prevalence of adverse pregnancy outcomes across different groups of women.

Composition

Groups do not necessarily comprise individuals who know or otherwise interact with each other, either prior to or while participating in a study. Also, individuals in the same group are not necessarily similar to each other. Group composition depends on a study's purpose and design.

One group. For a one-group design, the group is intended to represent the target population; thus its composition is determined by the target population's composition. A simple and logical strategy to achieve that goal is to include the entire target population in a study.

That approach may be reasonable when the population is relatively small and readily accessible, such as employees of one hospital. However, most target populations are large and may comprise millions of members. In most situations, including all members of a large population requires excessive resources and may even diminish data quality owing to the project management challenges it is likely to present. Therefore, most often participants for a one-group design are a **sample** that is selected to represent the target population (Chapter 7).

Multiple groups. For designs that include two or more groups, an important factor is how individuals are assigned to groups and how groups are assigned to study conditions. Similar to a one-group design, each group in a multiple-group design is intended to represent a target population, although the groups may not necessarily represent the same target population. Most often, however, each group is intended to represent the same population. In that situation, members of an entire population or a sample are assigned to the groups, preferably by an unbiased random process to create comparable groups. When a design involves comparing different populations, each population is represented by a group. For example, if populations are designated as birth cohorts, then the groups will comprise individuals from each cohort, such as separate samples of people aged 18–29, 30–44, and 45–60.

Intact groups are preexisting "naturally occurring" groups, such as students in the same classroom or employees in the same department. In such situations, each intact group may be assigned to a different condition. For example, to evaluate a conflict resolution program at a school with two seventh-grade classes, one class might be assigned to the treatment condition (program) and the other to the control condition (no program). If a design includes several intact groups, then more than one group would be assigned to each study condition. For example, an evaluation of a conflict resolution program across the population of all seventh-grade classes in a school district would assign more than one class to each study condition. Thus, the two study groups each would comprise several intact groups of seventh-grade classes.

CHECK YOUR UNDERSTANDING 4.3

- Describe how the number of groups influences how a study's results may be interpreted.

Conditions

Groups may be observed under two basic types of conditions. **Prevailing conditions** already exist at the time a study is conducted, and researchers do not exercise any control over them. **Manipulated conditions** may be either created entirely by researchers, or modifications of existing conditions.

One group

In a one-group design, all participants are observed under the same condition. Most often, one-group design observations are made under prevailing conditions that are determined by the study time frame and location. Such studies generally are described as **observational designs**. Although sometimes it is possible to manipulate conditions for a one-group design (Chapter 6), the validity of results from such designs to attribute causality is weak. For example, as discussed previously, observations about outdoor physical activity are likely to vary by the time of year and location, independent of any controlled intervention.

Multiple groups

Most often, groups are compared across different conditions. The basic approach is to compare two groups across two conditions, treatment and control.

Counterfactual model. Experimental research design is founded on the **counterfactual model**. Box 4.4 depicts the counterfactual model for five individuals (A, B, C, D, and E) who are observed *simultaneously* under two conditions, a **treatment condition** and a **counterfactual condition**. A treatment condition is a change in an independent variable manipulated by researchers. The counterfactual condition is the status of the *same* individuals when they *are not* exposed to an experimental treatment at the same time as they *are* exposed to it. Thus, the counterfactual model addresses the ultimate question for all experimental-type research designs: *What would be the treatment group's outcome if it were not exposed to the treatment?* Of course, it is not possible to observe the same individuals simultaneously under two conditions. However, if that were possible, then the treatment's effect could be assessed with all alternative explanations for a causal relationship ruled out. The only reasonable explanation for any difference in outcomes would be exposure to the treatment. Although most often the counterfactual condition is a no-treatment condition, it is not necessarily the absence of any treatment; it is the absence of the experimental treatment. Thus, an experimental treatment's effect may be compared with exposure to another treatment, such as standard care or an alternative experimental treatment.

> **Key Concept**
>
> *Experimental research design is founded on the counterfactual model.*

BOX 4.4: COUNTERFACTUAL MODEL

	Pretest		Posttest
Treatment Condition	A, B, C, D, E	X	A, B, C, D, E
Counterfactual Condition	A, B, C, D, E		A, B, C, D, E

A, B, C, D, and E are five individuals.
X is an experimental treatment.

Control group model. Because it is impossible to observe the same individuals simultaneously under two (or more) conditions in practice, research designs employ the **control group model** to simulate the counterfactual model. As depicted in Box 4.5, the counterfactual condition is simulated by a control condition, where the control group is designed to be as similar as possible to the treatment group. Random assignment (Chapter 7) is the most effective procedure for designating comparable groups.

A treatment's effect is assessed by comparing outcomes on the dependent variable across the treatment and control groups. However, as discussed in the **internal validity** section in Chapter 5, because the treatment and control groups are not identical, the validity of the control group model may be threatened in various ways.

> **Key Concept**
>
> *The control group model simulates the counterfactual model.*

BOX 4.5: CONTROL GROUP MODEL

	Pretest		Posttest
Treatment Condition	A, B, C, D, E	X	A, B, C, D, E
Control Condition	A', B', C', D', E'		A', B', C', D', E'

A, B, C, D, and E are five individuals.

A', B', C', D', and E' are five comparable individuals.

X is an experimental treatment.

Control conditions. In general, control conditions are the prevailing conditions individuals normally would experience during a study period. Implementing a study protocol to ensure that the control group is not exposed to the treatment does not constitute a manipulated condition. There are two basic approaches to specifying a control condition: The control group receives either no treatment or a standard treatment.

For a no-treatment control condition, treatment is withheld from the control group. If no treatment currently exists for the problem under study, then no treatment is the only control condition possible. In accordance with the beneficence ethical principle (Chapter 2), a no-treatment control condition should not involve selectively withholding a potentially beneficial treatment from research participants. In such a situation, after obtaining informed consent (Chapter 2) to be assigned randomly to a treatment or control condition, if the treatment demonstrates a positive outcome, then it should be provided to the control group participants under a **deferred-treatment** or **wait-list control condition**. While finding a positive treatment effect in a pilot study (Chapter 1) may support conducting an experimental trial, pilot study results do not provide reliable evidence of a treatment's effectiveness or safety. Aspects that may be taken into consideration regarding withholding an experimental treatment from control group participants are as follows:

- It might not be feasible to provide the treatment to all participants owing to limitations in costs, staffing, or other resources.
- Members of the control group will not be denied a treatment to which they otherwise would have access.
- In accordance with the justice principle (Chapter 2), if random assignment to conditions is employed, all participants are provided an unbiased opportunity to be assigned to the treatment condition.
- An experimental treatment's benefit is unknown until it is reliably tested.
- The control group will be protected from any unanticipated and yet to be identified adverse effects associated with an untested treatment.
- The control group will provided the treatment if it is demonstrated to be effective.

Also in accordance with the beneficence principle, a no-treatment control condition should not involve withdrawing a treatment individuals already are receiving. When a treatment already exists and the research purpose is to assess an experimental treatment's effect in comparison with a zero baseline, participants should be recruited from among individuals who are not receiving treatment, and their informed consent must be obtained to randomly assign them to a treatment or control condition. Using the wait-list control group strategy, if the treatment group demonstrates a positive outcome, then the experimental treatment should be provided to the control group participants. If the experimental treatment does not demonstrate a positive outcome, then all participants should be provided the existing standard treatment. The ethical aspects of not providing the standard treatment initially to either the treatment or control participants must be weighed carefully in terms of the nature and degree of potential risk of harm to them (Chapter 2).

A **placebo control** is a variation of a no-treatment control, where participants receive a bogus "treatment" that is an inactive agent. Comparing outcomes for treatment and placebo conditions provides an assessment of the extent to which an apparent treatment effect may be a **false positive** artifact (also called a "placebo effect") caused by treatment group participants expecting to experience a positive outcome. They might mistakenly report a positive outcome or even actually experience one that is not caused by the treatment. For example, being aware they are in a treatment condition, they might change a health behavior owing to the fact that they expect a change to occur. When comparing treatment and control outcomes, the exposure of control participants to a placebo takes into account potential change that might result from expecting a change.

A placebo-control condition must be credible, and as much as possible it should include the same aspects of study participation, such as duration and nature of effort, as the treatment condition. Also, placebo-control participants must not be told initially that they will be exposed to a placebo. Therefore, appropriate procedures must be implemented regarding informed consent and disclosure of a deception (Chapter 2). Placebo-control conditions often are used effectively in pharmaceutical trials. For example, an evaluation of the effectiveness of a transdermal patch as a smoking cessation aid might provide all participants with patches that appear identical, except the active agent is not present in those provided to the placebo-control group. It is difficult to employ a placebo control when evaluating cognitive-based programs to change health knowledge, attitudes, and/or behaviors. In such situations, an **attention-placebo** or an **informational-control** condition might be employed to simulate the basic features of the treatment condition. Box 4.6 presents an example of a study that implemented an attention-placebo control condition.

BOX 4.6: EXAMPLE OF IMPLEMENTING AN ATTENTION-PLACEBO CONTROL CONDITION
THE EFFECT OF A COUPLES INTERVENTION TO INCREASE BREAST CANCER SCREENING AMONG KOREAN AMERICANS

Lee et al. (2014) assessed a culture-specific educational program for Korean American couples to improve mammography uptake among Korean American women. A DVD-format video in the Korean language, guided primarily by the Health Belief Model, was designed to address culture-specific beliefs and promote spousal support for mammography screening. A total of 428 couples were assigned randomly to a treatment and an attention-control group. The treatment group viewed the video, engaged in a brief group discussion immediately afterward, and completed a discussion activity at home. Participants in the attention-control group followed the same procedures as those in the treatment group, with the exception that control participants viewed and discussed a video about improving their diet. Compared with the attention-control group, the treatment group showed a significant increase in mammography uptake at both six and fifteen months post intervention.

It is not necessary to include a placebo-control condition for every experimental treatment. Sometimes a potential placebo effect may reasonably be ruled out. For example, consider an evaluation of a community-level informational campaign to improve knowledge about warning signs for heart disease among African American men, where the research design includes a treatment community and a similar community as a control. If participants in the treatment community will not be aware that the informational campaign is part of an experimental study, then a placebo effect is not a threat to the study's validity.

There are two situations where a **standard-treatment control condition** may be employed. First, it may be deemed not ethical to withhold an existing treatment, even if it is considered to be not very effective. The second situation is when it is desirable to compare the effectiveness and/or efficiency of an experimental treatment with the normative condition in which a standard treatment is available. Moreover, implementing a standard-treatment condition provides a means for assessing whether the research environment is representative of its usual state. If a standard treatment does not have its usual effect, then that may indicate that the circumstances in which a study was conducted were atypical, and the study's result might not be valid. If both the experimental and standard treatments have no substantial effect, that may indicate a **false negative** outcome for the experimental treatment. If a substantial effect is found for the experimental treatment while the standard treatment's effect is atypically large, that may indicate either a false positive outcome for the experimental treatment or an overestimate of its true effect.

Treatment conditions. A treatment condition is a *change* in an independent variable. It may be the introduction of a new treatment or a modification of an existing treatment, such as its content, format, setting, timing, or duration. Research designs are not limited to assessing a single treatment at a time. A design may assess the relative effectiveness of two or more alternative treatments. For example, Box 4.7 depicts a randomized controlled trial design that includes a no-treatment control condition and two in-person presentation strategies for a program promoting HIV risk awareness among undergraduate college students: a health professional (P) and a student peer (S). This design provides the following outcome assessments:

- The health professional (P) and no-treatment control (C) difference (P − C) measures the health professional's total effect.

- The student peer (S) and no-treatment control (C) difference (S − C) measures the student peer's total effect.

- The health professional (P) and student peer (S) difference (P − S) measures the relative effectiveness of those treatments.

BOX 4.7: PRETEST–POSTTEST CONTROL GROUP DESIGN WITH TWO ALTERNATIVE TREATMENTS

R	O	P	O
R	O	S	O
R	O		O

P: Professional

S: Student

Moreover, treatments may comprise multiple components. A comparative evaluation to identify which components and combinations are most effective may lead to simplifying a treatment such that it is easier to deliver, less expensive, less time-consuming, and/or more receptive among the target population. A **factorial design** ensures that all possible conditions are considered for inclusion in a multiple-component evaluation. The design is derived as a cross-classification of all categories or levels for all treatment components (called factors). For example, Table 4.1 depicts a 2 × 2 (pronounced "two-by-two") factorial design for evaluating the relative effectiveness of an undergraduate HIV risk awareness program that is presented by either a health professional or a student peer, and whether the presentation is in-person or by a recorded video.

TABLE 4.1 ● 2 × 2 Factorial Design: Presenter by Mode

Presenter	Mode	
	In-person	Video
Health professional	A	B
Student peer	C	D

A: Health professional in-person
B: Health professional video
C: Student peer in-person
D: Student peer video

According to conventional notation, the number of factors is designated by the number of digits in a design's title. The number of categories/levels per factor is designated by the values of the digits. Thus, a 2 × 2 factorial design comprises two factors, with two categories/levels per factor. The number of possible treatment conditions is determined by multiplying the numbers in the design's notation. Thus, a 2 × 2 factorial design, as in Table 4.1, comprises four treatment conditions. A 2 × 3 factorial design would include two factors, with two categories/levels for the first factor, three for the second factor, and a total of six treatment conditions. Box 4.8 depicts the research design for the four treatment conditions specified in Table 4.1, plus a no-treatment control condition, which is not necessary to include in a factorial design configuration.

BOX 4.8: PRETEST–POSTTEST CONTROL GROUP DESIGN FOR A 2 × 2 FACTORIAL DESIGN

R	O	A	O	
R	O	B	O	
R	O	C	O	
R	O	D	O	
R	O		O	

Table 4.2 depicts a 2 × 2 × 2 factorial design that includes a third factor, presentation length. Thus, the design comprises eight possible treatment conditions.

TABLE 4.2 ● 2 × 2 × 2 Factorial Design: Presenter by Length by Mode

	Presentation Length and Mode			
	Short		Long	
Presenter	In-person	Video	In-person	Video
Health professional	A	B	C	D
Student peer	E	F	G	H

Although a factorial design ensures all possible conditions are considered, not all conditions necessarily are implemented in a study. For instance, some conditions might be considered too expensive or too difficult to implement in a study and/or in practice. In Table 4.2, for example, conditions C and G, which involve long in-person presentations, might be deemed not feasible for the target audience. Thus, instead of implementing a full factorial design (also called a fully crossed design), sometimes a partial factorial design may be implemented. The 2 × 2 design is the most common factorial design because the number of conditions increases dramatically as the factors and/or categories/levels per factor increase. For example, instead of a 2 × 2 design, with four conditions, adding one more category/level to each factor would result in a 3 × 3 design with nine conditions. In addition to making study management more challenging, if the analysis plan specifies a certain number of participants per condition, then expanding the design will require more participants. Thus, if 100 participants will be included per condition, then the total number increases from 400 for a 2 × 2 design to 900 for a 3 × 3 design.

CHECK YOUR UNDERSTANDING 4.4

- Describe the counterfactual model and explain its role.
- Describe the control group model and explain how it simulates the counterfactual model.

Observation Points

Observation points are the times when variables are measured. Their number, type, and timing vary according to a study's purpose, context, and resources. Ideally, at each observation point, all individuals would be measured simultaneously to avoid any time-related influence that might cause a difference between individuals measured early and late in the data collection process. For instance, individuals who are observed later in the data collection process might have access to new information related to the study topic that is not available to those who are observed earlier. Therefore, although it is not feasible to observe all participants simultaneously in most situations, data should be collected as quickly as possible at each observation point. That may be facilitated by strategies such as choosing an efficient data collection mode, employing adequate numbers of staff, minimizing the number of variables and instruments, and minimizing the number of research participants.

Treatment designs

Although some designs that include one or more treatment conditions include only a posttest (Chapter 6), most often treatment designs include both pretest and posttest observation points.

Pretest. A **pretest observation** point is employed to obtain baseline measurements of the dependent variable and other key variables. That information may be used to

- describe the population to whom a study's results apply,
- assess preexisting differences across study groups/conditions,
- provide a baseline for assessing change at the posttest observation point, and
- assess participant attrition between pretest and posttest observation points.

First, pretest observation provides data to describe the population to whom a study's results apply, and with whom results from other studies may be compared. Differences in participants' baseline status on the dependent variable may account for different treatment effects across studies. For instance, those at a low level on the dependent variable have more capacity to improve than those at a high level. Thus, a larger treatment effect might be observed for them than for others. It is especially important to develop a profile of participants before study conditions are implemented that may change their status on the dependent variable.

A second application of pretest observation is assessing preexisting differences across study groups/conditions to measure potential assignment bias prior to implementing study conditions. When individuals/groups are randomly assigned to study conditions, a **randomization check** assesses group comparability in terms of whether they differ on dependent variable and other key variables by more than would be expected due to random chance. Although random assignment is an unbiased procedure, it does not guarantee that all groups will be comparable. When groups differ significantly, either random assignment may be redone, or the difference may be taken into account when analyzing results. A randomization check is especially important when the number of participants is small (e.g., fewer than 100), because the potential for a substantial random difference is greatest under that condition (Chapter 7). Moreover, when participants/groups are not randomly assigned to study conditions, it is virtually certain there will be preexisting differences across study groups/conditions. In such situations, it is imperative to assess preexisting differences so they may be taken into account when assessing a treatment's effect.

Third, pretest observation provides a baseline for assessing change. To obtain a valid baseline, a pretest should be conducted as close as possible prior to implementing study conditions. Otherwise, posttest differences may be confounded with normal change in the dependent variable or influence from factors other than the treatment(s) during a long pretest–posttest interval.

Finally, pretest observation enables assessing the potential influence of **attrition** during the course of a study. Unless the loss of participants before outcome measurements are collected at posttest is random, those on whom a study's results are based are likely to differ from the target population. Also, group comparability may change due to a differential loss of participants across study groups. Both of those situations are potential threats to a study's validity and are discussed further in Chapter 5.

Sometimes the dependent variable is null at the pretest observation point, such as when evaluating a program for which the goal is for treatment participants to initiate a beneficial behavior. For example, in an evaluation of a program to teach young women how to perform breast self-examination, it would not be possible to assess their baseline performance of a procedure they have not been taught and do not perform. Nevertheless, a pretest observation still may be conducted to develop a profile of their background characteristics and measure variables that might moderate or mediate their response to the program.

Posttest. The main purpose of a **posttest observation** point is to assess change in the dependent variable. Box 4.9 presents a generic representation of a pretest–posttest control group design with subscript notation. Numeric subscripts indicate observation points (1 = pretest, 2 = posttest), and alphabetic subscripts indicate group/condition (A = treatment, B = control). The treatment's total effect is indicated by the posttest difference across groups ($O_{2A} - O_{2B}$).

> **BOX 4.9: GENERIC PRETEST–POSTTEST CONTROL GROUP DESIGN**
>
> | O_{1A} | X | O_{2A} |
> |---|---|---|
> | O_{1B} | | O_{2B} |

However, posttest differences do not take into account any pretest differences. A **difference-in-differences analysis** assesses within-group change for the treatment group relative to within-group change for the control group. For the design in Box 4.9, the difference in differences is $(O_{2A} - O_{1A}) - (O_{2B} - O_{1B})$. If the treatment is effective, the difference should be greater than zero, indicating that improvement within the treatment group exceeded any coincidental improvement observed in the control group. Thus, a difference-in-differences analysis adjusts for pretest differences across groups and differential change within groups that may be attributed to factors other than the treatment.

Sometimes it is not possible to compare a pretest–posttest difference directly. For instance, that may occur when evaluating a program for which the goal for treatment participants is to terminate a harmful behavior. In such a situation, the dependent variable may be measured using different metrics at pretest and posttest, such as measuring its frequency at pretest but whether it is stopped or continuing at posttest. For example, although all participants in a smoking cessation program evaluation must be smokers, the number of cigarettes they smoke per day on average is likely to vary (unless eligibility requires all participants to be at the same level). Typically, the outcome is classified dichotomously as smoking or not smoking, not the number of cigarettes smoked at posttest. Another view is that the outcome, smoking cessation, does not exist at the pretest observation point and may be measured only at posttest. Either way, it would not be possible to compute a direct pretest–posttest difference. However, participants' pretest smoking level may be analyzed as a moderator of the program's effect, such as whether the treatment is more effective among light, moderate, or heavy smokers.

The posttest observation should not necessarily occur as soon as possible after implementing study conditions is complete. Posttest timing depends on the nature of the treatment, the nature of the dependent variable, and the type of participants. If a posttest is conducted before sufficient time elapses for change to occur, or for change to be at or near its maximum, a treatment's effect will be underestimated. Posttest timing is especially important when a research design includes a single posttest observation because there is only one opportunity to assess a treatment's effect.

Posttest observations may include measurements for conducting a **process evaluation** to describe the implementation of study conditions. While some aspects of participation may be observed directly, such as training session attendance, other aspects may be measured only by self-report. For example, participants might be asked to report what sections of a self-help manual they read, if they practiced any skills they were taught, or if they discussed their participation in the study with family members and/or friends. Also, treatment condition participants may be asked to assess aspects of the treatment delivery, such as how well a health educator presented information, the attractiveness and clarity of reading materials or videos, the convenience and comfort of the site, and the amount of time and effort their participation required.

Potential **control group contamination** (also called "treatment diffusion") may be assessed by asking control group participants if they were exposed to any aspects of the treatment. For example, in a clinic-based setting, control group participants might obtain reading materials intended only for the treatment group if treatment participants leave them behind in a waiting room. In a school-based setting, treatment participants might discuss their experience with control participants who attend the same school and/or with whom they interact outside of school. In addition, posttest observation may assess whether treatment or control participants are exposed to any unintended competing treatments, such as viewing a television program or voluntarily searching the internet for information about the health problem a study addresses.

Observational designs

Observational designs do not involve manipulating conditions, such as assigning participants to treatment and control groups. Instead, they observe participants under prevailing conditions to describe a target population at a particular time point, or to describe change/stability longitudinally, over a particular time period. The terms *pretest* and *posttest* do not apply to observation points in such studies. Instead, multiple observation points in an observational design are called **waves**, as depicted for a panel design in Box 4.10.

BOX 4.10: PANEL DESIGN

Wave 1	Wave 2	Wave 3
O	O	O

Observation points in an observational design may be planned at a consistent interval, such as annually for the National Health Interview Survey (NHIS) conducted by the Centers for Disease Control and Prevention (2018e). However, it is not necessary for them to occur at equal intervals. Depending on a study's purpose, the nature of key variables, and the types of participants, an observation schedule may target key time points. For Add Health, the ongoing panel study initiated in 1994 with adolescents in Grades 7–12, the observation points are Wave I, 1994–1995; Wave II, 1996; Wave III, 2001–2002; Wave IV, 2007–2008; and Wave V, 2015–2018. For participants in Grade 7 when the study was initiated, Wave II was at the end of grammar school, Wave III was post–high school, and Wave IV was postcollege.

The length of observation intervals may affect the validity of results (Bradburn et al., 2004). For a repeated-measures design, such as a panel study, there may be a lack of independence across observation points when intervals are short. For example, if participants are asked repeatedly to provide self-reports about the same attitudes or behaviors, the shorter the interval, the more likely they are to recall their previous reports and repeat them. They might be motivated to do so in order to reduce their participation burden or to appear consistent even if they have changed. **Recall errors** may threaten validity when observation intervals are so long that participants may not recall certain experiences or details about them. That is especially likely for experiences that are of low salience. For example, over the past two years, participants are more likely to recall details about undergoing major surgery than they are to recall the number of servings of a certain food item they consumed. Finally, the longer the observation intervals, the greater the likelihood of attrition owing to inability to recontact participants, or some choosing not to continue participating in a study. Attrition reduces statistical power for the analysis. Moreover, attrition bias may be incurred if participants who do not continue differ on key variables from those who do continue (Chapter 5). Consequently, the degree to which the remaining participants represent the target population may be diminished.

CHECK YOUR UNDERSTANDING 4.5

- Describe how and why observation points may vary according to each of the following:
  - Number
  - Type
  - Timing

Key Points

Research Design Diagrams

- A research design is the pattern for how a study is conducted.
- A research design diagram is a graphic device for developing a design, assessing potential threats to validity, implementing a research plan, and guiding analyzing and interpreting results.
- There are four basic components in a research design diagram.
  - **Time:** the sequence in which other components will be implemented
  - **Groups:** one or more groups of participants
  - **Conditions:** the context in which participants will be observed
  - **Observations:** measurements of variables at predesignated time points

Research Design Components

- The **time frame** in which a research design is implemented may influence validity of conclusions.
- The **number of groups** influences how results may be interpreted.
- Groups may be observed under prevailing or manipulated **conditions**.
  - The counterfactual model is the status of individuals when they *are not* exposed to a treatment at the same time as they *are* exposed to it.
  - The control group model simulates the counterfactual model.
- The number, type, and timing of **observation points** vary according to a study's purpose, context, and resources.

Review and Apply

You have been asked to evaluate a substance use prevention program for adolescents that will be implemented during the next school year with students in seventh grade through the high school sophomore year in two adjacent suburban school districts. School district A includes six middle/junior high schools and two senior high schools; school district B includes eight middle/junior high schools and four senior high schools. Owing to an outbreak of heroin use among adolescents in the community, the program will focus on developing the motivation and skills to prevent heroin use. It will comprise eight weekly sessions that will be presented in school classrooms during normal school hours. The program will include the following components: slideshow presentations by school district social workers, a presentation by a health professional, a presentation by a former heroin user, student discussions, and role-playing.

Draw a research design diagram for your evaluation plan and draft a proposal to the school district administrators that addresses the following aspects of your plan.

1. What would you recommend regarding the timing for program implementation?
    a. What potential impact, if any, might there be on the program's effectiveness according to when it is implemented?
    b. How might the timing of the program affect your ability to collect data?
2. How many groups will your research design include, and to what condition would each one be exposed? Explain why.
3. How would you divide the schools into groups and assign them to study conditions? Explain why.
4. Will your design include a pretest observation point? If yes:
    a. When would you schedule the pretest observation? Explain why.
    b. What key variables would you measure at the pretest observation point?
    c. How would you collect pretest observation data? Explain why.
    d. Describe any ethical concerns regarding collecting pretest observations and the strategies you would employ to address them.
5. Will your design include one posttest observation point or more than one? Explain why.
    a. When would you schedule the posttest observation(s)? Explain why.
    b. What key variables would you measure at the posttest observation point?
    c. How would you collect posttest observation data? Explain why.
    d. Describe any ethical concerns regarding collecting posttest observations and the strategies you would employ to address them.
6. Describe your analysis plan.
    a. What is the independent variable?
    b. What is the dependent variable?
    c. What key difference(s) will your analysis assess?
    d. What factor(s) would you assess that might moderate the program's effect (Chapter 3)? Explain why.
    e. What factor(s) would you assess that might mediate the program's effect (Chapter 3)? Explain why.
    f. Draw a path diagram using methods from Chapter 3 to describe how you posit the key variables are related.

Study Further

Kahn Academy. (n.d.). *Correlation and causality*. Retrieved from https://www.khanacademy.org/math/statistics-probability/designing-studies/modal/v/correlation-and-causality

Shadish, W. R., Cook, T. D., & Campbell, D. T. (2002). *Experimental and quasi-experimental designs for generalized causal inference*. Boston, MA: Houghton Mifflin.

Trochim, W. M. (2006). *The research methods knowledge base* (2nd ed.). Retrieved from http://www.socialresearchmethods.net/kb/

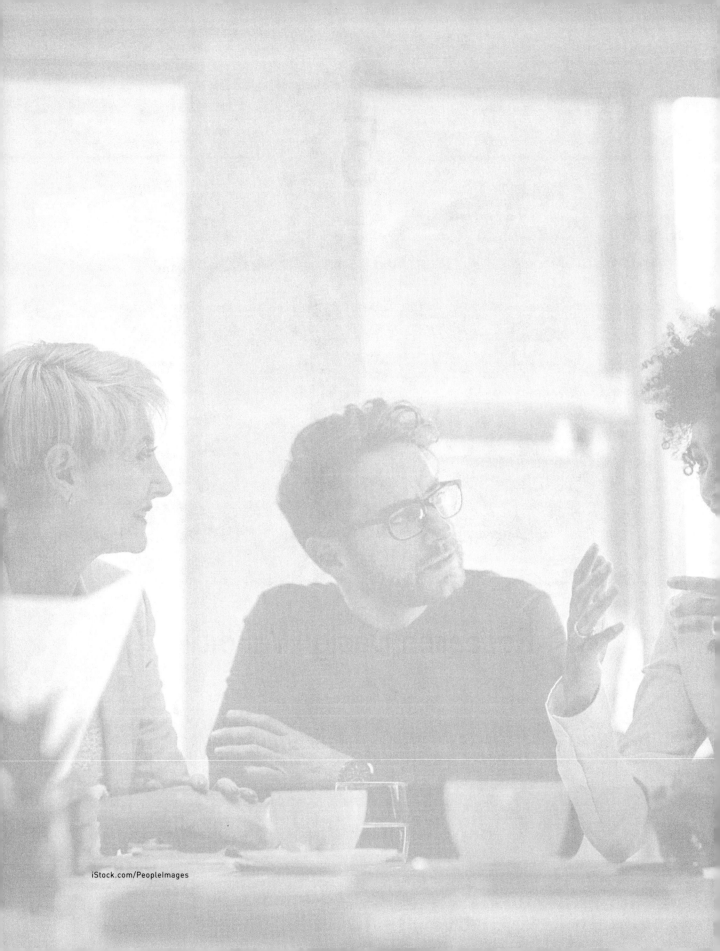
iStock.com/PeopleImages

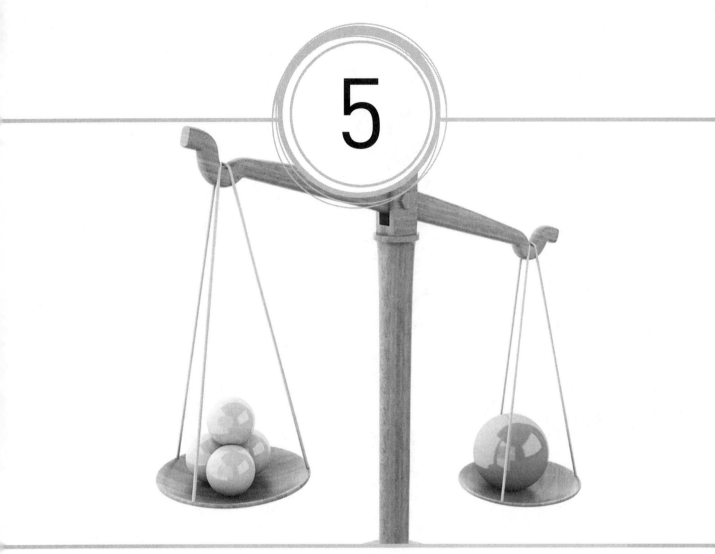

Research Design Validity

Chapter Outline

Overview
Learning Objectives
Observational Designs
Causal Designs
    Internal Validity
    External Validity
Internal Validity Threats and Strategies
    Design Threats
    Design Strategies
    Nondesign Threats
    Nondesign Strategies
External Validity Threats and Strategies
    Unrepresentative Units
    Unrepresentative Setting
    Unrepresentative Treatment
    Unrepresentative Outcome
Balancing Internal and External Validity
Key Points

Learning Objectives

After studying Chapter 5, the reader should be able to:

- Distinguish between observational and causal research design approaches
- Distinguish between internal and external validity of research designs
- Identify threats to internal validity and apply strategies to address them
- Identify threats to external validity and apply strategies to address them
- Apply guidelines for balancing priorities for emphasizing internal versus external validity

Overview

The factors that influence research design validity vary according to the research question and whether an observational or causal approach is employed. Choosing or developing the optimal design involves addressing a design's internal and external validity. It is essential to understand how each type of validity may be threatened and how a design may be developed to address those threats. The ultimate research design goal is to acquire evidence that is strong regarding both internal and external validity. Unfortunately, factors that enhance one type of validity often tend to diminish the other. In virtually all situations, a decision must be made regarding which type of validity to emphasize.

Observational Designs

Observational designs observe one or more populations under prevailing conditions to describe characteristics and relationships, and make comparisons across populations and/or within a population over time. Observational design validity is a function of two components:

- *Population*—how participants represent the target population
- *Conditions*—how well the observation point captures the intended study conditions

First, it is essential that a study includes representation of all population members in their appropriate proportions. As is described in Chapter 7, the most representative and trustworthy samples are obtained by employing random sampling procedures. Next, observation points must capture the conditions under which a study intends to observe a population. As discussed in Chapter 4, some variables are sensitive to seasonal fluctuations, such as the type, frequency, and intensity of outdoor physical activity in which individuals engage. Moreover, observations about relationships, such as between physical activity and health status, also may vary according to a study's timing. In addition to seasonal variation, other time-related factors that should be taken into consideration are special occasions, such as holidays and periods designated for observance of certain health issues (e.g., National Breast Cancer Awareness Month) (National Health Information Center, 2018). Although it is difficult or even impossible to anticipate some events, such as a weather-related disaster or a period of social unrest, when such factors are encountered, they must be taken into account when analyzing and interpreting a study's result. Of course, sometimes a study may be conducted deliberately to observe a population under such atypical conditions.

CHECK YOUR UNDERSTANDING 5.1

- Describe how observational design validity is a function of each of the following:
  - The population
  - Conditions

Causal Designs

Causal designs assess whether an independent variable causes a change in a dependent variable (Chapter 3). As discussed later in this chapter, not all causal designs are experimental designs. Causal design validity is assessed in terms of two aspects, internal validity and external validity.

Internal Validity

A causal design's internal validity is the extent to which there is confidence that an observed causal relationship is attributable to change in the independent variable rather than to an extraneous factor (Chapter 3). As discussed in following sections, a study's internal validity may be threatened by several factors. Internal validity is assessed as the extent to which plausible alternative explanations may be ruled out that a change in a dependent variable is not caused by the independent variable. The top panel of Box 5.1 illustrates the hypothesized causal relationship between an independent and a dependent variable. The bottom panel illustrates the internal validity assessment model, under which the possibility that the dependent variable is affected by an extraneous variable, rather than independent variable, is assessed. An extraneous variable may affect internal validity in two ways. One is that it might be the actual cause of change in the dependent variable, instead of the independent variable. For example, a health policy change that coincides with implementing a health education program may cause a change in health behavior instead of the

> **Key Concept**
>
> Internal validity is assessed as the extent to which plausible alternative explanations may be ruled out that a change in a dependent variable is not caused by the independent variable.

program. Other times, an extraneous variable may confound a study's result by moderating (Chapter 3) the independent variable's effect, such that it is enhanced or diminished compared to its effect in absence of the extraneous variable.

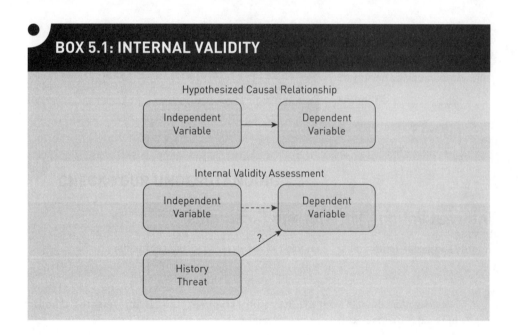

BOX 5.1: INTERNAL VALIDITY

External Validity

As depicted in Box 5.2, a causal design's **external validity** is the extent to which there is confidence that a study's result may be generalized to hold over variations in populations, settings, treatments, and outcomes. External validity is especially relevant to considering whether a result similar to that observed under research conditions may be expected under real-world,

> **Key Concept**
>
> External validity is assessed by comparing a study's features with those of situations to which its result might be generalized.

practice conditions. Even when using the same research design, external validity may vary across studies. Factors that may threaten a study's external validity are discussed in following sections. External validity is assessed by comparing a study's features with those of situations to which its result might be generalized. Although it is employed less often due to the need for additional resources, the most powerful external validity assessment strategy is replication (Chapter 1).

BOX 5.2: EXTERNAL VALIDITY

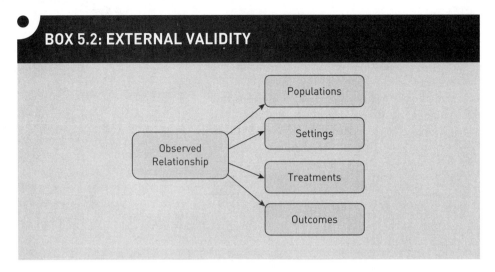

CHECK YOUR UNDERSTANDING 5.2

- In your own words, present a definition of each of the following:
  - Internal validity
  - External validity

Internal Validity Threats and Strategies

A study's internal validity may be affected by two general types of threats:

- *Design threats* arise from aspects of a study's design.
- *Nondesign threats* arise from the study context, how a study is implemented, and/or how participants or others react to a study.

The following sections describe these threats in detail and present strategies to eliminate or minimize them, drawing substantially on observations and recommendations by Campbell and Stanley (1963), Cook and Campbell (1979), and Shadish, Cook, and Campbell (2002).

Design Threats

Box 5.3 presents a summary of seven major design threats to internal validity.

Nonequivalent groups

When a research design includes two or more groups, the most serious internal validity threat arises when there is a systematic preexisting difference across groups on the dependent variable, or other variables that are correlated with it. If such preexisting differences are correlated with posttest differences, an incorrect conclusion about a treatment's effect

> **BOX 5.3: DESIGN THREATS TO INTERNAL VALIDITY**
>
> - **Nonequivalent groups:** There is a systematic preexisting difference across groups.
> - **History:** One or more events that affect the dependent variable occur concurrently with a treatment.
> - **Maturation:** A time-related change in participants affects the dependent variable.
> - **Attrition:** A systematic loss of participants during the course of a study reduces comparability within or across groups.
> - **Testing:** Repeated administration of a measurement instrument affects subsequent measurement outcomes.
> - **Instrumentation:** There is different dependent variable measurement within or across groups.
> - **Regression toward the norm:** Participants at an atypical pretest status on the dependent variable regress (return) to or toward their normal status at posttest.

may result. Other terms used to refer to this threat include *differential subject assignment*, *differential subject selection*, *differential selection*, and *selection*. Terminology that includes *selection* may be misleading by suggesting that nonequivalence is caused by the way participants are selected. While that is true in some situations (Chapter 7), it is not a general cause of nonequivalence. Regardless of how participants are selected, the key issue is how they are assigned to study groups/conditions. Terminology that includes *assignment* focuses on the process that leads to nonequivalence rather than its consequence. Therefore, *nonequivalent groups* is used here because it focuses on the condition that may threaten internal validity. Also, this terminology is consistent with common usage when referring to some research designs, such as the "nonequivalent control group design."

As described in Chapter 4, groups are truly **equivalent** only under the counterfactual model, where the same participants simultaneously are observed under two or more conditions. Because that is impossible, the control group model is used to simulate the counterfactual model and draw inferences about causal relationships. The more similar groups are before implementing a treatment, the greater the confidence that a study adequately simulates the counterfactual model. Accordingly, there is greater confidence in concluding that any posttest difference on the dependent variable is caused by the treatment.

Nonequivalence refers to a *systematic* difference that may bias a study's conclusion. For example, the validity of a result from an evaluation of a program to promote physical activity might be questioned if treatment and control groups differ markedly in terms of age. Engaging in physical activity tends to differ between younger and older individuals in terms of factors such as frequency and intensity. Random assignment (Chapter 7) is the most effective procedure for designating "equivalent" groups. However, even with that method, groups are not *identical*, as under the counterfactual model their differences are attributable to an unbiased random process.

There are several ways in which nonequivalence may bias results. For example, if the treatment group is at a more positive status than the control group on the dependent variable at the outset, most likely it will be at a more positive status at posttest, even if the treatment is not effective. Thus, it might be concluded incorrectly that the treatment is effective. Conversely, if the control group is at a more positive status at the outset and the treatment is effective, there might be little or no posttest difference across groups if the treatment group improves to the control group level. Thus, it might be concluded incorrectly that the treatment is not effective.

Moreover, even if the groups do not differ on the dependent variable, the result may be biased if they differ on a variable that is correlated with the dependent variable. For example, suppose for an evaluation of a program promoting physical activity, the treatment group participants are more motivated than the control group participants to increase their activity. Consequently, even if the treatment is not effective, at the posttest the treatment group might be more physically active than the control group. Another possibility is the treatment group's motivation might interact with the treatment such that these participants might experience a larger change in physical activity at posttest than would have occurred if they were less motivated.

History

A history threat is presented by one or more events that affect the dependent variable and occur concurrently with a treatment. It is one of the most common plausible alternative explanations for an observed relationship. There are two key characteristics for an event to pose a history threat:

- It occurs concurrently with treatment implementation.
- It is a plausible alternative explanation for change in the dependent variable.

A history threat does not necessarily refer to a recordable "historical" event. Indeed, a history threat may be posed by an otherwise unremarkable local event. Although factors such as participants' personal or family health "history" might moderate how they respond to treatment (Chapter 3), such factors do not pose a history threat because they *precede* treatment implementation. Also, a history threat is not posed by routine individual life events, such as going to school or work, which may occur concurrently with a treatment. Such events are aspects of the general conditions under which a study is conducted.

In addition, an event must be a plausible potential influence on the dependent variable. For example, an announcement that a major soft drink company is going out of business is not likely to be a plausible alternative explanation for how participants respond to an HIV prevention program. However, an announcement about a new HIV treatment would pose a history threat because it *might* affect how participants respond to the program. Nevertheless, that does not necessarily mean that it in fact accounts to any extent for a change in the dependent variable.

Consider an evaluation, using a one-group, treatment-only design, of a program conducted with women members of a church to encourage mammography screening. Suppose the women's ministries coordinator is diagnosed with breast cancer during the course of the study. If that information is shared with the study participants, it instead of the program might motivate them to get a mammogram. Another potential history effect is that learning about the coordinator's diagnosis might interact with the program, such as to increase the program's apparent effect.

Extending the example, suppose the evaluation design includes a second church to serve as a control site, which does not receive the program. Either control participants are not aware of the treatment church coordinator's diagnosis, or if they are aware of it, they might not be influenced by it because they do not know her. Thus, the coordinator's diagnosis might cause a greater proportion of treatment than control women to get a mammogram, leading to the same two potential incorrect conclusions: either a *false positive* that the program is effective, or *overestimating* the program's effect.

Now suppose the situation is reversed, whereby the women's ministries coordinator at the *control* church, rather than at the treatment church, is diagnosed with breast cancer. One possible incorrect conclusion is a *false negative* that the program has no effect. That is, even if the program causes treatment women to get a mammogram, if the coordinator's diagnosis motivates a similar proportion of control women to get a mammogram, there might be no treatment–control difference. Another possible incorrect conclusion is to *underestimate* the program's effect. That could happen if although the proportion of treatment women who get a mammogram is larger than for the control group, the treatment–control difference is diminished owing to more control women getting a mammogram than they would have done otherwise.

In yet another scenario, suppose both treatment and control participants are exposed to a history threat. For instance, during the course of the study, a national celebrity announces she has been diagnosed with breast cancer. That event might motivate *both* treatment and control women to get a mammogram. In that situation, a history effect could lead to a false negative conclusion or underestimating the treatment's effect, owing to finding either no significant treatment–control difference or a smaller difference than would be found in absence of the celebrity's announcement.

Maturation

A **maturation threat** is a potential change in the dependent variable caused by the passage of time during the course of a study instead of being caused by the independent variable/treatment. A maturation change may result from natural processes such as aging, a life-stage transition such as becoming a parent, or diurnal variation in a physiological factor such as blood pressure or appetite. A maturation threat also may be induced by research study participation, such as becoming anxious or fatigued while listening to a health education presentation.

A common source of maturational change is aging and factors correlated with aging, such as changes in weight, physical ability, cognitive ability, and social skills. The most noteworthy age-related changes generally occur among children and elderly. For example, an evaluation of a yearlong physical-fitness program for grade school children is virtually ensured to find improvement in their physical ability. However, physical fitness improves among children "naturally" as they age. Therefore, the change might be caused by maturation, independent of a physical-fitness program. Thus, maturation may lead to a false positive outcome, concluding that an ineffective program is effective. Another possible situation is that both a program and maturation affect the dependent variable, which would result in overestimating a program's effect.

Attrition

An attrition threat is a systematic loss of participants during the course of a study that reduces comparability across groups or within a group over time. Other terms used to refer to an attrition threat include *differential attrition, experimental mortality, subject mortality, differential subject loss,* and *differential subject mortality*. Attrition refers to losing participants at any time after the start of a study, including pretest observation, exposure to a treatment or control condition, and posttest observation. Potential causes of attrition include

- dropping out,
- being lost to follow-up at a subsequent observation point,
- a change in eligibility status, and
- being unable or unavailable to continue.

The main concern about attrition is whether it is *systematic*, such that it is correlated with differences in the dependent variable, which may lead to an incorrect conclusion about a treatment's effect. **Attrition bias** is a difference in a dependent variable that is a result of a systematic loss of participants across groups or within a group over time. Some degree of attrition is likely to occur in virtually any study that includes two or more observation points. If attrition is virtually a random event, it will have little or no effect on internal validity because the general characteristics of participants as a group will not change significantly. However, attrition rarely is a random event.

For example, attrition bias may affect internal validity if attrition is highest among the healthiest treatment participants, who might drop out of a program because they do not expect it will benefit them. Also, it might be more difficult to recontact the healthiest participants, who are likely to be more active than those who are least healthy. The least healthy participants who remain in the treatment group are most likely to experience a positive outcome, which might lead either to a false positive conclusion that the program is effective or to overestimating its effect. Attrition bias also may be introduced by a systematic loss of control group participants. For instance, those who are most in need of a treatment and are disappointed at not receiving one might drop out from a study. Meanwhile, participants who are most in need of a treatment and are assigned to the treatment condition are likely to remain in the study. Consequently, the validity of a treatment–control difference would be compromised.

An attrition threat sometimes is misunderstood as a differential in the rates of participant loss across treatment and control groups. However, that does not by itself result in biased group differences. Even when attrition is high, bias may be low if differences within or across groups are trivial. In general, when participant loss is small and differences in participant characteristics across groups and/or time are trivial, potential attrition bias is low and most likely ignorable. Potential attrition bias is greatest when participant loss is large and differences in participant characteristics across groups and/or time are substantial.

Testing

A testing threat occurs when repeated administration of a measurement instrument may affect subsequent measurement outcomes, which is called a **testing effect**. For example, a pretest measurement of the dependent variable may affect its posttest measurement. Participants' measurements may differ from pretest to posttest even if the independent variable has no effect on the dependent variable. Instead of changing in response to the independent variable, values of the dependent variable may change due to the influence of the pretest measurement experience.

In the general research context, testing refers to any measurement that involves active engagement of participants, such as an interview or a self-administered questionnaire. The term *testing* derives from experimental research, especially in educational contexts, where a participant's status on the dependent variable is assessed by administering a "test" of knowledge or skill. The terms *pretest* and *posttest* derive from administering such measurements (tests) before and after treatment implementation, respectively. Potential causes of a testing threat include the following:

- Participants learn to "take the test."
- The measurement experience changes the participants' status on the dependent variable.
- The measurement experience motivates participants to change.
- Posttest measurements are dependent on pretest measurements.

Participants may learn how to "take the test" by becoming familiar with the measurement protocol, format, task, content, and so on. For example, suppose at pretest participants are asked to view photographs of residential street scenes and identify aspects that indicate whether they depict safe or unsafe places for children to play outdoors. At posttest, they might identify more aspects of safety or risk because they have become familiar with the task of identifying those aspects of the scenes in the photographs. In other situations, a pretest measurement may act as an unintentional treatment that changes the participants' status on the dependent variable. For example, for an evaluation of a program that teaches women skills to negotiate with their partners to use condoms during sexual intercourse, their pretest negotiation skills might be assessed by observing their performance during role-playing sessions. However, the pretest sessions also may provide an opportunity for the women to practice their negotiation skills. Thus, they might be found to have improved at posttest independent of the treatment.

Another means for a testing effect to occur is if a pretest measurement motivates participants to change their status on the dependent variable. For example, in an evaluation of a program to increase knowledge about HIV risk factors, a pretest knowledge assessment might motivate participants to seek information about that topic independent of the study. Such motivation might be especially strong among control participants who will not receive the educational program. Finally, posttest measurements may be dependent on pretest measurements. For example, participants might recall their pretest responses to questions about attitudes or behaviors. Then they might deliberately respond differently at posttest if they believe they are being "tested" for a change in their attitudes or behaviors. In other situations, they might repeat their pretest responses if they believe they are being tested for stability.

Instrumentation

An instrumentation threat to internal validity may occur if the dependent variable measurement, either the instrument or the administration protocol, is different within or across groups. Although the term *instrument* implies the use of a physical device, such as a weight scale, in the general research context an instrument refers to any measurement method. In addition to physical devices, it includes questionnaires, interviews, focus groups, direct observations, records reviews, physical-fitness assessments, collecting biological specimens, and so on. Instrumentation threat sometimes is called "instrument decay," implying that it is a decline in measurement validity. However, sometimes it may be a measurement improvement, such as owing to staff gaining experience in administering a measurement. There are two basic types of instrumentation threat:

- Change in the instrument
- Change in the instrument's administration

Typically, an instrumentation threat is strongest if different measurement instruments or administration protocols are used to measure the dependent variable, either within or across groups. An example of using different instruments is to measure cigarette smoking behavior by self-report at one point and by a saliva specimen at another point. Although such a strategy might be beneficial in terms of one measurement, self-report, being more convenient and less expensive, it may introduce an **instrumentation bias/effect**, whereby a difference in a dependent variable is a result of a difference in how it is measured. In other situations, an instrument might be modified during the pretest–posttest interval with the intention of improving it, such as revising the content, wording, or format of a questionnaire. However, questionnaire design research has found that even small changes, especially in the wording of questions or response choices, may have substantial impacts on responses (Bradburn, Sudman, & Wansink, 2004). Finally, a physical measurement device might change in terms of its calibration, or it might malfunction.

An instrumentation threat also may be introduced by employing different administration protocols for the same instrument. An example is collecting pretest measurements by an in-person interview and collecting posttest measurements by a telephone interview. Another potential source of an instrumentation threat is if an instrument is administered differently from one observation point to another. One way that may occur is if different staff collect data at pretest and posttest. Another possibility is if staff performance changes from pretest to posttest (called "observer drift"). Their performance might improve as they become more experienced with an instrument over the course of a study. For example, they might become more proficient in distinguishing between observations of aggressive and nonaggressive behaviors. However, it also is possible for their performance to decline, such as becoming careless out of boredom with repeating the same measurement task or becoming frustrated with performing a difficult task. Finally, in addition, an instrumentation threat may be introduced by changing the measurement setting or protocol, such as from conducting face-to-face interviews at pretest with parents of high school children at the school, to conducting telephone interviews at posttest by calling parents at home (de Leeuw, 2005).

Regression toward the norm

When participants are selected because their pretest status on the dependent variable is atypical, internal validity may be threatened by participants regressing (returning) to or toward their normal status at posttest. Such a change might incorrectly be attributed to a treatment effect. A regression threat is strongest when participants are selected because their pretest status is extreme (either very high or very low). One reason is that there is virtually only one direction in which they may change. Another reason is that extremes tend to be unstable and are subject to change regardless of a treatment. For instance, consider situations where athletes occasionally deliver a subpar performance, but shortly thereafter they return to their normal level.

Sometimes the cause of **regression toward the norm** is attributed incorrectly to an unreliable pretest measurement that misclassifies participants as being in an extreme status. Instead, the cause is that participants' eligibility is reliably assessed at a point when their status is not normal. It is the participants' status that is unstable, not the measurement of their status.

As illustrated in Figure 5.1, suppose an evaluation of a blood pressure management program includes only participants who are screened at pretest as having the highest blood pressure readings and are deemed to be most in need of an intervention. If that is not their normal status, then they are likely to regress to their normal blood pressure status at posttest, independent of participating in the program. Thus, the evaluation might conclude incorrectly that the program is effective.

Other terms used to refer to this threat are *regression to the mean*, *statistical regression*, and *regression artifact*. This presentation uses regression to the *norm* because that term refers generally to a normal status, which for an individual is not necessarily the same as a population's mean value on the dependent variable. Also, the term *statistical* is not used here to avoid potential confusion about this threat being derived from conducting a statistical analysis rather than from how participants' eligibility is specified. Moreover, the *regression* aspect of this threat has no necessary relationship to whether a study's results are assessed using **regression analysis** methods. Instead, in this context, regression indicates a return to a previous/normal status, independent of a treatment.

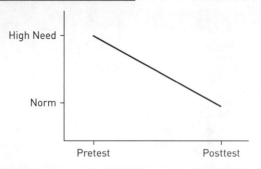

FIGURE 5.1 ● Regression to the Norm

Design Strategies

Designing a study to maximize internal validity sometimes presents a dilemma, such that a strategy to address one threat may increase a design's vulnerability to another threat. In such situations, a decision must be made about which threat is more likely and more serious. Some design strategies are specific to a single internal validity threat, while others address more than one. Designs that include only one group are more vulnerable to internal validity threats than ones that include a control group to simulate the counterfactual condition. Random assignment is the single design strategy that substantially addresses most of the internal validity threats.

> **Key Concept**
>
> *Sometimes a strategy to address one threat may increase another threat.*

Nonequivalent groups

Random assignment, which also is called "randomization" (Chapter 7), is the most effective strategy for designating "equivalent" groups. A simple example of random assignment is tossing a coin for each participant, such as heads designates treatment and tails designates control. Although randomly assigned groups are not identical, any differences between them are attributable to an unbiased random process. They are considered **statistically equivalent groups**, meaning that if a test of statistical significance is applied after random assignment, it will find no significant difference across groups on the dependent variable or any other variable. Moreover, any initial random variation across groups may be taken into account by applying inferential statistical procedures when analyzing results.

As depicted in Figure 5.2, in addition to designating equivalent groups, with random assignment any effect on the dependent variable from any other internal validity threat (history, maturation, attrition, testing, instrumentation, or regression toward the norm) will be experienced simultaneously and similarly by all participants regardless of the condition to which they are assigned. Accordingly, the treatment's effect is assessed net the effect of any and all internal validity threats. Thus, random assignment is a powerful internal validity strategy. However, using path diagram terminology (Chapter 3), random assignment controls only for any *direct effect* of an internal validity threat. It does not control for interactions among the other internal validity threats, or between them and study conditions.

Sometimes it is not feasible to randomly assign individuals. For example, in an evaluation of a program to increase high school students' knowledge about HIV risk factors, it might not be feasible to assign students randomly to treatment and control conditions. One possible reason is that school administrators might require making the program available

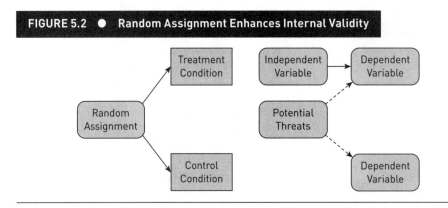

FIGURE 5.2 • Random Assignment Enhances Internal Validity

to all students. Also, there is a potential for *control group contamination* if students assigned to the treatment group share program information with friends in the control group. In such a situation, nonrandom assignment must be employed.

For example, a "comparable" high school might be designated as the control group. There are no standard criteria for specifying a minimal degree of comparability for nonrandom assignment. Identifying a comparable school is likely to be based on institutional and aggregate factors, such as school size and location, and the demographic and academic profile of the student body. Notably, it is not likely to be based on information about students' preexisting status on the dependent variable, knowledge about HIV risk factors, because that typically would not be available at that point.

Including a pretest measurement in the research design will enable assessing preexisting differences on the dependent variable so they may be taken into account when analyzing results. However, it will not be possible to take into account group differences on other variables that are not measured but may be correlated with the dependent variable. Moreover, as discussed in the following sections, including a pretest may make a design vulnerable to testing, instrumentation, and/or attrition. The great advantage of random assignment is it designates groups that may be considered equivalent on *all* variables, regardless of whether they are measured prior to treatment implementation. Nonrandom assignment is limited to designating comparability only on information that is available for certain variables at the point of assignment. Thus, the potential remains for groups to differ in unknown ways on many other variables.

Self-assignment, whereby participants choose their group/condition, should be avoided because virtually always it will result in **nonequivalent groups**. Participants who are most motivated to experience the potential treatment benefit are both most likely to choose that condition and most likely to experience a positive treatment outcome. Those who are less motivated to experience the potential treatment benefit and/or prefer not to invest their time and/or effort to participate in the treatment condition are likely to select the control condition. Consequently, **self-selection bias** will be introduced that enhances the likelihood of finding a positive treatment outcome and threatens internal validity.

A related issue is that participants' study group/condition should not be determined by an agent (e.g., parent, teacher, health care provider, or employer) acting on their behalf. For example, a teacher who hopes a program will be successful might assign or nominate for the treatment group students he or she expects are most likely to demonstrate a positive outcome.

History

As described in the preceding section, random assignment is the first line of defense against a history threat because participants' exposure to any such influence is expected to be similar across groups/conditions. Nevertheless, even with random assignment, an event might interact with study conditions. Returning to the mammography screening program example, if all participants are aware that a celebrity announced she has been diagnosed with breast cancer, their reaction to that event might vary according to group assignment. For instance, exposure to both the treatment and the announcement might interact to enhance treatment participants' intention to get a mammogram beyond being exposed to the treatment alone.

Other history threat strategies that are recommended even when participants are randomly assigned are

- avoiding anticipated events,
- minimizing the study time period,
- using multiple sites,
- monitoring the study context, and
- debriefing participants.

A study should be planned to avoid times and locations where events that may threaten internal validity are expected to occur. For example, an evaluation of an outdoor physical activity program should be conducted during a season and in a location to avoid severe weather conditions. The likelihood of a history threat increases with time. Therefore, the study time period from group assignment through posttest should be minimized. This strategy may include not conducting a pretest observation, as well as implementing the treatment promptly and collecting all data efficiently. When feasible, including multiple sites reduces the chance that a local history event will affect all participants. The study context should be monitored to detect any potential history threat. Monitoring may include on-site observation, interviewing site staff and administrators, and tracking media sources. Finally, participants may be debriefed at a study's end to determine if they were exposed to any event that influenced their participation in the study.

Maturation

Random assignment is the first line of defense against a maturation threat because equivalent groups are expected to experience similar maturational change. Other maturation threat strategies are

- minimizing the study time period,
- not studying participants when they are likely to change in response to factors other than the independent variable, and
- minimizing the participation burden.

The likelihood of a maturation threat increases with time because more time enhances the potential for change owing to factors other than an experimental treatment. Therefore, the study time period should be minimized to reduce the opportunity for maturation change to occur. That is especially important when nonrandom assignment is employed.

A maturation threat may be reduced by not studying participants at a time when their status on the dependent variable, and/or variables correlated with it, is likely to change during the study time period. Times of life-stage transitions, such as graduating from high school and entering college, generally should be avoided. For example, an evaluation of a youth alcohol abuse prevention program among high school seniors is likely to be threatened by maturation if pretest measures prior to graduation in spring are compared with posttest measures months later in fall after many or all participants have entered college. Such a study may reduce maturation by conducting the program and its evaluation early during the students' senior high school year, for instance, starting in fall and ending in spring. An alternative strategy is to study high school juniors, thus avoiding potential senior year maturational changes as well as the postgraduation life-stage transition.

Maturation owing to diurnal variation may be reduced by collecting pretest and posttest measurements at approximately the same time of day. So-called experimental fatigue that may be induced by study participation may be reduced by minimizing participants' burden in terms of the amount of time and effort requested of them. This strategy includes minimizing treatment demands, implementing the treatment efficiently, minimizing measurement demands, arranging comfortable environmental conditions, providing breaks, and employing methods to engage and maintain participants' interest.

Attrition

With random assignment, the nature and degree of participant losses are expected to be similar across groups/conditions. Nevertheless, several factors may cause a differential loss of participants such that groups *become* nonequivalent and internal validity is threatened by attrition bias. Moreover, when nonrandom assignment is employed, differential attrition may exacerbate preexisting group differences. Strategies for addressing a potential attrition threat are

- avoiding times when participants may not be willing or available to participate,
- minimizing the study time period,
- tracking participants,
- minimizing the participation burden,
- offering a participation incentive,
- emphasizing the importance of the research and encouraging full participation,
- blinding participants to group assignment, and
- employing a wait-list control condition.

An attrition threat may be reduced by conducting a study at a time when participants are expected to be willing and available to participate. In particular, times that generally should be avoided include vacation and holiday periods. The likelihood of attrition increases with the length of the study time period because participants are more likely to lose interest the longer a study continues. Also, attempts to make contact with participants for posttest measurements may become less productive owing to changes in contact information. The impact of such problems may be reduced by minimizing the study time period.

Also, when a study extends over a substantial time period, proactive tracking procedures should be employed, whereby interim contacts with participants should be made to verify that their contact information is up to date and to sustain their motivation to participate fully. In addition, at the outset, it is helpful to ask participants to provide third-party contact information (e.g., family member or friend) for someone who is not a member of their household and is likely to know how to contact them.

Of particular concern is the loss of participants who have participated in a study up to but not including the posttest. In addition to an internal validity threat, a substantial loss of participants wastes resources, reduces statistical power, and presents a missing data problem for the analysis (Chapter 15). The combined impact of nonequivalence and loss of analytical power owing to attrition may be devastating to a study. Generally, the most effective strategies for reducing such problems are minimizing the participation burden, as described in the maturation section, and offering an incentive for full participation (monetary or a gift). Also, the importance of the research and full participation should be emphasized throughout a study. Assurance of confidentiality should be emphasized, especially when studying a sensitive topic, and to the extent possible, measurement methods should be employed that are engaging and clearly relevant to the study's purpose.

Finally, when a treatment is highly desirable, participants who are assigned to a control condition might drop out if they are disappointed that they will not receive the treatment. In such a situation, attrition may be reduced by blinding (Chapter 1) participants to their study condition and placing control participants on a wait-list status, whereby they will receive the treatment after the study is completed (Chapter 4).

Testing

With random assignment, the nature and degree of any testing effects are expected to be similar across groups/conditions. In addition to random assignment, particularly when nonrandom assignment is employed, strategies for addressing a potential testing threat are employing

- nonreactive measurements,
- unobtrusive measurements,
- benign deception, and
- alternative measurements.

Whenever feasible, measurements that are not likely to sensitize participants to their status on the dependent variable should be employed. Assessing participants' pretest knowledge by a series of questions that may imply they are being tested should be avoided. For example, questions with multiple-choice or true/false formats may imply there are correct and incorrect answers to them (Chapter 11).

When possible, employing an **unobtrusive measurement** that does not involve interacting with participants may reduce a testing threat. For example, instead of asking participants to complete a questionnaire about their health history, that information might be obtained from records. A related strategy is to employ a benign deception (Chapter 2). For instance, consider the previously described example where participants are asked to view photographs of residential street scenes and identify aspects that indicate whether they depict safe or unsafe places for children to play outdoors. Participants' attention to safety aspects might be diffused by informing them that the purpose of the activity is to measure their perceptions about various aspects of community quality of life. That claim might be reinforced by embedding questions about child safety among other questions about the street scenes, such as housing style preferences and maintenance.

Finally, a strategy that may reduce the potential for participants "learning the test" or repeating pretest responses at the posttest is to employ alternative measurements at pretest and posttest. For example, participants might be asked to assess different but "equivalent" sets of residential community photographs at the two observation points. A strategy to avoid introducing an instrumentation threat (discussed in the next section) is to randomly assign which version of an instrument will be administered to each participant at the pretest. Then, at the posttest, each participant would be measured using the respective alternative instrument. For example, with two equivalent sets of photographs, A and B, each participant would be randomly assigned to assess either set A or set B at the pretest. At the posttest, those who assessed set A at the pretest would assess set B, and those who assessed set B at the pretest would assess set A. That procedure would distribute any potential instrumentation threat equally and randomly across both time and groups.

Instrumentation

With random assignment, the nature and degree of instrumentation effects are expected to be similar across groups/conditions. Nevertheless, strategies always should be employed to avoid differences in instruments or the way an instrument is administered across time and/or groups. Key strategies for addressing a potential testing threat are

- administering the same instrument the same way throughout,
- minimizing the study time period,
- maintaining the instrument for optimal performance (as appropriate),
- training and monitoring data collection staff,
- using experienced data collection staff, and
- minimizing data collection staff turnover.

The most effective strategy to prevent an instrumentation threat is to administer the same instrument the same way with every participant at every observation point. Minimizing the study time period reduces the opportunity for an instrumentation threat to occur. When an instrument is a mechanical or electronic device, it should be maintained in optimal functioning condition. Data collection staff should be trained and their performance monitored to ensure they are administering an instrument reliably. Whenever feasible, experienced staff should be employed when administering an instrument is particularly challenging and/or a high level of precision is required. Finally, staff turnover should be minimized by recruiting staff who are expected to be available throughout a study, providing appropriate compensation, minimizing the staff burden, and implementing appropriate procedures to ensure staff safety.

Regression toward the norm

Even when specifying eligibility criteria such that participants will be at a relatively extreme status on them, random assignment will distribute a pool of participants across groups equitably (Chapter 7). Other strategies for addressing potential regression toward the norm are

- classifying participants' baseline status reliably, and
- not conducting a study when participants' status may be expected to be atypical.

Classifying participants' baseline status as reliably as possible (Chapter 8) reduces the chance that "extreme" observations are not atypical instances. One strategy for achieving that goal is employing a trustworthy instrument and administration procedure. Another strategy is assessing participants on multiple occasions and under various conditions, as appropriate. In addition, when feasible, convergence of results from more than one instrument and/or administration mode may enhance classifying participants reliably. Finally, a study should not be conducted at a time when participants' status on the criterion variable may be expected to be atypical owing to a temporary deviation from their normal status. For example, a study involving dietary patterns should avoid major holiday periods.

Nondesign Threats

Box 5.4 presents a summary of six nondesign threats to internal validity. They may arise from the study context, how a study is implemented, and/or how participants or others react to a study. These threats sometimes are called "reactive," "reactivity," or "social interaction" threats. Although such terminology applies to most of them, it does not apply to them all. Therefore, they are presented here under the more general and inclusive heading of nondesign threats.

> **BOX 5.4: NONDESIGN THREATS TO INTERNAL VALIDITY**
>
> - **Treatment diffusion/control group contamination:** Control group participants are exposed to part or all of a treatment.
> - **Treatment imitation:** Control participants independently adopt the same or a similar treatment as the experimental treatment.
> - **Compensatory equalization:** A third party provides control participants an alternative treatment.
> - **Compensatory rivalry:** Control participants strive to achieve positive outcomes despite not receiving a treatment.
> - **Demoralization:** Control participants' performance and outcomes are reduced by disappointment at not receiving a treatment.
> - **Participant reactivity:** Participants change their performance in response to being aware they are being studied.

Treatment diffusion/control group contamination

Treatment diffusion, also called "control group contamination," occurs when control group participants are exposed to part or all of a treatment, which may change their posttest status on the dependent variable from what it would be otherwise. Consequently, an incorrect conclusion about a treatment's effect may be made. Treatment diffusion is most likely to occur when experimental and control condition participants are in close proximity during the course of a study. One way diffusion may happen is by communication across conditions, where treatment participants share information and/or materials with control participants. For example, such sharing might occur among students or coworkers during lunch periods. Another way is through incidental treatment exposure. For instance, if treatment and control participants receive services at the same site, control participants might encounter materials left inadvertently by treatment participants or staff in a common area, such as a clinic waiting room. A third way is through erroneous treatment exposure, where treatment administrators do not follow the study protocol reliably. For example, if the same staff serve both treatment and control participants, they might erroneously provide the treatment to control participants.

Treatment imitation

Treatment imitation threatens internal validity when some or all control participants independently adopt the same or a similar treatment as that to which the treatment group is exposed. Treatment imitation is most likely to occur when the treatment is highly desirable and it may be imitated easily (e.g., inexpensive, does not require special expertise). For example, control participants in an evaluation of a clinic-based smoking cessation program that provides counseling and nicotine replacement therapy might independently obtain the same or an alternative form of nicotine replacement therapy.

Compensatory equalization

Compensatory equalization is similar to treatment imitation in that control participants are exposed to an unintended alternative treatment. Instead of the participants seeking to imitate a treatment, a third party provides them a treatment to compensate for a situation they might regard as unfair because they are deprived of a potential benefit. Typically, the third party is someone who normally operates in the research context in a role that involves interacting with the participants, such as a schoolteacher or health care provider. Like treatment imitation, compensatory treatment equalization is most likely to occur when the treatment is highly desirable and it may be duplicated or simulated easily.

Compensatory rivalry

Compensatory rivalry occurs when control participants are aware they are being denied treatment and are motivated to compete with the treatment group by striving to achieve positive outcomes despite not receiving the treatment. This threat also is called the "John Henry effect," after a legendary manual steel driver who died of overexertion from striving to outperform a steam drill.

Demoralization

Demoralization, also called "resentful demoralization," is the opposite of compensatory rivalry. It may occur when control participants' disappointment at not receiving a treatment leads to a decline in their level of performance on the dependent variable from what it would be otherwise. Consequently, the control group would not reliably represent the target population's typical status at posttest.

Participant reactivity

Participant reactivity refers to participants changing their performance in response to being aware they are being studied. This threat is also called the "Hawthorne effect," which derives from occupational productivity experiments conducted at Western Electric's Hawthorne Works plant in Cicero, Illinois (Roethlisberger & Dickson, 1939). Although contested (Jones, 1992), the findings suggested that participants' performance might be influenced by knowing they are being observed. For example, instead of a response to a treatment, participants might change their behavior because they believe they are expected to demonstrate a change. Shadish et al. (2002) include this threat under the heading of "novelty and disruption effects," which may result in either a false positive conclusion, typically in response to a novelty, or a false negative conclusion, typically in response to a disruption.

Nondesign Strategies

Table 5.1 presents a summary of strategies for addressing nondesign internal validity threats. The most notable aspect of the table is that isolating treatment and control participants reduces all nondesign threats except participant reactivity.

TABLE 5.1 ● Nondesign Internal Validity Threat Strategies

Strategy	Treatment Diffusion	Treatment Imitation	Compensatory Equalization	Compensatory Rivalry	Demoralization	Participant Reactivity
Isolate groups	✓	✓	✓	✓	✓	
Monitor control environment	✓	✓	✓			
Train and monitor staff	✓					
Assign different staff to conditions	✓					
Minimize treatment period	✓	✓	✓			
Participant blinding		✓		✓	✓	✓
Placebo control		✓		✓	✓	✓
Wait-list control		✓	✓	✓	✓	
Staff blinding			✓			
Collaborate with staff			✓			
Minimize treatment awareness						✓

Treatment diffusion/control group contamination

Isolating participants, such as by implementing treatment and control conditions at different sites, reduces the likelihood that they will communicate. Also, it reduces the risk of both incidental treatment exposure and erroneous treatment exposure. In addition, the control environment should be monitored to ensure the participants do not have access to any treatment materials. This strategy is especially important when both treatment and control conditions are implemented at the same site(s). The chance of erroneous treatment exposure may be reduced by carefully training and monitoring staff, and assigning different staff to implement the treatment and control conditions when feasible. Finally, minimizing the treatment implementation period reduces the risk of treatment diffusion, which generally increases with time.

Treatment imitation

The treatment imitation threat may be reduced by isolating treatment and control participants, monitoring the control condition, and minimizing the treatment implementation period. In addition, motivation to imitate a treatment may be diminished by blinding participants to their study condition, employing a placebo control condition, or placing control participants on a treatment wait-list status.

Compensatory equalization

Implementing treatment and control conditions at different sites reduces the chance that control site staff will be aware of and have access to the treatment. In addition, the control environment should be monitored to detect any compensatory initiatives, and the treatment implementation period should be minimized to reduce the opportunity to implement an alternative treatment. Concern about unfairness may be addressed by placing control participants on a treatment wait-list status. When both treatment and control conditions are implemented at the same site, staff blinding may be employed where feasible. Otherwise, staff motivation to compensate control participants might be diminished by developing a collaborative relationship to gain their support of the research goal and commitment to comply with the research plan.

Compensatory rivalry and demoralization

Isolating treatment and control participants reduces the opportunity for communication across conditions, whereby control participants might learn about the treatment. In addition, control participants' reaction to not receiving a treatment may be diminished by blinding participants, employing a placebo control condition, or placing them on a treatment wait-list status.

Participant reactivity

The primary strategies for addressing participant reactivity are blinding participants and employing a placebo control condition. Also, this threat may be minimized by implementing a treatment in a manner that draws as little attention to it as possible.

Box 5.5 presents an example of implementing internal validity strategies.

BOX 5.5: EXAMPLE OF IMPLEMENTING INTERNAL VALIDITY STRATEGIES

THE EFFECT OF A COUPLES INTERVENTION TO INCREASE BREAST CANCER SCREENING AMONG KOREAN AMERICANS

Lee et al. (2014) (see Box 4.6) employed the following strategies to enhance internal validity:

- Recruited participants from multiple sites (50 Korean American religious organizations)
- Randomly assigned participants to treatment and control groups at the organizational level to avoid within-organization contamination
- Implemented treatment and control conditions immediately after pretest
- Implemented conditions and collected data at participants' religious organization
- Trained and monitored a staff of social workers from a Korean American community service agency to implement conditions and collect pretest data
- Trained treatment and control staff separately to avoid contamination
- Trained and supervised a separate staff to collect posttest measurements
- Blinded posttest staff to participants' study condition

CHECK YOUR UNDERSTANDING 5.3

- List the internal validity threats that are related to **time**.
  - For each threat, describe how it might threaten internal validity.
  - For each threat, describe how it might be avoided or minimized.
- List the internal validity threats that are related to **measurement**.
  - For each threat, describe how it might threaten internal validity.
  - For each threat, describe how it might be avoided or minimized.

External Validity Threats and Strategies

External validity is evaluated in terms of the extent to which a study is representative of the population, setting, treatment, and outcome to which an experimental treatment may be applied under real-world, practice conditions. In general, external validity is enhanced by conducting a study such that the research context is as similar as possible to the practice context. Box 5.6 presents a summary of four external validity threats.

BOX 5.6: EXTERNAL VALIDITY THREATS

- **Unrepresentative units:** The units of study do not represent the units of generalization.
- **Unrepresentative setting:** The setting differs from the setting to which results will be generalized.
- **Unrepresentative treatment:** An experimental treatment cannot be implemented similarly outside the research context.
- **Unrepresentative outcome:** The outcome is not similarly observable outside the research context.

Unrepresentative Units

Threats

Although units of study most often are individuals, they may be entities such as families, schools, workplaces, or health clinics. The more similar the units of study are to the external units to which a study's results might be applied, the stronger is a study's external validity. Figure 5.3 illustrates two levels of generalizability based on the units of study. The first level is how well they represent the target population. The second level, which is conditional on the first one, is how similar the target population is to other populations. If a valid inference cannot be made from the units of study to the target population, then there is no point in considering how similar the target population may be to one or more other populations. Returning to the example of a program conducted with women in one church to encourage mammography screening, the target population would be women affiliated with the study church. A secondary level of generalizability might be to consider how similar women at the study church

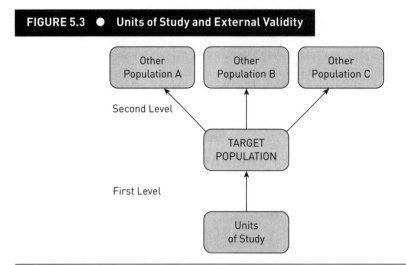

FIGURE 5.3 • Units of Study and External Validity

are to other populations of women, such as at other churches, local community-based organizations, or community health clinics.

Strategies

Strategies for addressing **unrepresentative units** as an external validity threat are

- selecting participants the same way target population members would come to receive a treatment in practice,
- specifying a target population that is as diverse as possible,
- studying more than one population, and
- minimizing inclusion and exclusion criteria.

At the first level of generalizability from the units of study (Figure 5.3), external validity is higher the more similar the selection of participants is to how members of the target population would come to receive a treatment in practice. As described in Chapter 7, random sampling generally is the most valid sample selection procedure because it eliminates potential selection bias that might derive from judgments about which units to select, or from self-selection, whereby target population members volunteer. However, results from a random sample might not be generalizable if random selection is not employed in practice, where administrators or staff might select individuals they deem to be most in need of treatment, or where individuals volunteer to participate in a program. Furthermore, sometimes random sampling is not feasible in either research or practice. For example, if a random sample of cigarette smokers is enrolled in a smoking cessation program, those who are not motivated to stop smoking are not likely to participate. Instead, volunteers who are motivated to stop smoking should be recruited. Viewed from the target population perspective, instead of selecting participants from among cigarette smokers at-large, external validity would be enhanced by recruiting cigarette smokers who are motivated to stop smoking.

At the second level of generalizability, external validity is higher the more similar the target population is to other populations. A target population is not selected randomly. Instead, it is specified based on theory, previous research, policy issues, and practical considerations such as feasibility to access a particular population. External validity may be enhanced by specifying a target population that is as diverse as possible. Moreover, whenever possible, generalizability may be increased by studying more than one population. For example, instead of studying women of one racial/ethnic group, women in two or more racial/ethnic groups would be included. Finally, inclusion and exclusion criteria should be minimized to include a broad spectrum of study units.

Unrepresentative Setting

Threats

External validity is stronger the more similar the research setting is to settings in which a treatment might be delivered in practice. The research setting comprises two key aspects: time and place. Time characteristics include the time of year, day of the week, and time of day. Furthermore, atypical conditions and/or special events as discussed earlier regarding a history threat to internal validity may cause a research setting to be unrepresentative of its normal state.

Site characteristics include geographic location, type of place, and space. Site location may be specified in terms of common geographic units such as city, state, or region. In addition, it may be specified in terms of geopolitical units, such as school districts, police precincts, and ZIP code areas. Type of place includes a wide variety of venues, such as institutions and agencies (e.g., schools, hospitals, churches, health clinics, and community-based service organizations), private companies and work sites, retail businesses, public places (e.g., street intersections, parks, and libraries), and private residences. Type of space also may vary widely, such as a private office, a clinic examination room, a school classroom, a community center conference room, or a grocery store produce section. Typically, site characteristics are combined in a nested manner. For example, for a study with students in urban high schools, likely site selection factors would include the city (or cities), school district(s), school(s), and within-school space(s).

Strategies

Research site selection typically is determined by practical considerations, such as established relationships with administrators, convenient geographic location, and available project resources. Such factors may lead to selecting a site that not only is unrepresentative of practice but may be atypical in a broader sense, such as a school where the overall level of academic achievement is superior to other schools in the district. Strategies for addressing an **unrepresentative setting** as an external validity threat are

- selecting a research site that is as similar as possible to where a treatment would be delivered in practice;
- employing multiple, diverse sites; and
- avoiding atypical time settings.

First, the research site(s) should be as similar as possible to where a treatment would be delivered in practice. Second, to the extent possible, a study should be conducted at multiple, diverse sites, which may vary in terms of aspects such as administration, staffing, clientele, physical features, and location. Finally, the time setting should be selected to avoid atypical times of year, days of the week, and/or times of day.

Unrepresentative Treatment

Threats

In the context of experimental research, a treatment is any manipulation of an independent variable, either by introducing it where it is absent, or by changing it when it already is present. In addition to assessing a treatment's effect in a research context, it is important to generalize its effect to other instances in which the treatment might be implemented, particularly in practice. External validity is threatened when treatment differences between the research and practice contexts lead to different treatment effects. The more similarity there is between how a treatment is implemented in the research context and how it may be implemented in practice, the stronger is a study's external validity. The main factors in treatment variation between research and practice contexts are content, format, and administration.

Treatment variation typically occurs when more control is exercised over a treatment in the research context than in practice. For instance, in practice, it might not be feasible to duplicate the number, length, or timing of treatment sessions. In other situations, the mode of delivering a treatment might vary. For example, in the research context a treatment might be delivered in-person by a health educator, but in practice the intervention might be delivered by a video presentation. When incentives are employed to recruit and retain research participants, in practice it often is not feasible to duplicate them. Also, external validity may be threatened by differences in staff who implement a treatment in the research and practice contexts that may contribute to different treatment effects. For example, in the research context a treatment might be delivered by staff who are trained and monitored extensively to ensure the treatment is implemented as intended. However, in practice the treatment might be delivered by staff (e.g., schoolteachers, nurses, or volunteers) with minimal training and monitoring.

Strategies

Although in the research context a substantial degree of control typically is exercised over treatment implementation, adherence to a treatment protocol may vary substantially under practice conditions. Sometimes it will not be feasible in practice to implement all of the treatment content, or some treatment content might be implemented with less fidelity than in the research context. Strategies for addressing an **unrepresentative treatment** as an external validity threat are

- assessing a treatment with content and format that are feasible to implement in practice,
- avoiding incentives for participation in research if it is not likely that they will be employed in practice,
- employing the same type of staff who would administer a treatment in practice, and
- permitting the same degree of flexibility in treatment implementation in the research context as is likely to occur in practice.

First, a treatment's generalizability may be enhanced by assessing a treatment with content and format attributes that are feasible to implement in practice. For instance, in a research context, it might be possible to employ a treatment that involves multiple, lengthy sessions, especially if participants are paid a cash incentive. However, in practice, staff and/or treatment recipients might not be willing or able to engage in such an "optimal" treatment protocol. Second, incentives for participation in research should be avoided if it is not likely that they will be employed in practice as well. Another strategy is to employ the same type of staff who would administer a treatment in practice, instead of employing research staff with little or no experience with the target population and the practice setting. Finally, although standardization of treatment implementation is a hallmark of experimental research, external validity may be enhanced by permitting the same degree of flexibility in treatment implementation across units, settings, and staff in the research context as is likely to occur in practice.

Unrepresentative Outcome

Threats

External validity is threatened when a treatment's effect is assessed differently in the research and practice contexts. If the research outcome measurement cannot be duplicated in practice, a treatment's effect might not be generalized outside the research context. There are four ways in which external validity may be threatened by an **unrepresentative outcome**:

- The outcome measurement is not feasible outside the research context.

- The outcome criterion defining treatment success differs between the research and practice contexts.

- It is not feasible to measure the outcome at the same observation point(s) outside the research context.

- The ultimate outcome is not observable directly in the research context.

First, it may not be feasible to employ the same outcome measurement in practice as in a research context. Such a situation may occur if the most valid measurement of a dependent variable is employed in the research context but that measurement is not feasible in practice. For instance, a study might have access to equipment, material, and staff resources that are not available in practice. Thus, it might employ an outcome measurement that is more expensive to collect, physically invasive, or complex to administer in practice. Therefore, in practice, it might be necessary to employ an alternative outcome measurement, which may indicate a treatment effect that is different from the effect observed in a research context. For example, a cigarette smoking cessation intervention's effect might be assessed by a biochemical indicator of tobacco consumption, such as saliva cotinine (SRNT Subcommittee on Biochemical Verification, 2002; Velicer, Prochaska, Rossi, & Snow, 1992). However, in practice, the outcome for the same intervention delivered by staff at a community-based organization might be assessed by self-reports about smoking behavior, which may result in discrepant interpretations of the treatment's effect (Caraballo, Giovino, Pechacek, & Mowery, 2001).

A second way external validity may be threatened is if treatment success in a research context is defined by an outcome criterion that differs from how success would be defined outside the research context. Such a difference might result from applying a more stringent criterion in the research context than in practice out of a concern by researchers to be conservative when concluding that an experimental treatment appears to be effective (see the discussion of type I and type II errors in Chapter 15). For example, a smoking cessation program evaluation might define a successful outcome as not smoking at all, even one puff, during the first four weeks postprogram. However, in practice, the program might be considered successful even if participants experience occasional slips but do not smoke an entire cigarette during that time period.

Third, access to participants in a research context may enable measuring the outcome more often and/or at times that are not feasible in practice. For example, when evaluating a weight reduction program, each participant's body weight might be measured within one to three days after the program ends. However, when the program is implemented in a community context, it might take one to two weeks or longer to measure each participant's postprogram weight.

Finally, for some treatments, especially ones that involve a behavior change, the ultimate outcome might not be observable within a study's time period. For example, the long-term goal (distal outcome) of a smoking cessation program is that participants will not smoke for the rest of their lives. However, in the typical research context, it is feasible only to measure short-term or midterm outcomes over a period from several months to a few years.

Strategies

In general, an unrepresentative outcome threat is addressed by specifying an outcome that is as similar as possible to the outcome that will be assessed in practice. The criterion for defining treatment success should coincide with that in practice. Whenever possible, the same treatment-to-outcome time interval(s) should be employed in the research context as in practice.

Box 5.7 presents an example of implementing external validity strategies.

BOX 5.7: EXAMPLE OF IMPLEMENTING EXTERNAL VALIDITY STRATEGIES

THE EFFECT OF A COUPLES INTERVENTION TO INCREASE BREAST CANCER SCREENING AMONG KOREAN AMERICANS

Lee et al. (2014) (see Box 4.6) employed the following strategies to enhance external validity:

- They collaborated with a Korean-owned media company to develop treatment and control videos designed around Korean American cultural values.
- Social workers from a Korean American community agency implemented treatment and control conditions.
- Social workers from a Korean American community agency collected data.
- Treatment and control conditions were implemented at participants' religious organizations.

CHECK YOUR UNDERSTANDING 5.4

- List the four external validity threats, and for each one, describe how it might do each of the following:
    - Reduce external validity
    - Be avoided or minimized

Balancing Internal and External Validity

The ultimate research design goal is to acquire evidence that is strong regarding *both* internal and external validity. However, designing and conducting a study to maximize both internal and external validity presents a dilemma. Strategies that enhance one type of validity tend to diminish the other one. Strategies for enhancing internal validity generally involve exercising a high degree of control over participants, settings, treatment protocols, and outcome measurements to eliminate or minimize potential alternative explanations of results. However, the more such aspects are controlled, the more a study's results are restricted to a specific context, which reduces external validity. Conversely, the less control a study exercises, the more similarity there may be between the research and practice contexts.

> **Key Concept**
>
> *Strategies that enhance one type of validity tend to diminish the other one.*

For example, conducting a study in one site may enhance internal validity because more control may be exercised over a single site as opposed to multiple sites. However, studying only one site diminishes the generalizability of results to other sites. While including multiple, diverse sites may enhance external validity, that strategy might diminish internal validity. For instance, it might result in nonequivalence across groups/sites and introduce internal threats such as history, maturation, attrition, and instrumentation. Thus, for all studies, a decision must be made regarding which type of validity to emphasize. Then strategies to enhance the other validity type should be employed to the extent they are feasible.

As described in Chapter 1, each study is a component for developing a body of evidence that comprises results from many studies, some of which emphasize internal validity while others emphasize external validity. In general, studies that emphasize internal validity assess a treatment's **efficacy**, which is its beneficial effect when it is delivered under optimum conditions. Studies that emphasize external validity assess a treatment's **effectiveness**, which is its beneficial effect when it is delivered under real-world, practice conditions (Flay, 1986). If a treatment's efficacy is not substantial, there is no point in assessing its effectiveness in practice. Thus, internal validity is a prerequisite for external validity. However, little if anything is gained by identifying a treatment that is effective in the research context but is not deliverable and not similarly effective in practice.

As illustrated in Figure 5.4, research about a particular problem typically progresses sequentially, whereby **efficacy trials** are followed by **effectiveness trials** (Flay, 1986; Flay et al., 2005; Mercer, De Vinney, Fine, Green, & Dougherty, 2007; Steckler & McLeroy, 2008). However, as discussed in Chapter 1, developing a body of trustworthy evidence about a problem is an iterative process. Accordingly, as depicted in Figure 5.4, effectiveness trial results may engender subsequent efficacy trials with modified or alternative treatments and/or protocols. Then the cycle regenerates.

FIGURE 5.4 ● The Relationship Between Internal and External Validity (Efficacy and Effectiveness Trials)

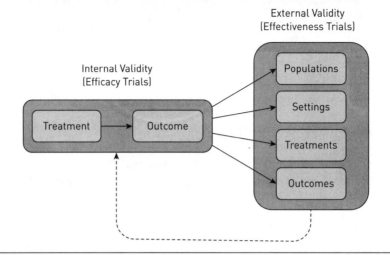

CHECK YOUR UNDERSTANDING 5.5

- Why is it virtually not possible for a research design to be strong in terms of *both* internal and external validity? Explain in your own words.

Key Points

Observational Designs

- Observational designs observe one or more populations under prevailing conditions.
- Observational design validity is a function of two components:
  - **Population:** how well participants represent the target population
  - **Conditions:** how well the observation point captures the intended study conditions

Causal Designs

- Assess whether an independent variable causes a change in a dependent variable.
- **Internal validity** is the extent to which plausible alternative explanations may be ruled out that a change in a dependent variable is not caused by the independent variable.
- **External validity** is the extent to which there is confidence that a study's result may be generalized to hold over variations in populations, settings, treatments, and outcomes.

Internal Validity Design Threats

- **Nonequivalent groups:** There is a systematic preexisting difference across groups.
- **History:** One or more events that affect the dependent variable occur concurrently with a treatment.

- **Maturation:** A time-related change in participants affects the dependent variable.
- **Attrition:** A systematic loss of participants during the course of a study reduces comparability within or across groups.
- **Testing:** Repeated administration of a measurement instrument affects subsequent measurement outcomes.
- **Instrumentation:** There is different dependent variable measurement within or across groups.
- **Regression toward the norm:** Participants at an atypical pretest status on the dependent variable regress (return) to or toward their normal status at posttest.

Internal Validity Nondesign Threats

- **Treatment diffusion:** Control group participants are exposed to part or all of a treatment.
- **Treatment imitation:** Control participants independently adopt the same or a similar treatment as the experimental treatment.
- **Compensatory equalization:** A third party provides control participants an alternative treatment.
- **Compensatory rivalry:** Control participants strive to achieve positive outcomes despite not receiving a treatment.
- **Demoralization:** Control participants' performance and outcomes are reduced by disappointment at not receiving a treatment.
- **Participant reactivity:** Participants change their performance in response to being aware they are being studied.

External Validity Threats

- **Unrepresentative units:** The units of study do not represent the units of generalization.
- **Unrepresentative setting:** The setting differs from the setting to which results will be generalized.
- **Unrepresentative treatment:** An experimental treatment cannot be implemented similarly outside the research context.
- **Unrepresentative outcome:** The outcome is not similarly observable outside the research context.

Balancing Internal and External Validity

- A decision must be made regarding which type of validity to emphasize. Then strategies to enhance the other validity type should be employed to the extent they are feasible.
- Studies that emphasize internal validity assess a treatment's **efficacy**, which is its beneficial effect when delivered under optimum conditions.
- Studies that emphasize external validity assess a treatment's **effectiveness**, which is its beneficial effect when delivered under real-world, practice conditions.
- Research about a particular problem typically progresses in a cyclical manner.

Review and Apply

1. For each internal validity strategy presented in Box 5.5 from the study by Lee et al. (2014), identify which internal validity threat(s) it might avoid or minimize, and explain why.

2. For each external validity strategy presented in Box 5.7 from the study by Lee et al. (2014), identify which external validity threat(s) it might avoid or minimize, and explain why.

3. Developing a research design often involves trade-off decisions about whether to prioritize strengthening a design against threats to internal validity or external validity. Present some guidelines for deciding which type of validity a study should emphasize.

Study Further

Glasgow, R. E., & Emmons, K. M. (2007). How can we increase translation of research into practice? Types of evidence needed. *Annual Review of Public Health, 28,* 413–433.

Green, L. W., & Glasgow, R. E. (2006). Evaluating the relevance, generalization, and applicability of research: Issues in external validation and translation methodology. *Evaluation & the Health Professions, 29*(1), 126–153.

Tunis, S. R., Stryer, D. B., & Clancy, C. M. (2008). Practical clinical trials: Increasing the value of clinical research for decision making in clinical and health policy. *JAMA, 290*(12), 1624–1632.

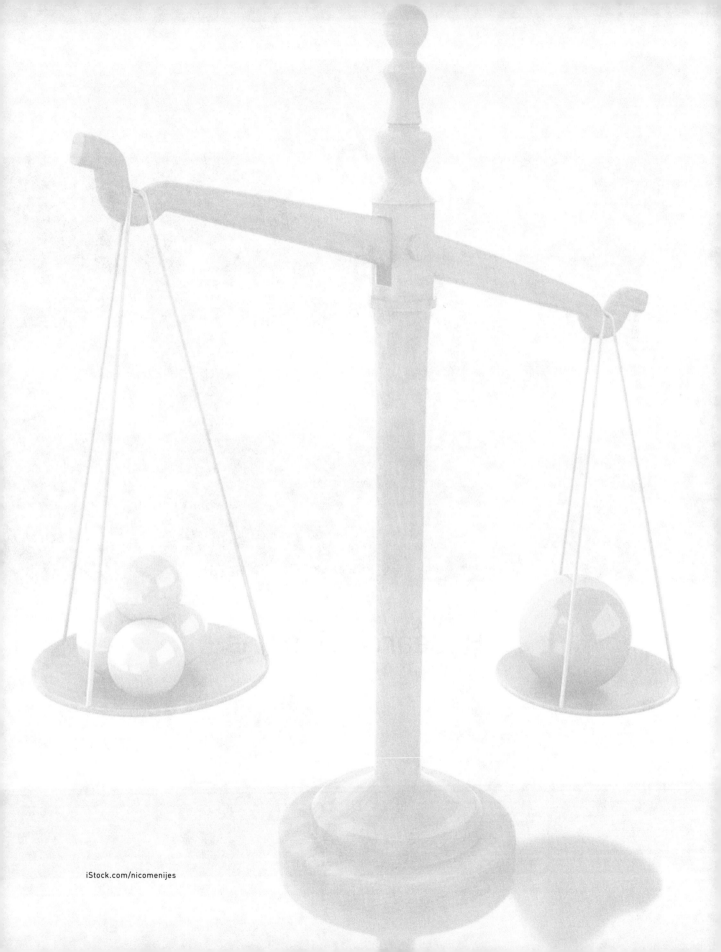
iStock.com/nicomenijes

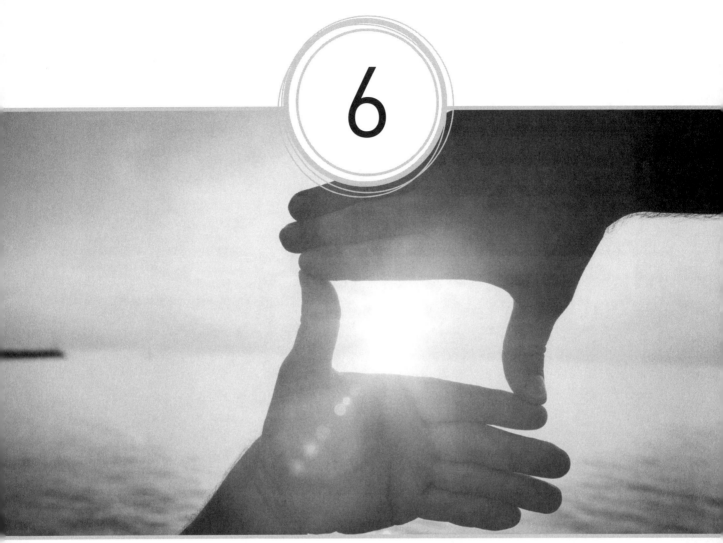

6

Research Designs

Chapter Outline

Overview
Learning Objectives
Observational Designs
    Cross-sectional Designs
    Longitudinal Designs
Causal Designs
    Nonexperimental Designs
    Experimental Designs
    Quasi-experimental Designs
    Design Variations
Key Points

Learning Objectives

After studying Chapter 6, the reader should be able to:

- Distinguish between observational and causal research designs
- Classify causal research designs as nonexperimental, experimental, or quasi-experimental
- Draw and interpret a research design diagram
- Assess strengths and weaknesses of a research design
- Apply design variations to enhance validity and efficiency

Overview

Research is conducted for many purposes, such as

- describing one or more populations at a particular point in time,
- exploring relationships among variables,
- identifying factors that account for differences across populations,
- monitoring stability/change within and across populations over time, and
- assessing causal relationships to evaluate the impact of interventions.

Moreover, factors such as the types of research participants, timing, conditions, key variables, and resources vary widely across studies. Typically, it is not adequate simply to plan a study by choosing from a menu of designs in a book or an online source. A research design often must be custom-fit to a study's purpose and circumstances. The way a design is structured and implemented directly influences the validity of results. Therefore, it is essential to understand how to combine, modify, and deploy design most effectively.

Observational Designs

Observational designs are used to observe populations under prevailing conditions to describe key characteristics and relationships. They are not appropriate for assessing causality because they do not involve introducing or modifying a treatment. Thus, observational design diagrams do not include an "X" symbol. The designs may include one or more populations, and one or more observation points. Observations may be compared across populations and/or within populations over time. When an observational design includes more than one group, participants are not randomly assigned to groups. They are studied as representatives of the populations of which they already are members. A major concern about validity of observational designs is how well participants represent the target population(s). Random sampling procedures (Chapter 7) generally provide the most representative and trustworthy samples.

> **Key Concept**
>
> *Observational designs observe populations under prevailing conditions.*

Cross-sectional Designs

Cross-sectional designs collect data from or about one or more populations at one observation point (O). Although the primary focus of most cross-sectional studies is to measure participants' current status on variables such as health knowledge and beliefs, and health-related behaviors, they may collect retrospective measures, such as health history and past behavior, as well.

Box 6.1 depicts the one-group cross-sectional design, which is the most common observational design. To indicate whether participants are selected as a random or nonrandom sample, the symbols "RS" and "NR," respectively, may be inserted to the left of the observation point. Thus, the design would be represented as "RS O." Another option is to insert a time-frame label above the observation point to indicate when data are collected. Examples of research questions that might be addressed using a cross-sectional design are as follows:

- What proportion of the children under age 6 in the Uptown community currently are not up-to-date on their immunization schedule?

- What is the current knowledge about risk factors for heart disease among African American men age 40 and older in the North Lawndale community?

BOX 6.1: ONE-GROUP CROSS-SECTIONAL DESIGN

O

The one-group cross-sectional design often is referred to as a *survey design*, which is an unfortunate misnomer for three reasons. First, although survey methods (Chapter 12) often are employed with this design, a survey itself is not a research design. A survey is a *method* for collecting data through self-reports in a standardized format. Second, the application of survey methods is not restricted to a cross-sectional design. Third, data for a cross-sectional design may be collected by methods other than a survey, such as focus groups, unstructured interviews, nonparticipant observation, and records review.

A multiple-group cross-sectional design collects data from two or more populations at the same observation point to make comparisons across populations. Box 6.2 depicts an example that includes three groups/populations. The dashed horizontal line indicates participants are from different groups/populations.

BOX 6.2: MULTIPLE-GROUP CROSS-SECTIONAL DESIGN

O
- - -
O
- - -
O

Longitudinal Designs

Longitudinal designs involve collecting data from or about one or more populations at multiple observation points, typically called "waves." They are employed to study variation in variables and relationships under prevailing conditions over a specific time period. Although it is not essential, typically observation intervals are equal, such as every six months or annually. The expected rate of change for key variables is the primary factor that determines observation points. When change is expected to occur more often, observation intervals should be relatively short, and vice versa. Longitudinal designs are expensive, time-consuming, and logistically challenging.

Trend study (sequential cross-sectional design)

A **trend study** design, depicted in Box 6.3, is used to monitor a population over time and obtain up-to-date profiles regarding certain characteristics, such as health status and health behaviors. Such data are useful for identifying emerging health problems and tracking progress toward health policy objectives. An example of a research question that might be addressed using a trend study design is as follows:

> Over the next five years, will the proportion of women aged 20–25 who regularly smoke cigarettes decrease, stay about the same, or increase?

A trend study design comprises a series of cross-sectional studies with *separate* samples selected from the *same* population at each observation point. In most cases, samples are

BOX 6.3: TREND STUDY DESIGN

Wave 1	Wave 2	Wave 3
O		
	O	
		O

Note: Waves may also be identified by date.

selected randomly, which generally is the preferred method. The key feature of this design is that selecting a new sample at each wave adjusts for changes in population composition between waves, such as becoming younger or older overall, owing to some members leaving it (e.g., out-migration or death) and others entering it (e.g., in-migration or birth). By collecting data from separate samples, the results are not vulnerable to attrition bias or a testing effect (Chapter 5). However, strategies should be employed to avoid an instrumentation effect.

Box 6.4 presents an example of a trend study.

BOX 6.4: EXAMPLE OF A TREND STUDY
U.S. NATIONAL HEALTH INTERVIEW SURVEY

The National Health Interview Survey (NHIS) has been conducted annually since 1957 by the Centers for Disease Control and Prevention to monitor the health of the U.S. civilian noninstitutionalized population on a broad range of health-related topics. The surveys are conducted by trained interviewers during in-person household interviews (Chapter 12). Information is collected continuously throughout each year about approximately 87,500 individuals of all ages, from approximately 35,000 households. The data track changes in health status, health behaviors, and health care utilization. Results are analyzed to identify health trends, evaluate health policies and programs, and monitor progress toward achieving national health objectives.

Source: Centers for Disease Control and Prevention. (2018e). *National Health Interview Survey.* Retrieved from https://www.cdc.gov/nchs/nhis/index.htm

Panel study

A panel study design comprises a series of observations from or about the *same* participants, called "the panel," at multiple points, as depicted in Box 6.5. Repeated observations of the same participants provide insight to the dynamics of change. For instance, while a trend study might indicate that the prevalence of engaging in regular physical activity has changed at the population level, it is difficult to specify the factors (e.g., demographic characteristics, health knowledge, and health beliefs) that might account for the change in different individuals who are observed at each point. However, panel data may be analyzed at the individual level, and the order of change among variables may be specified within the same individuals across observation points. For example, it might be observed that individuals whose knowledge changes at one point change their behavior at a subsequent point.

BOX 6.5: PANEL STUDY DESIGN

Wave 1	Wave 2	Wave 3
O	O	O

In particular, a panel design is useful for studying health issues over the life course as related to factors such as life events, technological developments, and policy changes.

An example of a research question that might be addressed using a panel study design is as follows:

> How does internet use for obtaining health-related information vary over the course of a calendar year? (To investigate this question, the observation intervals might be monthly.)

By collecting repeated observations from the same individuals, differences across waves are not confounded with changes in population composition as they would be for a trend study. However, a panel increasingly is likely to become unrepresentative of the population owing to several factors. First, a basic panel study design does not adjust for changes in population composition. Second, even if the population is relatively stable, the panel will age. For example, suppose the mean (arithmetic average) age of both the population and a random sample (the panel) of adults is 35 at wave 1. Five years later, the panel's mean age would be 40 while the population's mean age still might be 35. Third, panel studies are highly vulnerable to attrition bias (Chapter 5) when individuals are asked to participate repeatedly in the same data collection activities. Moreover, loss of participants across waves presents analytical issues regarding missing data and reduces analytical power (Chapter 15). In addition to strategies described in Chapter 5 for addressing attrition, those issues may be addressed by refreshing a panel, which is called **"panel maintenance,"** whereby supplemental samples are selected to update a panel's representativeness and maintain analytical power (Stafford, 2010). Panel studies also may be influenced by testing effects, called **"panel conditioning,"** and instrumentation effects (Chapter 5).

Box 6.6 presents an example of a panel study.

BOX 6.6: EXAMPLE OF A PANEL STUDY
NURSES' HEALTH STUDIES

The Nurses' Health Studies (NHS), initiated in 1976 and now in their third generation, have collected biennial data to repeatedly assess health and lifestyle factors from a total of more than 280,000 participants. In addition, data about special topics are collected from subgroups of participants. NHS began as a prospective cohort study of 121,700 married registered nurses. NHS II was launched in 1989 and enrolled 116,430 nurses; NHS3 began in 2010 and has ongoing enrollment (Bao et al., 2016). The range of lifestyle and health outcome data collected has increased over time. In addition to data collected by questionnaires, the study has collected biological specimens. Results have made significant contributions to health policy and practice, especially regarding chronic diseases in women.

Source: Nurses' Health Study. (2018). Retrieved from http://www.nurseshealthstudy.org/

CHECK YOUR UNDERSTANDING 6.1

- Under what conditions and for what reasons would a *trend study* be preferred instead of a panel study?
- Under what conditions and for what reasons would a *panel study* be preferred instead of a trend study?

Causal Designs

Causal designs assess whether an independent variable (*treatment*) causes change in a dependent variable (*outcome*). This section presents three types of causal designs:

- Nonexperimental
- Experimental
- Quasi-experimental

Although nonexperimental designs are vulnerable to substantial internal validity threats, they are presented under the "Causal Designs" heading for two reasons. First, sometimes they are employed in practice settings, where employing an experimental or quasi-experimental design is not feasible. Second, understanding the limitations of nonexperimental designs provides insight to the advantages of experimental and quasi-experimental designs. In general, experimental designs are preferred for assessing causality. Quasi-experimental designs are employed in situations where random assignment to groups is not feasible.

> **Key Concept**
>
> *Causal designs assess whether an independent variable (treatment) causes change in a dependent variable (outcome).*

Nonexperimental Designs

A **nonexperimental design** (also called "preexperimental") does not include a control group, *or* it includes a control group without random assignment *and* without a pretest observation point. Typically, nonexperimental designs are employed in situations where it is not feasible to include a control group or when evaluating a program that already is under way and a pretest observation is not possible.

One-group posttest-only design

Also called the "one-shot case study design," the one-group posttest-only design is depicted in Box 6.7. Although it appears similar to the cross-sectional observational design (Box 6.1), it differs in that it includes a treatment (X) that is followed by a posttest observation (O). For example, a college might require students during their first term to complete a web-based relationship abuse prevention course and then measure their knowledge, attitudes, and behavior related to that issue.

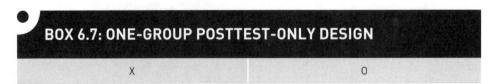

BOX 6.7: ONE-GROUP POSTTEST-ONLY DESIGN

| X | O |

This design might be appealing because five of the seven design threats to internal validity (Chapter 5) do not apply, as summarized below:

- Nonequivalent groups—there is only one group.
- Attrition, testing, and instrumentation—there is only one observation point.
- Regression toward the norm—there is no pretest to select atypical participants.

However, the design does not include a pretest observation to assess whether there is a difference in participants' pretest versus posttest status. Also, it does not include a control group to simulate the counterfactual model (Chapter 5). Thus, this design provides no means to assess whether the treatment is effective. Moreover, it is vulnerable to history and maturation threats. For example, it would not be possible to know if students' knowledge, attitudes, or behavior changed after completing an abuse prevention course. If they generally score high on such factors at the posttest observation point, it would not be known whether their status is attributable to the course or a history or maturation effect, or if that was their status prior to taking the course and it did not change.

One-group pretest–posttest design

The one-group pretest–posttest design depicted in Box 6.8 adds a pretest observation to the one-group posttest-only design. The pretest enables assessing whether participants change regarding the dependent variable after being exposed to a treatment. When analyzing results for the one-group pretest–posttest design, participants are considered as serving as *their own controls*. The underlying logic is that the pretest observation provides an estimate of their posttest status under the counterfactual model, whereby they would not have been exposed to a treatment. That assumption is more tenable the shorter the pretest–posttest interval, during which results might be influenced by history, maturation, attrition, instrumentation, or regression toward the norm. However, as the pretest–posttest interval becomes shorter, the threat of a testing effect generally increases.

BOX 6.8: ONE-GROUP PRETEST–POSTTEST DESIGN

O	X	O

Comparing the one-group pretest–posttest design with the one-group posttest-only design provides a striking illustration of how a single modification may significantly impact a design's internal validity. Adding one design component, a pretest observation, enhances information about the treatment group's posttreatment change. However, it also increases the number of internal validity threats. First, the one-group posttest-only design still is vulnerable to history and maturation because there is no control group to assess potential change in absence of a treatment. Moreover, adding a pretest observation extends the study period, which may exacerbate the history and maturation threats. In addition, a pretest observation makes the design vulnerable to attrition, testing, and instrumentation. If participants are selected based on atypical pretest scores, the design may be vulnerable to regression toward the norm. Without a control group, the design is not vulnerable to a nonequivalent-groups threat. However, there is no reliable means for assessing the influence of the six other internal validity threats:

- History
- Maturation
- Attrition
- Testing
- Instrumentation
- Regression toward the norm

It is important to be mindful that being *vulnerable* to an internal validity threat does not mean the threat necessarily influences a study's result. Nevertheless, if a threat cannot be ruled out, its potential impact always must be taken into consideration when interpreting a study's result.

Nonequivalent-groups posttest-only design

Box 6.9 depicts the nonequivalent-groups posttest-only design, also called the "static-group comparison design" and the "ex post facto design" (derived from Latin meaning "after the fact"). In contrast with the one-group posttest-only design, this design adds a control group without random assignment. The dashed horizontal line indicates participants are from different groups/populations or are different subsets of the same population. This design often compares intact groups selected based on similarity in their overall characteristics. For example, the control group for an evaluation of a relationship abuse prevention course might be students at a college where the course is not available, and that is similar in terms of factors such as student demographic characteristics and college size and location. However, without a pretest observation about relationship abuse knowledge, attitudes, and behavior, preexisting group differences on those variables could not be taken into account. Thus, it would not be possible to reliably attribute any posttest differences to treatment exposure.

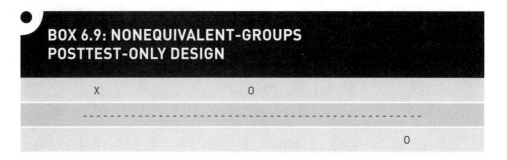

The nonequivalent-groups posttest-only design is not vulnerable to attrition, testing, instrumentation, or regression to the norm because it includes only one observation point. Ironically, although the purpose for adding a control group is to assess the potential influence of history and maturation, that addition actually might exacerbate those threats. That could occur if the two groups do not experience and react to history and/or maturation factors similarly. Thus, as the design's name implies, nonequivalent groups is the main internal validity threat to this design.

CHECK YOUR UNDERSTANDING 6.2

- The one-group pretest–posttest design may be viewed as adding a pretest observation point to the one-group posttest-only design. Explain how adding a pretest observation point
    - enhances the one-group pretest–posttest design in comparison with the one-group posttest-only design, and
    - introduces additional internal validity threats to the one-group pretest–posttest design. Be specific about which internal validity threats are introduced, and explain why.

Experimental Designs

Experimental designs, sometimes called "true experimental designs," include two key features: a control group and random assignment. As discussed in Chapter 5, those design features address most internal validity threats and provide the strongest foundation for ruling out alternative explanations for a treatment effect.

> **Key Concept**
>
> *An experimental design includes a control group and random assignment.*

Pretest–posttest control group design

Box 6.10 depicts the pretest–posttest control group design, which also is called the "classical experimental design" and "randomized controlled trial (RCT)." It comprises two groups to which participants are randomly assigned (RA, which may be omitted as understood in some contexts). The treatment group is exposed to an experimental treatment (X), while the control group is not exposed to the treatment. The control group may be assigned to a no-treatment condition, an alternative-treatment condition, or a placebo condition (Chapter 5). Pretest and posttest observations (O) are made for both groups at the same time points.

BOX 6.10: PRETEST–POSTTEST CONTROL GROUP DESIGN

RA	O	X	O
RA	O		O

The pretest–posttest control group design generally is regarded as the gold standard causal design because it provides strong protection against internal validity threats. Random assignment (Chapter 7) minimizes initial group differences, which addresses the nonequivalent-groups threat. Moreover, although randomly assigned groups are not identical as in the counterfactual model, group differences are not systematic. Instead, they are attributable to an unbiased random process and may be taken into account by applying inferential analysis procedures (Chapter 15). Furthermore, with random assignment, any effect on the dependent variable from other internal validity threats (history, maturation, attrition, testing, instrumentation, or regression toward the norm) will be experienced similarly by all participants regardless of the condition to which they are assigned. Therefore, any posttest difference between groups is most likely attributable to a treatment effect. However, the pretest–posttest control group design is vulnerable to an *interaction* between testing and treatment exposure that might cause the treatment group's posttest observation to differ from what it would be in absence of a pretest. For example, a pretest prior to completing a relationship abuse prevention course might increase students' concern about the issue and cause treatment participants to be more attentive and responsive to the course than they would be otherwise.

Box 6.11 presents an example of a study that used a pretest–posttest control group design.

Posttest-only control group design

The simplest strategy for addressing a potential testing × treatment interaction is to omit the pretest observation and employ the posttest-only control group design, depicted in Box 6.12. Moreover, this design is less expensive, requires less time, and is logistically simpler than the pretest–posttest control group design. Indeed, it is the simplest experimental design, yet it is very effective.

> **BOX 6.11: EXAMPLE OF A PRETEST–POSTTEST CONTROL GROUP DESIGN STUDY**
>
> THE EFFECT OF A COUPLES INTERVENTION TO INCREASE BREAST CANCER SCREENING AMONG KOREAN AMERICANS
>
> Lee et al. (2014) (see Box 4.6) employed the following pretest–posttest control group design:
>
> | | | | 6 mos. | 15 mos. |
> |----|---|---|--------|---------|
> | RA | O | X | O | O |
> | RA | O | AP| O | O |
>
> Couples were randomly assigned to intervention (X) or attention-placebo (AP) control conditions. The treatment and attention-placebo conditions were employed immediately following the pretest observation. Posttest observations were made at six and fifteen months postintervention.

The main concern about omitting a pretest observation is that it excludes performing a randomization check to verify group similarity, such as applying a *t* test for differences in mean age across groups. However, a randomization check is necessary only when the number of participants is small and random variation may result in substantial group differences. The key to employing the posttest-only control group design is to include a large number of participants to increase confidence that any pretreatment differences are trivial (Chapter 7). Furthermore, pretreatment group differences may be taken into account by inferential analysis procedures to assess whether posttest differences are larger than expected owing to random assignment. When differences exceed that expectation, they are deemed to be **statistically significant**, and it may be concluded within a certain margin of error (called type I or alpha error; Chapters 7 and 15) that the difference most likely is attributable to treatment exposure.

> **BOX 6.12: POSTTEST-ONLY CONTROL GROUP DESIGN**
>
> | RA | X | O |
> |----|---|---|
> | RA | | O |

Solomon four-group design

Another experimental design that addresses a potential testing × treatment interaction is the Solomon four-group design. As presented in Box 6.13, it combines the pretest–posttest control group and the posttest-only control group designs. Because the Solomon four-group design is expensive and logistically challenging to implement, it is reasonable to employ it only when it is important to assess participants' pretreatment status on the dependent variable *and* the threat of a testing × treatment interaction is substantial.

This design enables measuring the testing "main effect" and the testing × treatment interaction effect. The testing main effect (without interacting with the treatment) is the

BOX 6.13: SOLOMON FOUR-GROUP DESIGN

RA	O_1	X	O_2
RA	O_3		O_4
RA		X	O_5
RA			O_6

(Subscripts are included to supplement the text.)

difference between posttest observations O_4 and O_6, in Box 6.13, which under random assignment differ only in that O_4 is preceded by a pretest observation (O_3). If there is no main effect of testing, then O_4 and O_6 should not differ beyond random variation. The testing × treatment interaction effect is the difference between O_2 and O_5, which under random assignment differ only in that O_2 is preceded by a pretest observation (O_1).

Separate-sample designs

Separate-sample designs address threats from testing and attrition by making pretest and posttest observations separately for two randomly assigned groups.

Separate-sample two-group design. The separate-sample two-group design, depicted in Box 6.14, makes pretest and posttest observations from two separate, randomly assigned groups. This design may be viewed as an extension of the one-group posttest-only control group design (Box 6.7) by adding a randomly assigned pretest-only group to estimate participants' pretreatment status. Because different participants are measured at pretest and posttest, it is not possible for the pretest to have an effect on the posttest observation. For the same reason, this design is not vulnerable to attrition. However, because there is no posttest observation for an untreated group, the design is vulnerable to internal validity threats from history, maturation, and instrumentation.

BOX 6.14: SEPARATE-SAMPLE TWO-GROUP DESIGN

RA	O		
RA		X	O

Separate-sample three-group design. The separate-sample three-group design addresses the history, maturation, and instrumentation threats to the separate-sample (two-group) pretest–posttest design by including a randomly assigned posttest-only control group, as depicted in Box 6.15. The posttest-only control group provides an estimate of the treatment group's status at posttest if it had not been exposed to the treatment. This design is effective in addressing all seven internal validity threats.

- Nonequivalent groups—this threat is addressed by random assignment.
- History—the posttest-only control group is affected similar to the treatment group; any historical influence is taken into account by $O_1 - O_3$.

- Maturation—the posttest-only control group is affected similar to the treatment group; any maturational influence is taken into account by $O_1 - O_3$.
- Attrition—no group is measured more than once.
- Testing—no group is measured more than once.
- Instrumentation—the posttest-only control group is affected similar to the treatment group; any instrumentation influence is taken into account by $O_1 - O_3$.
- Regression toward the norm—if atypical participants are studied, the posttest-only control group will regress similar to the treatment group; any regression influence is taken into account by $O_1 - O_3$.

BOX 6.15: SEPARATE-SAMPLE THREE-GROUP DESIGN

RA	O_1		
RA		X	O_2
RA			O_3

The separate-sample three-group design measures the treatment effect in two ways: $O_2 - O_1$ is the pretest–posttest difference; $O_2 - O_3$ is the posttest difference. Moreover, this design is much less expensive and more feasible to implement than the Solomon four-group design, and it is only slightly more expensive and challenging to implement than the separate-sample (two-group) pretest–posttest design.

CHECK YOUR UNDERSTANDING 6.3

- What are the two key features of an experimental research design? Explain how each one enhances internal validity.

Key Concept

Quasi-experimental designs assess causality when it is not feasible to employ random assignment or include a control group.

Quasi-experimental Designs

Quasi-experimental designs assess causality when it is not feasible to employ random assignment or include a control group. They use other strategies to address internal validity threats and rule out alternative explanations of a potential treatment effect. Although they are not as strong as experimental designs, they may be effective when research is conducted in real-world practice settings.

Nonequivalent pretest–posttest control group design

Box 6.16 depicts the nonequivalent pretest–posttest control group design. It is similar to the pretest–posttest control group design except random assignment is not employed, as is indicated by a dashed horizontal line between groups. As discussed previously, having nonequivalent groups renders a design vulnerable to all internal validity threats because it is difficult to determine whether posttest differences are attributable to a treatment effect or preexisting group differences. The effectiveness of this design is maximized by selecting groups that are as similar as possible so they will experience and respond similarly to extraneous influences. In contrast with the nonequivalent-groups posttest-only design (Box 6.9), this design adds pretest observations to assess preexisting group differences.

BOX 6.16: NONEQUIVALENT PRETEST–POSTTEST CONTROL GROUP DESIGN

O	X	O
O		O

When feasible, this design may be enhanced by including *multiple pretest observations* to describe any within-group trends in the dependent variable that might be misinterpreted as a treatment effect. Box 6.17 depicts an example of that strategy, where three pretest observation points are represented for illustrative purposes. However, adding pretest observations might increase the likelihood of threats from testing, instrumentation, attrition, and regression toward the norm. In addition, it is expensive and logistically challenging.

BOX 6.17: NONEQUIVALENT PRETEST–POSTTEST CONTROL GROUP WITH MULTIPLE PRETESTS DESIGN

O	O	O	X	O
O	O	O		O

Interrupted time-series designs

Interrupted time-series designs comprise a series of observations of the dependent variable that is *interrupted* by a treatment. Alternatively, such designs may be viewed as comprising both multiple pretest and posttest observations. The number and timing of observations depend on the nature of the dependent variable. A *discontinuity* in the pattern of a treatment group's pretreatment status that coincides with treatment exposure most likely may be attributed to a treatment effect. Multiple pretest observations are employed to identify any pretreatment trend in the dependent variable that might be misinterpreted as a treatment effect. Multiple posttest observations assess whether a posttreatment change endures as would be expected according to the nature of the dependent variable and the conceptual approach on which the treatment is based. However, including multiple observations is expensive and logistically challenging.

Box 6.18 includes three pretest and posttest observation points for illustrative purposes. The top panel depicts the one-group interrupted time-series design. As with the one-group pretest–posttest design (Box 6.8), the analysis of results for the one-group interrupted time-series design considers participants as serving as their own controls. The validity of that

BOX 6.18: INTERRUPTED TIME-SERIES DESIGNS

One-Group Interrupted Time-Series Design

| | O | O | O | X | O | O | O |

Nonequivalent Control Group Interrupted Time-Series Design

| | O | O | O | X | O | O | O |
| | O | O | O | | O | O | O |

approach is enhanced by monitoring participants' pretreatment status over multiple pretest observation points to provide a more reliable estimate of their posttest status under the counterfactual model. However, adding multiple pretest observations increases the likelihood of threats from testing, instrumentation, and attrition. Those threats are reduced by adding a nonequivalent control group to create the nonequivalent control group interrupted time-series design, which is depicted in the bottom panel of Box 6.18. Moreover, the multiple pretest observations enhance the validity of comparing the treatment group to the nonequivalent control group.

Figure 6.1 illustrates how results from the nonequivalent control group interrupted time-series design might indicate a treatment effect. Suppose alcoholic beverage consumption by new students at two similar colleges is assessed in terms of a risky behavior scale every week, six weeks before and after they are exposed to a responsible drinking program. During the six-week pretest observation period, risky behavior at both colleges increases similarly. However, while that trend continues among the control group, it is *disrupted* among the treatment group and declines during the six-week posttest period. If the one-group design were employed instead of the two-group design, results would be represented only by the treatment group trend line. Although a discontinuity still would be observed, there is less confidence in attributing the change to a treatment effect in absence of a control group comparison. For instance, the discontinuity might coincide with a history effect,

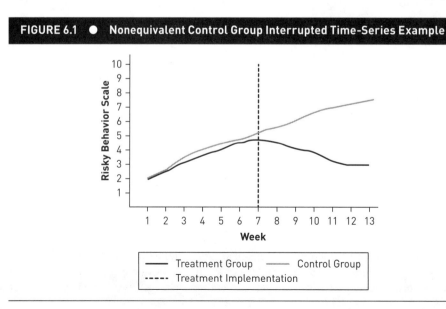

FIGURE 6.1 • Nonequivalent Control Group Interrupted Time-Series Example

such as a media report about a tragic outcome associated with alcoholic beverage consumption at another college.

Case-control design

Sometimes a study is conducted to identify the cause of a change in an independent variable that already has occurred. An example is to identify the cause of a disparity in the prevalence of low birth weight pregnancy outcomes across different groups of women. Another example is to assess whether a particular adverse health outcome is attributable to a supposed cause, such as whether childhood cognitive development is impaired by exposure to lead-contaminated drinking water. The **case-control design** often is employed in such situations, especially by epidemiologists, to identify the primary factor(s) that caused one group, called *cases*, to experience a particular adverse outcome while a similar group, called *controls*, did not experience it.

The case-control design sometimes is referred to as an "analytical design." In contrast with the causal designs discussed previously, the case-control design does not implement a treatment. Instead, observations (e.g., records review and/or interviews) are collected retrospectively to assess differential exposure to potential causal factors that might account for why a certain outcome occurred among the cases but not the controls. In addition, this design may identify factors that might be protective against an adverse outcome. That is, it may identify factors whose presence or absence might account for why controls did not experience it. As depicted in Box 6.19, the case-control design is similar to the nonequivalent groups posttest-only design (Box 6.9), except the observations are retrospective in an attempt to identify the presence and absence of factors that account for the case-control difference.

BOX 6.19: CASE-CONTROL DESIGN

Cases	X	O
Controls		O

It is not feasible or ethical to randomly assign which participants will or will not experience an adverse health outcome. Therefore, cases and controls are nonequivalent groups. The key to implementing a case-control design is to select cases and controls that are as similar as possible in all respects other than having been exposed to the supposed causal factor(s). Typically, participants are selected using a **matching** strategy (Chapter 7). Matching cases and controls is fairly straightforward when a study is focused on a single supposed cause, such as to assess the effect of exposure to lead-contaminated drinking water. However, it is challenging to specify the appropriate matching characteristics when the full range of likely causes is not identifiable in advance, such as for a study about a disparity in the prevalence of adverse pregnancy outcomes.

Cohort studies

Instead of studying a sample of the general population, sometimes a research question focuses on a **cohort**, which is a group that shares an event-based characteristic that usually is anchored at some time point, such as date of

- birth,
- entry into college,

- marriage,
- delivering first live birth,
- diagnosis, or
- retirement.

Cohorts often are employed to study patterns of relationships prospectively over relatively long time periods. Cohorts also are employed when it is not feasible to randomly assign participants to experience a particular event, such as an infectious disease diagnosis, because it already has occurred or it would not be ethical. In most situations, the timing of the defining event is specified as having occurred during a particular year or range of years. Observations for a cohort study may be collected prospectively or retrospectively.

Typically, a cohort study collects multiple observations from or about one or more cohorts, and may be conducted using various research designs. For example, using a panel study (Box 6.5) approach, children born during a certain year (a birth cohort) might be monitored from birth through age 20 to identify risk factors for adolescent obesity. In other situations, cohorts might be compared using a nonequivalent control group approach. For example, instead of, or in addition to, assessing the effect of a responsible drinking program at one college by comparing alcoholic beverage consumption at a similar college, a comparison might be made at the treatment college between the treated cohort of first-year students and the preceding untreated cohort of first-year students. Using that approach, college type and location would be controlled more effectively by comparing cohorts at the same college. However, it would be vulnerable to a history threat. Therefore, when feasible, making both comparisons would be most effective.

CHECK YOUR UNDERSTANDING 6.4

- Quasi-experimental research designs may be employed when it is not feasible to employ random assignment or include a control group.
- Describe some of the strategies that quasi-experimental designs employ to address internal validity threats, and explain the logic underlying each strategy.

Design Variations

Staggered starts

When it is anticipated that a disruptive history event (e.g., a weather-related disaster or civil unrest) might occur during the study period but it is not possible to predict its occurrence reliably, a design may be partitioned into a series of *replicates*. This strategy may prevent an entire study from being affected by such an event. If an event is highly disruptive of a study's conditions, the study might be suspended and restarted with any replicates that have not been initiated. Moreover, the replicates may strengthen validity by serving as separate replication studies. A staggered starts strategy may be employed by randomly dividing individual participants into two or more replicate groups, or by designating intact groups of participants (e.g., all students at certain schools) as replicates that are randomly assigned to different starting points. Although staggered starts may be employed with many research designs, Box 6.20 illustrates the strategy for the pretest–posttest control group design (three replicates are depicted for illustrative purposes).

BOX 6.20: PRETEST–POSTTEST CONTROL GROUP DESIGN WITH STAGGERED STARTS

First Replicate
RA O X O
RA O   O

Second Replicate
RA O X O
RA O   O

Third Replicate
RA O X O
RA O   O

Switching replications

A switching replications strategy may be employed to increase the number of treatment participants when the number of participants is small. Also, it provides an immediate replication with a randomly assigned group of participants. Although this strategy may be incorporated into other causal designs, it is most feasible with the pretest–posttest control group design (Box 6.10) and the nonequivalent pretest–posttest control group design (Box 6.16). Box 6.21 depicts the basic switching replications approach as an extension of the pretest–posttest control group design. The design is particularly effective when a wait-list control condition (Chapter 4) is employed. After the initial treatment assessment, the treatment is switched to the initial wait-list control group, followed by a second posttest observation for that group. Thus, the initial treatment effect ($O_2 - O_1$) is replicated by $O_5 - O_4$.

BOX 6.21: PRETEST–POSTTEST CONTROL GROUP WITH SWITCHING REPLICATIONS DESIGN

RA	O_1	X	O_2		
RA	O_3		O_4	X	O_5

When the treatment effect is extinguishable or is self-extinguishing, a full switching replications design, typically called a "crossover design," may be employed, as depicted in Box 6.22. This design adds a second posttest observation for both groups to verify that the initial treatment group has returned to its pretest observation status, and to provide a fresh

BOX 6.22: PRETEST–POSTTEST CONTROL GROUP CROSSOVER DESIGN

RA	O	X	O	O		O
RA	O		O	O	X	O

baseline for the initial control group. The timing of the second posttest is determined by when the initial treatment effect is expected to have been extinguished and there will be no or minimal carryover effects from treatment exposure. In some situations, it may be necessary to conduct more than one such posttest check. Then group conditions are switched, or participants are said to *cross over*, such that the initial treatment group becomes the second-round control and the initial (wait-list) control becomes the treatment group.

Counterbalancing

When a treatment includes two or more components and there is no inherent order in which they must be implemented, **counterbalancing** may be employed to assess the treatment order effect. Counterbalancing randomly assigns equal numbers of treatment participants to receive all components but in different order. For example, Box 6.23 depicts a counterbalanced pretest–posttest control group design for assessing a responsible drinking program for college students that includes two components, an in-person session and an online video. The first order presents the in-person session followed by viewing the online video. The second order is the reverse, viewing the online video first followed by the in-person session.

BOX 6.23: COUNTERBALANCED PRETEST–POSTTEST CONTROL GROUP DESIGN

RA	O	IP + V	O
RA	O	V + IP	O
RA	O		O

IP: In-person session
V: Video

CHECK YOUR UNDERSTANDING 6.5

- What is the difference between a "crossover" design and a "counterbalanced" design?

Key Points

Observational Designs

Observational designs observe one or more populations under prevailing conditions.

One-Group Cross-Sectional Design	Trend Study Design	Panel Study Design
O	O	O O O
	O	

Nonexperimental Designs

Nonexperimental designs do not include a control group, or include a control group without random assignment and a pretest observation point.

One-Group Posttest-Only Design	One-Group Pretest–Posttest Design	Nonequivalent-Groups Posttest-Only Design
X O	O X O	X O --------- O

Experimental Designs

Experimental designs address most internal validity threats by including a control group and random assignment.

Pretest–Posttest Control Group Design	Solomon Four-Group Design	Separate-Sample Three-Group Design
RA O X O RA O O	RA O X O RA O O RA O X O RA O O	RA O RA O X O RA O O

Posttest-Only Control Group Design
RA   O   X   O RA   O   O

Quasi-experimental Designs

Quasi-experimental designs assess causality when it is not feasible to employ random assignment or include a control group.

Nonequivalent Pretest–Posttest Control Group Design	One-Group Interrupted Time-Series Design
O X O ------------ O O	O O O X O O O

Nonequivalent Control Group Interrupted Time-Series Design
O   O   O   X   O   O   O ------------------ O   O   O   O   O   O

Design Variations

- Staggered starts
- Switching replications
- Counterbalancing

Review and Apply

1. Review the research plan you developed in the "Review and Apply" section of Chapter 1 or 3. If you did not do that previously, either do it now or identify a health-related problem that interests you.

   a. Briefly describe a treatment that you propose might improve outcomes for the target population.

   b. Develop a causal research design to assess the treatment's effectiveness, and present your design in a diagram.

   c. Consider each potential design threat to internal validity, and explain why it is or is not likely to influence results from your design.

   d. For each potential design threat that applies, describe how you would address it in your study.

   e. Would you describe your study as an efficacy or effectiveness trial? Explain why.

2. Suppose you have been asked to evaluate the relationship abuse prevention course that was presented as an example in this chapter. The research plan will use a nonequivalent pretest–posttest control group design (see Box 6.16) to compare pretest and posttest observations from students who complete the course and students at a control college. The course must be implemented during the fall semester. However, owing to administrative reasons, it is discovered that data may not be collected at the control college until spring semester. It is too late to identify and negotiate access to a substitute control college. Thus, the research design must be modified as depicted in the diagram below, with only a single control group observation at posttest.

   ```
   O     X     O
   - - - - - - - - - - - - - - - - - - - - - - - - - - - -
                       O
   ```

   In addition to nonequivalent groups, identify the internal validity threats to this modified design, and describe how you would take them into consideration when assessing the study's results.

3. You have been asked to evaluate an ongoing health education program that was initiated two years ago. Describe the research design you would employ, and assess its internal and external validity.

4. A county health department in a metropolitan area will implement a health behavior intervention program starting six months from now. Because of ethical and political concerns, the program will be available to all county residents, although it is expected that not all residents for whom the program is appropriate will participate in it.

   a. What research design would you recommend to evaluate the program's impact over the first two years during which it is provided?

   b. Explain why you recommend that design.

   c. Assess the design's internal validity.

   d. Assess the design's external validity.

Study Further

CONSORT. (2010). *The CONSORT statement.* Retrieved from http://www.consort-statement.org/ (CONSORT stands for *Consolidated Standards of Reporting Trials.*)

Creswell, J. W. (2014). *Research design* (4th ed.). Los Angeles, CA: Sage.

Mercer, S. L., De Vinney, B. L., Fine, L. J., Green, L. W., & Dougherty, D. (2007). Study designs for effectiveness and translation research: Identifying trade-offs. *American Journal of Preventive Medicine, 33*(2), 139–154.

Shadish, W. R., Cook, T. D., & Campbell, D. T. (2002). *Experimental and quasi-experimental designs for generalized causal inference.* Boston, MA: Houghton Mifflin.

Trochim, W. M. (2006). *The research methods knowledge base* (2nd ed.). Available from http://www.socialresearchmethods.net/kb/

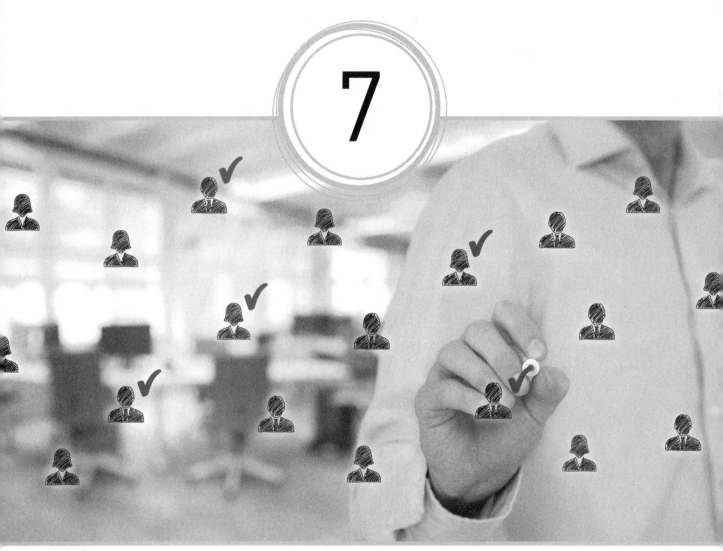

7

Random Sampling and Assignment

Chapter Outline

Overview
Learning Objectives
Random Sampling
    Reasons for Sampling
    Random Sampling Concepts
    Random Sampling Procedures
    Stratified Random Sampling
    Cluster Random Sampling
    Sample Size
Random Assignment
    Separate Random Samples
    Simple Random Assignment
    Stratified Random Assignment
    Block Randomization
    Matching
Key Points

Learning Objectives

After studying Chapter 7, the reader should be able to:

- Describe the principles of random sampling and how they enhance a sample's representativeness of a population
- Select and apply a sampling design appropriate for a specific research question, population, and study design
- Assess a sample's representativeness of a population
- Select and apply an appropriate method for randomly assigning subjects to study conditions

Overview

After developing a research design, *subjects* is the next stage in the research process as presented in Chapter 1 (Figure 1.5). Virtually all research involving human subjects is conducted with a *sample* that is a representative subset of a target population. Taking into consideration a study's particular circumstances, a key aspect of external validity is whether the sample selection strategy optimizes a sample's representativeness. When a research design includes a comparison across conditions (Chapter 6), whether the assignment strategy yields equivalent groups is a major factor that affects internal validity. Sample selection and assignment to conditions are not necessarily related. For instance, a nonrandom sample, such as volunteers in response to recruitment advertising, may be assigned to groups randomly. As illustrated in the diagram below, all studies involve selecting subjects, regardless of whether they are a sample or an entire target population. If a research design includes a comparison across conditions, assignment to conditions is done subsequent to selection.

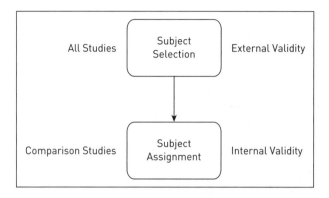

Random Sampling

There are two basic subject selection approaches, random sampling and nonrandom sampling, which also respectively are called **probability sampling** and **nonprobability sampling**. **Random sampling** is the key component of the inference process introduced in Chapter 1 (Figure 1.4). Based on **probability theory**, inferential statistical methods may be applied to a **random sample** to assess confidence in population estimates derived from them. Random sampling is not influenced by subjective decisions of researchers or potential participants that may cause **selection bias**, which results in an unrepresentative sample. **Nonrandom sampling**, which is not based on probability theory, is vulnerable to selection bias, and it is not appropriate to apply inferential statistical methods to assess confidence in population estimates derived from a nonrandom sample. Nevertheless, nonrandom sampling may be employed when random sampling is not feasible. Moreover, it may be preferred in some situations, particularly for qualitative research. Therefore, nonrandom sampling methods are described in Chapter 13, which addresses qualitative research methods.

> **Key Concept**
>
> Random sampling is the key component of the inference process.

Reasons for Sampling

The primary reasons for studying a sample instead of an entire target population are to

- minimize costs,
- minimize time,
- improve access to subjects,
- improve data quality, and
- minimize population exposure.

Unless it is small, collecting data from an entire population generally is prohibitively expensive and time-consuming. Also, studying a sample generally shortens the data collection time period, which reduces a study's vulnerability to a history threat (Chapter 5) and enhances the timeliness of results. Studying a sample may improve access to participants and data quality by reducing the administrative burden, and focusing resources on recruiting and interacting with fewer individuals. A sample restricts risks and burdens associated with study participation to a proportion of the population (Chapter 2). Finally, a sample leaves available a pool of potential participants who are not influenced by prior exposure to a study protocol.

Random Sampling Concepts

Terms and notation

A random sample is a subset of n sampling units selected to represent a population of N elements. Although most often sampling units are individual people, they also may be groups (e.g., households or school classes) or institutions (e.g., schools or health clinics). Box 7.1 presents definitions of key sampling terms.

Table 7.1 presents basic random sampling notation. *Capital* Roman or Greek characters designate population parameters; *lowercase* Roman characters designate a sample's characteristics, called statistics. A sample's statistics are used to estimate corresponding population parameters. For example, a sample's mean (arithmetic average) age is an estimator of the population's mean age; the proportion of a sample that smokes cigarettes is an estimator of the population proportion that smokes cigarettes.

BOX 7.1: KEY SAMPLING TERMS

- **Population:** the total set of entities targeted for a study
- **Element:** an individual population entity
- **Parameter:** a population characteristic, designated by a capital Roman or Greek character
- **Population size:** the number of population elements, N
- **Sample:** a subset of a population selected for a study
- **Sampling unit:** a population element selected in a sample
- **Statistic:** a sample characteristic, designated by a lowercase Roman character, used to estimate a corresponding population parameter
- **Sample size:** the number of sampling units, n, selected in a sample

TABLE 7.1 • Basic Random Sampling Notation

Attribute	Population	Sample
Size	N	n
Mean	μ	$\bar{x}$
Proportion	P	p
Variance	σ^2	s^2
Standard Deviation	σ	s

Random selection

There are two key features of random sampling. First, each population element has an *independent* chance to be selected. That is, the selection probability for each population element is > 0, and the selection of an element is not contingent on selection of another one. Second, the selection probability for each element is known, or may be calculated.

Key Concepts

- *Each element has an independent chance to be selected.*
- *The selection probability for each element is known, or may be calculated.*

Simple random sampling

Simple random sampling (SRS) is the basic random sampling design. With simple random sampling, for a sample of size n selected from a population of size N, the probability (chance) of selection is *equal* for all elements. The probability of selection is expressed as the **sampling fraction** (f), which is also called the "sampling rate," where $f = n/N$. A sampling design for which each element has the same selection probability is called an **EPSEM design** (derived from **Equal Probability Selection Method**). For example, for a random sample of 100 elements selected from a population of 1,000, each element has a 1-in-10 chance of selection ($f = 100/1{,}000 = 1/10$). Simple random sampling is not the only type of EPSEM design. Although it is not essential for the selection probability to be equal for all elements, an EPSEM design is desirable because it does not require calculating weights to adjust for unequal selection probabilities. Nevertheless, in some situations, designs that are not EPSEM may be preferred if they are more cost and time efficient, and/or otherwise better serve a study's purpose.

Simple random sampling with replacement. When an element is selected using **simple random sampling with replacement**, it is returned to the population before making the next selection. Thus, an element may be selected more than once. Although simple random sampling with replacement is the model on which random sampling theory is founded (Cochran, 1963; Kish, 1965), it rarely is used in practice, especially when studying human populations. Selecting the same element more than once is undesirable because the resulting redundancy does not provide n unique points of information about a population. Moreover, sampling with replacement typically is not feasible when data collection or a treatment implementation involves interacting with participants who likely would be unwilling to participate in the same activities more than once, or for whom repeated treatment exposure would be inappropriate. Furthermore, repeated participation experience likely would influence subsequent participation. Therefore, the remaining discussions of random sampling methods focus on selection *without* replacement.

Simple random sampling without replacement. With **simple random sampling without replacement**, when an element is selected, it is *not* returned to the population. Each element may be selected only once. Other elements are selected until a sample comprises n unique elements. Despite the procedural difference between simple random sampling with and without replacement, both are EPSEM designs. As illustrated in Box 7.2, the selection probability is the same for each element at each draw ($1/N$) and overall (n/N).

Sampling distribution. A **sampling distribution** is the distribution of a sample statistic for all possible random samples of size n from a population of size N. It is the foundation for applying inferential statistical methods to estimates of population parameters. Many simple random samples comprising different combinations of n elements may be

BOX 7.2: SIMPLE RANDOM SAMPLING SELECTION PROBABILITIES $N = 12$, $n = 4$

$N = 12$, $n = 4$, $f = n/N = 4/12$

With replacement

$f = n/N = 1/N + 1/N + 1/N + 1/N$

$f = 4/12 = 1/12 + 1/12 + 1/12 + 1/12$

Without replacement

$f = n/N = 1/N + [(N - 1/N) \times (1/N - 1)] + [(N - 2/N) \times (1/N - 2)] + \ldots$

$f = 4/12 = 1/12 + [(11/12) \times (1/11)] + [(10/12) \times (1/10)] + [(9/12) \times (1/9)]$

$f = 4/12 = 1/12 + (1/12) + (1/12) + (1/12)$

selected from a population of size N. For example, using simple random sampling without replacement, more than 17 trillion combinations are possible for a sample of 10 from a population of 100. With simple random sampling, in addition to population elements having the same chance of selection, all possible combinations of n elements have the same chance to be selected as the sample. If all possible random samples were very similar to the target population and to each other, it would matter little which sample was selected. However, there may be considerable variation across samples. The sampling distribution provides a means for assessing confidence in a particular random sample's estimate of a population parameter.

> **Key Concept**
>
> With simple random sampling, all possible combinations of n elements from a population of size N have the same chance to be selected.

Although a parameter's value typically is unknown, for the purpose of illustrating a sampling distribution, suppose a random sample is selected to estimate the mean age of a population of adults, for which the mean (μ) is 45. Further, suppose all possible random samples of the same size are selected from the population and their mean ages are plotted in a graph of the sampling distribution of the mean, for which a simulation is depicted in Figure 7.1.

FIGURE 7.1 ● **Sampling Distribution Illustration**

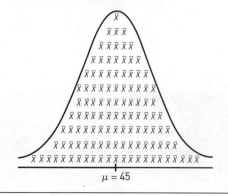

Owing to random variation, the sample means do not all have the same value, and the differences between sample means and the population mean vary. The sampling distribution is symmetrical, unimodal, and centered on the population parameter. That is, there is an equal number and similar distribution of sample means above and below the population mean, and the most frequent sample outcome is equal to the population mean. Moreover, most samples will be reasonably representative of the population. According to the **central limit theorem**, if repeated simple random samples of the same size are selected from a large population, the sampling distribution will approach a **normal distribution**, which is described by the normal curve imposed over the plot of sample means in Figure 7.1. Moreover, that will happen regardless of the shape of the population distribution.

Sampling error. **Sampling error** does not refer to a mistake when designing or selecting a sample. It is the difference between a random sample statistic and its corresponding population parameter, expressed as $\bar{x} - \mu$ for a mean and $p - P$ for a proportion. As illustrated in Figure 7.1, with simple random sampling, the sampling distribution mean (the mean of all possible sample means) equals the population parameter, which is its **expected value**. Although the mean age for an individual sample is not necessarily equal to the population mean, random sampling is **unbiased** because sampling error *overall* is zero. That is, if the sampling error were calculated for all samples in a sampling distribution, their sum would be zero because there would be an equal number of samples at the same distance above and below the sampling distribution mean.

Standard error. Sampling error often is assessed in terms of the **standard error (SE)**, which is a special name for the standard deviation (square root of the variance) of a sampling distribution. The standard error is calculated by dividing the population variance for a parameter by the sample size (σ^2/n), which often is expressed as $SE = \sigma/\sqrt{n}$. As Figure 7.2 depicts, as the sample size increases, there is less variation across samples. Thus, the standard error decreases and parameter estimates are more reliable as sample size increases. Moreover, as the sample size increases, the standard error decreases at a decreasing rate, which suggests there is an optimum sample size beyond which it is not worth investing more resources (that aspect will be addressed further in the "Sample Size" section).

> **Key Concept**
>
> As the sample size increases, the standard error decreases.

FIGURE 7.2 ● **Hypothetical Sampling Distributions of a Mean for Random Samples of Different Size From the Same Population**

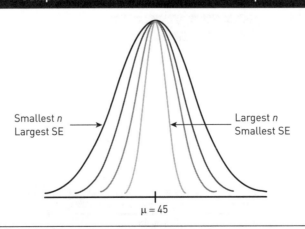

BOX 7.3: CONFIDENCE INTERVAL AROUND A SAMPLE MEAN

General structure of a confidence interval (*CI*)

CI = Statistic ± (Confidence Level × Standard Error)

Confidence interval about a sample mean

$CI_x = \bar{x} \pm z\, SE_{\bar{x}} = \bar{x} \pm z\,(s/\sqrt{n})$

95% Confidence interval about a sample mean

$CI_{95} = \bar{x} \pm 1.96\,(s/\sqrt{n})$

90% confidence level $z = 1.65$.
99% confidence level $z = 2.58$.

Point and interval estimates. A sample statistic such as the mean age (or proportion who smoke cigarettes) is a **point estimate** of a corresponding population parameter. In practice, it is not possible to calculate the sampling error for a point estimate because the population parameter's value typically is not known. Instead, sampling error is taken into account by calculating a **confidence interval (CI)** around a point estimate as the product of a confidence level and the standard error, as shown in Box 7.3. The **confidence level** is indicated by a standard score (z) from the normal distribution. Most often that value is set at ±1.96, corresponding to the 95% confidence level ($z = \pm1.96$ includes 95% of a normal distribution). Because the population variance (σ^2) for a parameter typically is unknown, the standard error is estimated using the *sample standard deviation* (*s*). Thus, $SE = \sigma/\sqrt{n} \cong s/\sqrt{n}$. As shown in Box 7.3, the width of a 95% confidence interval around a sample mean is $\pm1.96(s/\sqrt{n})$.

A 95% confidence interval has a 95% chance of including the population parameter because *overall*, if all possible random samples of size *n* are selected from a population of size *N*, 95% of such intervals are expected to include the population parameter. Nevertheless, there is a 5% chance that any particular such interval will *not* include the population parameter.

CHECK YOUR UNDERSTANDING 7.1

- Describe the main reasons for selecting a sample instead of studying an entire target population.
- Identify the two key features of random sampling.
- Explain why it is important to understand simple random sampling without replacement.
- Explain why simple random sampling without replacement is used in practice instead of simple random sampling with replacement.
- Describe the concept of a sampling distribution and how it is used.
- Describe sampling error and explain how it is taken into account.

Random Sampling Procedures

Sampling frame

The first step in selecting a random sample is to obtain or develop a **sampling frame**, which is a source that identifies population elements and is a vehicle from which a sample may be selected. The generally preferred type of sampling frame is a list of population elements that may be available in hard-copy or digital format, such as a student roster, an employee directory, or a roster of health clinic patients. Before using a sampling frame, it should be assessed regarding

- coverage
- duplicates, and
- ineligibles.

Coverage. **Coverage** of the target population generally is the most important sampling frame issue because it may introduce **noncoverage bias** if some elements systematically are not included. A sampling frame should be assessed for currency to ensure it is up to date so the most recent population members are not excluded. Another key aspect is a frame's inclusiveness. For example, health professionals in a particular field might belong to either or both of two professional organizations. If the membership directory of only one organization (e.g., the largest) is used as the sampling frame, it might underrepresent or even exclude entirely professionals who work in certain types of practice settings. In such a situation, a **dual frame** strategy may be employed that merges directories to create a more inclusive sampling frame. Nevertheless, if some in the target population are not members of either organization, they still will not be included in the dual frame. The nature and degree of noncoverage bias should be taken into consideration when interpreting and reporting a study's results.

Duplicates. If a sampling frame includes duplicate or multiple entries, those elements will have an increased chance of selection. Even a single-source sampling frame might include some elements more than once, such as a directory of university faculty listing someone as both a professor and an administrator. When compiling a dual frame, some elements might be included in both sources. When feasible, duplicates should be deleted before selecting a sample so the sampling frame includes only one entry per element.

When duplicates are identified at the point of selection (e.g., consecutive entries appear for the same person in an alphabetical directory), they may be given a second random chance to remain in the sample that is the *inverse* of the number of times they are listed in the sampling frame. For an element with two entries, that probability would be 1/2 and could be implemented by a coin toss, for instance. The element's *overall* selection probability would be the product of the initial chance of selection and the chance of remaining in the sample. For example, if a sample of 100 is selected from a population of 1,000, the sampling fraction is 100/1,000, or 1/10. An element that is included twice in the sampling frame has an initial selection probability of 2/10, but its chance of remaining in the sample would be 1/2; thus, its overall selection probability would be $(2/10)(1/2) = 1/10$. An initial sample larger than if there were no duplicates must be selected to account for duplicate elements that will not be retained.

Sometimes duplicates may be identified during data collection. For example, it is common practice for a telephone interview survey to ask participants whether they could have been contacted at more than one telephone number. The usual procedure is to conduct an interview rather than pass up an interview opportunity. Data from duplicates are weighted by the inverse of the number of telephone numbers at which they could be contacted. For example, data for a participant who reports being able to be contacted at two telephone numbers would be weighted by a factor of 1/2 or .5.

Ineligibles. If a sampling frame includes information about eligibility criteria, when feasible, ineligible elements should be deleted before selecting a sample. An alternative strategy is to ignore ineligibles when they are encountered. However, that strategy requires selecting a sample larger than if there were no ineligibles so as not to reduce the final sample size. The procedure for calculating an adjusted sample size is described in the "Field Sample Size" section.

Random selection

In addition to simple random sampling, the other main sampling designs are stratified sampling and cluster sampling. The random selection methods described in the following sections may be applied to select elements within strata, clusters, elements within clusters, or subsamples from samples already selected. Regardless of the sampling design and selection method, the best practice is not to select a substitute for a duplicate or ineligible element. In particular, it is not appropriate to select substitute elements by judgment or convenience. For instance, if a duplicate or ineligible element is selected, an element immediately above or below it in the sampling frame should not be used as a substitute. That procedure would give such elements an additional chance for selection, which violates the principle that each element has an independent chance of selection.

Basic random selection. Perhaps the most familiar random selection method is a lottery drawing, where each element has one entry and a blind selection process is used, such as selecting cards with names or numbers mixed in a container. However, a lottery is cumbersome and inefficient for selecting a large sample from a large population. Most often, **random number selection** is employed, which is a three-step procedure (also known as **basic random selection**):

1. Assign numbers from 1 through N to all elements in the sampling frame.
2. Use a random number source to select n unique numbers.
3. Identify the elements on the sampling frame corresponding to the n unique randomly selected numbers.

First, assign numbers from 1 through N to all elements in the sampling frame, including duplicates and ineligibles if they have not been deleted. Next, use a random number source to select n unique numbers from 1 to N. Without replacement, each element may be selected only once, and its number is ignored if it is selected again. The random number source may be a random number table (e.g., The RAND Corporation, 2001) or a random number generator (e.g., **Research Randomizer** at www.randomizer.org). Finally, identify the elements on the sampling frame corresponding to the n unique randomly selected numbers. When feasible, especially when the sampling frame is in digital format, it is most efficient to implement random selection using data processing software, such as Excel, IBM SPSS Statistics, SAS, and Stata. Also, online sampling programs are available, sometimes free, such as Research Randomizer.

Systematic random selection. A **systematic random sample** uses a systematic process, whereby population elements are selected using a fixed selection interval (k) from a random starting point in a sampling frame. Systematic random selection is more convenient and efficient than the basic random selection methods.

There are three steps in the systematic random selection procedure:

1. Determine the selection interval: $k = N/n$.
2. Select a random starting point between 1 and k.
3. Select the element at the random starting point and every kth element thereafter.

First, determine the **selection interval** (k) by dividing the population size by the sample size: $k = N/n$. Next, select a **random starting point** within the first instance of the selection interval in the sampling frame, located between elements 1 and k, inclusive. Third, select the element at the random starting point and every kth element thereafter, passing through the sampling frame once.

Table 7.2 illustrates systematic random selection for a sample of 5 selected from a population of 20 employees, where the selection interval is 4 ($k = 20/5$) and 2 is selected

TABLE 7.2 ● **Systematic Random Selection of a Sample of 5 From a Population of 20 ($n = 5$, $N = 20$, $k = 4$)**

Selection Points	Number	Employee
	1	Jorge
RSP	2	Priya
	3	Camille
	4	Francesca
	5	Daniel
	6	Brandon
	7	Vijay
	8	Martin
	9	Yuka
	10	Leslie
	11	Shalini
	12	Robin
	13	Jamil
	14	Franklin
	15	Katherine
	16	Stacy
	17	Amanda
	18	Miguel
	19	Nakia
	20	Rosalba

RSP: random starting point

as the random starting point between elements 1 and 4. The sample comprises element 2 plus every fourth element thereafter (2, 6, 10, 14, and 18), passing through the sampling frame once.

Periodicity. Unlike the basic random selection methods, systematic random selection does *not* give all possible samples of size n from a population of size N the same chance of selection. Using one of the basic random selection methods, 15,504 random samples of 5 are possible from a population of 20. However, using systematic random selection, the number of possible samples is equal to the selection interval, k, which is 4 in Table 7.2. Thus, with systematic random selection, the entire sample is determined by a single random selection that identifies the starting point, $1/k$. All elements in the sample are determined by their location in the sampling frame relative to the random starting point and the selection interval. Nevertheless, the selection probability for individual elements using systematic random selection is the *same* as when a sample of size n is selected from a population of size N using a basic random selection method: $1/k = 1/(N/n) = n/N$.

In general, the reduced number of possible samples with systematic random selection is not an issue except when the sampling frame is arranged in a cyclical pattern that coincides with the selection interval. That condition is called periodicity, which may introduce **periodicity bias** if the selected elements differ systematically from the rest of the population. For example, Table 7.3 presents a roster for a population of 100 employees arranged by teams, with the supervisors listed first. If systematic random selection is used to select a sample of 20 and the random starting point (RSP) is 1, with a selection interval of 5 ($k = 100/20$), the sample will consist only of supervisors. If the random starting point is 2, 3, 4, or 5, then the sample will consist only of team members. In either situation, the result would be devastating because the sample would not represent the population that includes both supervisors and team members.

> **Key Concept**
>
> With systematic random selection, the entire sample is determined by a single random selection to identify the starting point.

TABLE 7.3 ● **Systematic Random Selection From a Sampling Frame With Periodicity ($N = 100$, $n = 20$, $k = 5$, RSP = 1)**

Sample	Number	Employee
1	1	Supervisor A
2	2	Team Member A1
3	3	Team Member A2
4	4	Team Member A3
5	5	Team Member A4
1	6	Supervisor B
2	7	Team Member B1
3	8	Team Member B2
4	9	Team Member B3
5	10	Team Member B4

(Continued)

TABLE 7.3 ● (Continued)

Sample	Number	Employee
1	11	Supervisor C
2	12	Team Member C1
3	13	Team Member C2
4	14	Team Member C3
5	15	Team Member C4
...	...	...
1	96	Supervisor T
2	97	Team Member T1
3	98	Team Member T2
4	99	Team Member T3
5	100	Team Member T4

Periodicity solutions. When periodicity is known or suspected to be present in a sampling frame, if feasible, the sampling frame may be arranged in random or quasi-random order. For example, if the sampling frame is a roster in digital format, a software program might arrange elements in order based on employee identification numbers or alphabetically. For instance, if the sampling frame in Table 7.3 is arranged alphabetically, there is no reason to expect every fifth employee would be a supervisor or a team member. In general, it is unlikely every *k*th entry in an alphabetical list would share any attribute(s) that might bias a sample, such as sex, education, or race.

When periodicity is known to be present, the sampling frame may be partitioned into subgroups from which separate random samples are selected. This strategy is a form of stratification, which will be discussed further in the next section. For example, the population in Table 7.3 may be partitioned into subgroups of 20 supervisors and 80 team members. To ensure the subgroups will be represented according to their proportions in the population, the subgroup sample size is determined by multiplying the subgroup size (N_h) by the overall sampling fraction, *f*. For a sample of 20 from a population of 100, the sampling fraction is 20/100 = 1/5 = .20. Accordingly, 20% (.20 × 100) would be selected from each subgroup to obtain a total sample of 20 that includes 4 (.20 × 20) supervisors and 16 (.20 × 80) team members.

CHECK YOUR UNDERSTANDING 7.2

- Identify the three main aspects of a sampling frame that must be assessed before selecting a sample from it.
- Describe how systematic random selection differs from basic random selection.
- Describe periodicity bias and present strategies for addressing it.

Stratified Random Sampling

Stratified random sampling divides a population into subgroups, called strata, and a random sample is selected from each **stratum** (note: *stratum* is singular; *strata* is plural). Samples may be selected within strata using one of the basic random selection methods or systematic random selection. Moreover, different selection methods may be used within strata depending on which one is most feasible and efficient. Although stratification requires investing additional resources and effort, when it is done effectively, its rewards almost always exceed its costs.

Conditions

There are four conditions under which stratification may be most beneficial:

1. The population is highly diverse (variance is large).
2. The analysis will focus on population subgroups rather than the population as a whole.
3. Data collection resource requirements differ substantially across subgroups.
4. The value of information differs across subgroups.

First, when the population is highly diverse in terms of key characteristics, stratifying ensures representation at all levels of diversity. Second, if the analysis will focus on population subgroups rather than the population as a whole, and subgroups differ substantially in size, stratification may ensure an adequate size sample is selected from each subgroup to conduct meaningful analyses within and/or across subgroups. Third, if data collection resource requirements differ substantially across subgroups, stratification facilitates allocating the sample size to avoid resources being depleted by the most resource-intensive subgroup(s). Fourth, if the value of information differs across subgroups, stratification may ensure an adequate size sample is selected from the subgroup(s) about which the need for information is greatest.

Impact

Stratification reduces sampling error by eliminating the least representative samples that could be selected using simple random sampling. As illustrated in Figure 7.3 (based on Figure 7.1), without stratification it is possible that the sample will mostly include the youngest or oldest population members. Those unrepresentative samples are highlighted in the left panel of the figure. However, if the population is stratified by age, then some elements will be selected from each age group. Thus, as depicted in the right panel, it will not be possible to select a sample comprising predominantly the youngest or oldest population members.

> **Key Concept**
>
> *Stratified random sampling reduces sampling error by eliminating the least representative samples.*

From a graphic perspective, stratification crops the tails of the sampling distribution, which contain the least representative samples. Compared with a simple random sample of the same size (n) from a population of the same size (N), the standard error for a stratified random sample will be smaller, and the width of confidence intervals around parameter estimates will be reduced. It is especially noteworthy that stratification reduces the standard error without increasing the sample size. Although stratification does not give all possible samples under simple random sampling a chance of selection, all possible stratified samples

FIGURE 7.3 ● **Sampling Distribution of Mean Age Without and With Stratification**

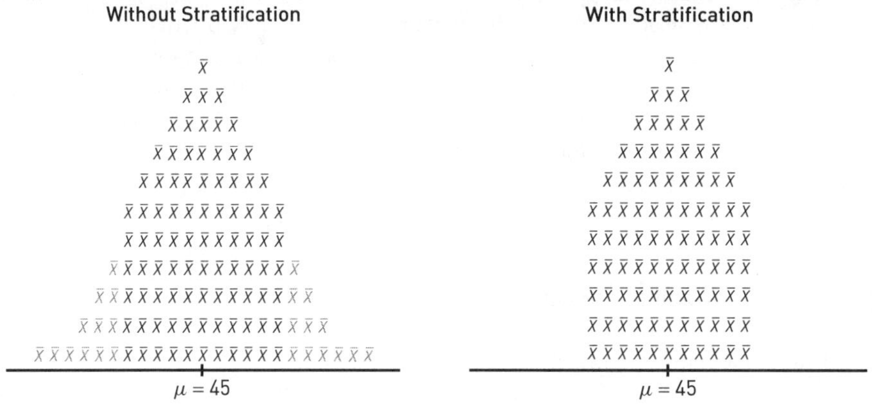

```
          Without Stratification                          With Stratification

                    x̄                                              x̄
                  x̄ x̄ x̄                                          x̄ x̄ x̄
                x̄ x̄ x̄ x̄                                       x̄ x̄ x̄ x̄
              x̄ x̄ x̄ x̄ x̄ x̄                                  x̄ x̄ x̄ x̄ x̄ x̄ x̄
            x̄ x̄ x̄ x̄ x̄ x̄ x̄ x̄                              x̄ x̄ x̄ x̄ x̄ x̄ x̄ x̄ x̄
          x̄ x̄ x̄ x̄ x̄ x̄ x̄ x̄ x̄ x̄                          x̄ x̄ x̄ x̄ x̄ x̄ x̄ x̄ x̄ x̄
          x̄ x̄ x̄ x̄ x̄ x̄ x̄ x̄ x̄ x̄                          x̄ x̄ x̄ x̄ x̄ x̄ x̄ x̄ x̄ x̄
        x̄ x̄ x̄ x̄ x̄ x̄ x̄ x̄ x̄ x̄ x̄ x̄                        x̄ x̄ x̄ x̄ x̄ x̄ x̄ x̄ x̄ x̄
      x̄ x̄ x̄ x̄ x̄ x̄ x̄ x̄ x̄ x̄ x̄ x̄ x̄ x̄                      x̄ x̄ x̄ x̄ x̄ x̄ x̄ x̄ x̄ x̄
    x̄ x̄ x̄ x̄ x̄ x̄ x̄ x̄ x̄ x̄ x̄ x̄ x̄ x̄ x̄ x̄                    x̄ x̄ x̄ x̄ x̄ x̄ x̄ x̄ x̄ x̄
  x̄ x̄ x̄ x̄ x̄ x̄ x̄ x̄ x̄ x̄ x̄ x̄ x̄ x̄ x̄ x̄ x̄ x̄ x̄ x̄ x̄ x̄          x̄ x̄ x̄ x̄ x̄ x̄ x̄ x̄ x̄ x̄
  ─────────────┼─────────────                          ─────────────┼─────────────
                 μ = 45                                                μ = 45
```

of size n from a population of size N have the same chance of selection. Moreover, with stratification the sampling distribution still is symmetrical and unimodal, and the expected value of a sample statistic is the population parameter. Thus, a stratified random sample is unbiased.

Specifying strata

In order to divide a population into strata, information about every population element's status on a stratifying variable must be known. Thus, it is not always possible to employ stratification or to stratify on a particular variable. Instead, strata most often are specified using information about demographic characteristics available from the sampling frame or records, such as age, education, sex, year in school, years of employment, or number of clinic visits. Strata may be specified using a single variable, or two or more variables in combination, such as age and education. However, each population element must be assigned to one and only one stratum.

Three guidelines for specifying strata are as follows:

1. A stratification variable must be correlated with key study variables.
2. Strata should group elements that are similar in ways that are relevant to the analysis.
3. Do not specify more strata than will be beneficial.

First and foremost, a stratification variable must be correlated with key study variables. Stratification should not be done simply because information is available for a particular variable. If a sample is stratified on a variable that is not correlated with key study variables, there will be little if any gain from investing resources to stratify the sample. Second, strata should group elements that are similar in ways that are relevant to the analysis, such as specifying age strata according to periods when significant life changes typically occur. Third, do not specify more strata than will be beneficial. For example, in most situations, the impact of stratifying a population ranging in age from 20 to 89 using five-year intervals (14 strata) is not likely to be substantially different from not stratifying at all. Moreover, the more strata, the greater will be the investment of resources and complexity to select the sample, collect and analyze data, and report results.

Proportionate allocation

Proportionate allocation of a sample among strata ensures the number of elements selected from each stratum is proportionate to the stratum's size in the population. Thus, when the analysis will focus on the population as a whole, proportionate allocation yields a sample that reflects the population composition on the stratifying variable(s). However, it does not ensure a sample will be similarly reflective of the population regarding other variables unless they are highly correlated with the stratifying variable(s). Proportionate allocation is an EPSEM design (sometimes called "self-weighting") and does not require applying stratum weights for analysis.

The total number of population elements in a stratum is designated as N_h, and the stratum sample size is n_h, where h indicates individual strata. The sample size for each stratum may be calculated by multiplying the stratum size by the overall sampling fraction: $n_h = N_h(n/N)$. Thus, the same sampling rate is applied within each stratum. Table 7.4 presents an illustration for a stratified random sample of 100 students selected with proportionate allocation from a population of 1,000. The overall sampling fraction, n/N, is .10; therefore, 10% of the students in each stratum will be selected. Consequently, the proportion of the total sample selected from each stratum (p_h) is identical to the proportion of the population in each stratum (P_h). An alternative method for calculating the stratum sample size is to multiply the total sample size by the proportion of the population in each stratum ($n_h = n \times P_h$).

TABLE 7.4 ● Stratified Random Sampling With Proportionate Allocation ($N = 1,000$, $n = 100$)

Stratum	Stratum Population Size N_h	Stratum Population Proportion P_h	Stratum Sample Size n_h	Stratum Sample Proportion p_h	Sampling Fraction
Freshman	400	.40	40	.40	40/400 = .10
Sophomore	200	.20	20	.20	20/200 = .10
Junior	300	.30	30	.30	30/300 = .10
Senior	100	.10	10	.10	10/100 = .10
Total	1,000	1.00	100	1.00	100/1,000 = .10

Disproportionate allocation

Disproportionate allocation of a sample among strata is employed when the analysis will focus on the strata rather than the population as a whole. It ensures that the number of elements selected from each stratum is adequate to conduct a meaningful analysis within a stratum and/or to compare results across strata. Stratum weights are not necessary for analyses within or across strata. In both situations, samples within strata may be analyzed as independent random samples. However, because stratification with disproportionate allocation is not an EPSEM design, stratum weights must be applied when combining results across strata to represent the population as a whole. Applying stratum weights in an analysis is greatly facilitated by data processing software.

Equal allocation. Equal allocation selects the same size sample from each stratum. The stratum sample size (n_h) is calculated by dividing the total sample size (n) by the number of strata (L): $n_h = n/L$. Equal allocation is optimal when the analysis will focus on comparisons across strata because it minimizes the standard error of differences, which maximizes statistical power to detect differences across strata. Table 7.5 illustrates equal allocation for a stratified sample of 100 students from a population of 1,000. The cells that differ from

Table 7.4 for proportionate allocation are highlighted. The proportion of the total sample that will be selected from each stratum (p_h) differs from the proportion of the population in each stratum (P_h). If results from all four strata are combined to represent the total population, without applying stratum weights the analysis would underrepresent the freshman class, which is the largest stratum. The senior class, which is the smallest stratum, would be overrepresented.

TABLE 7.5 ● Stratified Random Sampling With Disproportionate (Equal) Allocation (N = 1,000, n = 100)

Stratum	Stratum Population Size N_h	Stratum Population Proportion P_h	Stratum Sample Size n_h	Stratum Sample Proportion p_h	Sampling Fraction
Freshman	400	.40	25	.25	25/400 = .0625
Sophomore	200	.20	25	.25	25/200 = .125
Junior	300	.30	25	.25	25/300 = .0833
Senior	100	.10	25	.25	25/100 = .25
Total	1,000	1.00	100	1.00	

The basic stratum weight is the reciprocal of the selection probability within the stratum, $1/f_h$. Although that approach will bring the strata into their proper proportions, it inflates the sample size to equal the stratum population size and introduces an artificial increase in statistical power. Instead, stratum weights should be calculated so they adjust the stratum sample sizes relative to their population proportions without changing the total sample size. A simple method to appropriately calculate a **stratum weight** (w_h) is the ratio of the stratum population proportion (P_h) to the stratum sample proportion (p_h): $w_h = P_h/p_h$. Conceptually, it is the ratio of the proportion of the sample that would have been selected from a stratum with proportionate allocation (P_h), to the proportion that is selected with disproportionate allocation (p_h). If a stratum's proportion is smaller than its population proportion, the stratum's weight will be greater than 1.00. If a stratum's proportion is larger than its population proportion, the stratum's weight will be less than 1.00.

Table 7.6 presents stratum weights for the sample of students. The weighted total sample size equals the actual total sample size, and the weighted stratum sample sizes are the same as if the sample had been allocated proportionately (Table 7.4).

Purposive allocation. Purposive allocation selects stratum sample sizes that are disproportionate but not equal. It may be employed when one or more subgroups merit special attention

TABLE 7.6 ● Calculation of Stratum Weights for Disproportionate (Equal) Allocation (N = 1,000, n = 100)

Stratum	Stratum Population Size N_h	Stratum Population Proportion P_h	Stratum Sample Size n_h	Stratum Sample Proportion p_h	Stratum Weight w_h	Weighted Sample Size n_{wh}
Freshman	400	.40	25	.25	.40/.25 = 1.6	40
Sophomore	200	.20	25	.25	.20/.25 = 0.8	20
Junior	300	.30	25	.25	.30/.25 = 1.2	30
Senior	100	.10	25	.25	.10/.25 = 0.4	10
Total	1,000	1.00	100	1.00	4.0	100

in the analysis. For example, a stratum might be *oversampled* (a disproportionately large sample) if it has a large variance, it has a small population size (to ensure an adequate sample size is selected from it), or it is in a special need status. A stratum might be *undersampled* (a disproportionately small sample) if it has a small variance, there is substantial information already known about it, or resource requirements to select a sample and/or collect data from it are excessive. Similar to when equal allocation is used, stratum weights must be applied to analyze results if strata are combined.

CHECK YOUR UNDERSTANDING 7.3

- Identify the conditions for selecting a stratified random sample and explain why each one is important.
- Describe the impact of selecting a stratified random sample and explain why it happens.
- Present guidelines for specifying strata.
- Describe the difference between selecting a stratified random sample with proportionate versus disproportionate allocation of the sample.

Cluster Random Sampling

Cluster random sampling involves at least two stages. First, **clusters** of elements (e.g., households, schools, classes, health clinics, or community areas) are selected randomly. Then, individual elements are selected randomly within those clusters. Although both strata and clusters are groups of population elements, they are constituted differently. Also, whereas stratified sampling selects elements from all strata, cluster sampling selects elements within a random sample of clusters. In general, cluster designs are the most complex sampling designs. When planning to use a cluster design, it is recommended to seek consultation from a sampling professional, such as at an academic or commercial survey research organization.

Conditions

There are two conditions for employing cluster random sampling:

1. It is not feasible to obtain or develop a sampling frame.
2. Data will be collected on-site from a population distributed over a large geographic area.

The first condition applies when it is not feasible, or possible, to obtain or develop a sampling frame, such as for the population of all students in a large public school system or all adult residents of a city. However, it may be feasible to obtain or develop a sampling frame of individuals within a sample of clusters, such as a roster of students enrolled in several randomly selected schools, instead of at all schools. The second condition applies when the data collection plan requires staff to be present on-site (e.g., to conduct in-person interviews, focus groups, or direct observation) and the target population is distributed over a large geographic area. It is more efficient to conduct such data activities within a sample of representative clusters instead of across an entire population. Moreover, resources might render it not feasible to collect data from individuals across such a population.

Specifying clusters

Four guidelines for specifying clusters are as follows:

1. Clusters should be relevant to a study's purpose.
2. Cluster boundaries must not overlap.
3. Maximize variance within clusters.
4. Minimize variance across clusters.

First, clusters are specified by identifying preexisting units that are relevant to a study's purpose. For instance, to select a sample of health care workers, clusters might be clinics, hospitals, and/or private companies that employ such workers. Clusters may differ in size in terms of geographic area and/or population. Second, it is essential that cluster boundaries do not overlap so each population element is included in only one cluster. Third, to the extent possible, clusters should be specified to maximize variance within clusters. Maximizing variance within clusters enhances data collection efficiency by capturing as much of a population's diversity as possible within each cluster. Fourth, clusters should be specified to minimize variance across clusters. Minimizing variance across clusters enhances efficiency and minimizes sampling error. The more similarity there is across clusters, the fewer clusters that must be selected because the less it matters which clusters are selected.

Selecting clusters

The basic cluster sampling design comprises two stages: a random sample of clusters and a random sample of individuals within those clusters. A design may include more than one stage of cluster selection, such as selecting first a random sample of school districts, then schools within those districts, then eighth-grade classes within those schools. For simplicity of presentation, a two-stage design is assumed here.

The ultimate goal is to select a sample of individuals, not merely a sample of clusters. Therefore, the number of individuals within clusters, called the **cluster size**, must be taken into account so individual selection probabilities will be equal. That is achieved by selecting clusters with **probabilities proportionate to size (PPS)**. For instance, a cluster containing twice as many individuals as another will be given twice the chance to be selected in the first stage of a cluster sample design, and so forth. A simple approach to selecting clusters with PPS is to weight one of the basic random selection methods according to each cluster's **measure of size (MOS)**.

For example, applying a lottery drawing to a sample of Illinois counties, Cook County, with a population of 5.2 million people, would have 5.2 million entries; Hardin County would have 4,256 entries. Using simple random sampling without replacement, when *any* of a cluster's entries is drawn, the cluster is included in the sample and set aside until all other clusters are selected. Although this procedure initially gives individuals in a large cluster a higher selection probability than individuals in a small cluster, overall individual selection probabilities are equalized when the second stage of a cluster sample design is implemented.

The most efficient strategy for selecting clusters with probabilities proportionate to size is systematic random selection. Suppose the goal is to select three clusters from the population of twelve clusters in Table 7.7. The number of clusters to be selected is designated as m; thus $m = 3$. The systematic random selection interval (s) is determined by dividing the population size by the number of clusters to be selected, $s = N/m$, so $s = 60,000/3 = 20,000$. A random starting point is selected between 1 and s, which in the example is between 00,001

TABLE 7.7 ● Systematic Random Selection of Three Clusters With Probabilities Proportionate to Size

Cluster	MOS	Within-Cluster Number Range	Selection Points[a]
1	15,000	00,001–15,000	
2	8,000	15,001–23,000	18,500
3	7,000	23,001–30,000	
4	6,000	30,001–36,000	
5	5,000	36,001–41,000	38,500
6	4,000	41,001–45,000	
7	4,000	45,001–49,000	
8	3,000	49,001–52,000	
9	3,000	52,001–55,000	
10	2,000	55,001–57,000	
11	2,000	57,001–59,000	58,500
12	1,000	59,001–60,000	
Total	60,000		

[a]Random starting point = 18,500; s = 20,000

and 20,000. As illustrated in Table 7.7, if the random starting point is 18,500, cluster 2 will be in the sample. Applying the selection interval of 20,000, clusters 5 and 11 also will be selected. When selecting clusters with PPS, the selection points designate clusters, not individuals within them. Thus, the example did not select individuals 18,500, 38,500, and 58,500; it selected their cluster.

Although the largest cluster (1) had the best chance to be selected, it was not selected in the example. If not including that cluster is of concern for potential sample representativeness (e.g., not including Cook County, which contains about 40% of the Illinois population), clusters may be stratified by size. For example, cluster 1 might constitute one stratum, and a second stratum might comprise the 11 smaller clusters. In that situation, the probability of selecting cluster 1 is 1.00 because it is the only cluster in that stratum. A cluster whose probability of selection is 1.00 is called a **certainty cluster**. The number of elements selected from a certainty cluster is proportionate to its size. Accordingly, since cluster 1 contains 25% (15,000/60,000) of the population, 25% of the sample of individuals would be selected from cluster 1. Then two clusters would be selected randomly from the 11 smaller clusters, and the remaining 75% of the sample would be selected from them.

Another way in which a certainty cluster may be encountered is when a cluster's measure of size is greater than or equal to the selection interval (MOS ≥ s). Regardless of the random starting point, such a cluster is certain to be selected. Moreover, when a cluster's MOS is greater than the selection interval, more than one selection point might occur within it. A certainty cluster should be treated similar to a stratum, and the appropriate proportion of the sample should be allocated to it. After setting aside a certainty cluster, the other clusters are selected, and the remaining sample is allocated among them.

Selecting individuals within clusters

In the second stage of a two-stage cluster sample design, individuals are selected within the clusters selected in the first stage. Sometimes, when feasible, in the interest of convenience and efficiency, all individuals within a cluster may be included in a sample. For example, self-administered questionnaires might be distributed to an entire class of students in a single session. Moreover, in such a situation, it would not be necessary to obtain or develop a sampling frame of individuals. However, except in the rare situation where clusters are the same size, such a design requires weighting the data to adjust for unequal selection probabilities, the calculation and application of which may be complex.

Most often, a random sample of individuals is selected within the clusters selected in the first stage. That strategy is particularly effective when the typical cluster size is large, such as counties, and it is not feasible to select all individuals. As with a stratified sample, individuals may be selected using one of the basic random selection methods or systematic random selection. Moreover, different selection methods may be used within clusters depending on feasibility and efficiency.

When a cluster sample is selected with PPS, the *same* number of individuals is selected within each cluster. That strategy results in an EPSEM design overall. In the first stage, individuals' selection probabilities are *directly proportional* to their cluster's MOS. Thus, an individual in a large cluster has a higher chance of selection than an individual in a small cluster. In the second stage, an individuals' selection probability is *inversely proportional* to their cluster's MOS. Thus, an individual in a small cluster has a higher chance of selection than an individual in a large cluster.

The overall selection probability (P_O) is the product of the selection probability of a cluster in the first stage (P_1) and the probability of an individual being selected within the cluster in the second stage (P_2): $P_O = P_1 P_2$ (for three or more stages, the overall selection probability is the product across all stages). In the first stage, the selection probability for a cluster is the product of the number of clusters selected (m) and the ratio of the cluster's MOS to the population size (MOS/N): $P_1 = m(\text{MOS}/N)$. This expression may be rewritten to relate it directly to systematic random selection of clusters: $P_1 = \text{MOS}/(N/m) = \text{MOS}/s$. In the second stage, the selection probability for an individual within a cluster is the ratio of the number of individuals selected within each cluster (n_c) to the cluster's MOS: $P_2 = n_c/\text{MOS}$. Accordingly, allocating the sample of individuals equally across clusters, where $n_c = n/m$, an individual's overall selection probability is $P_O = m(\text{MOS}/N) \times n_c/\text{MOS}$. Substituting n/m for n_c, the overall selection probability, P_O, for each individual in a PPS cluster sample may be reduced to n/N, the overall sampling fraction. Thus, it is an EPSEM design.

Impact

Individuals within the same cluster are likely to be similar on many characteristics, such as students who experience the same learning and community environments. The more similarity there is among individuals within a cluster, the less there is within-cluster variance. **Within-cluster homogeneity** reduces the number of independent observations in a sample, which is called the **design effect (deff)**. Consequently, the *effective sample size* for a cluster sample will be smaller than for a simple random sample of the same size. Also, sampling error will be larger for a cluster sample than for a simple random sample of the same size selected from the same population.

The design effect for a cluster sample design is defined as the ratio of the variance of the sampling distribution for a cluster sample (VAR_C) to the variance

Key Concept

The design effect of a cluster sample reduces its effective sample size and increases sampling error.

of the sampling distribution for a simple random sample (VAR_{SRS}) of the same size: deff = (VAR_C)/(VAR_{SRS}). For example, a design effect of 2.3 indicates the variance of a parameter estimate from a cluster sample is 2.3 times larger than it would be for a simple random sample of the same size. Similarly, the standard error, which is the square root of the variance of an estimate, also would be 2.3 times larger.

When planning a study, an initial sample size estimate may be multiplied by the design effect, $n \times$ deff, to determine the sample size necessary for a cluster sample to have the same precision and statistical power as a simple random sample. For example, if the initial sample size is 200 and the design effect is estimated to be 1.90, the cluster sample size should be $200 \times 1.90 = 380$. After data are collected from a cluster sample, the effective sample size may be calculated by multiplying the actual sample size by the inverse of the design effect: n/deff. For example, if a sample of 400 elements is selected in a cluster design and the design effect is 1.60, the effective sample size that would be comparable in precision and statistical power to a simple random sample would be $400/1.60 = 250$. Thus, data for each individual in a cluster sample should be weighted by the inverse of the design effect. For a cluster sample with a design effect of 1.60, the data would be weighted by a factor of $1/1.60 = 0.625$.

CHECK YOUR UNDERSTANDING 7.4

- Identify the conditions for selecting a cluster random sample.
- Present guidelines for specifying clusters and explain why each one is important.
- Describe the impact of selecting a cluster random sample and explain why it happens.
- Explain why selecting a cluster random sample with probabilities proportionate to size yields an EPSEM design.

Sample Size

The main concern for determining the sample size is that it is sufficient to provide a trustworthy answer to the research question. There is no standard sample size for any particular population or research design. Moreover, contrary to some misconceptions, the proportion or percentage of a population that will be selected is *not* relevant to determining sample size. When a random sample design is employed, the sample size is assessed in terms of statistical aspects such as precision and power that are based on probability theory. Although it is not appropriate to apply such concepts to nonrandom sampling designs, logistical aspects of sample size apply to both random and nonrandom sampling. The statistical approaches presented in the following sections assume a simple random sample without replacement. The references and resources for further study cited at the end of this chapter should be consulted regarding strategies for complex stratified or cluster sample designs. Also, it is recommended to consult a sampling statistician.

Population estimates

The basic sample size formula to calculate the sample size for estimating a population parameter is derived from the confidence interval formula, for which the general expression is CI = Statistic ± (Confidence Level × Standard Error). The value of a sample statistic may be ignored at this point because it will be determined after selecting a sample and collecting data. A confidence interval also is called the **margin of error (MOE)**, which commonly is cited when political poll results are reported, for instance. Thus, the confidence interval formula may be expressed as MOE = ±$z(\sigma/\sqrt{n})$, which may be solved for the sample size as $n = z^2\sigma^2/\text{MOE}^2$ or $n = (z\sigma/\text{MOE})^2$. Conceptually, the formula may be expressed as Sample Size = Confidence Level² × Variance/Margin of Error², from which it may be observed that a larger sample size is required

- the higher the desired confidence level,
- the larger the population variance, or
- the smaller the desired margin of error.

This formula may be used to calculate the sample size for an entire study or for subgroups. Technically, the sample size formula should be calculated for every variable in a study. However, only one sample size can and will be selected. In most situations, the best practice is to determine the minimum acceptable sample size to address the research question and increase it as resources allow. Alternatively, the sample size may be calculated for several key variables, and then the average, smallest, or largest sample size may be selected, depending on resources and a study's purpose.

Sample size for a proportion. Most often, especially for studies in which many variables will be measured, a conservative and comprehensive approach is employed whereby the population variance is set at maximum, which is the worst-case scenario. The maximum variance is determined most conveniently when the sample size is calculated for a proportion. When treated as a dichotomy (e.g., the proportion that smokes cigarettes vs. does not smoke), the variance of a proportion is $P(1 - P)$, which also is expressed as PQ, where $Q = 1 - P$. The maximum possible value for the variance of a proportion occurs when $P = .5$; thus, PQ = .5 × .5 = .25. By substitution in the basic sample size formula, the sample size is $n = z^2(.25)/\text{MOE}^2$.

For many studies, confidence is set at the 95% level, which corresponds to $z = \pm1.96$. Also, the margin of error often is set at ±.05, independent of the 95% confidence. Note that MOE = .05 is not derived as 1 − .95. For instance, the sample size may be calculated where confidence is set at the 95% level, and the margin of error may be set at .10, or .01 instead of .05. Ignoring ± signs, setting the confidence level at 95% ($z = 1.96$), variance at maximum (PQ = .25), and the margin of error at .05, the sample size is $n = 1.96^2(.25)/.05^2$ = 384. Thus, if variance is maximum, a sample of 384 elements will enable estimating a population proportion within a margin of error of ±.05 (or 5%) with 95% confidence ($z = 1.96$). Moreover, for any variable for which variance is less than maximum, a population proportion will be estimated within a smaller margin of error and/or greater than 95% confidence.

Adjustment for population size. The basic sample size formula is derived from probability theory, which assumes an infinite size population. Accordingly, it does not include the population size, N. However, in practice, most populations are of a finite size. In particular, it will not be possible to select a sample size of 384 elements if the population is smaller than that number. Therefore, especially when planning to select a sample from a relatively small population, an adjustment for population size, called the **finite population correction (fpc)**, may be included when calculating the sample size as follows: $n = n'/[1 + (n' - 1/N)]$, where n' is the initial sample size calculated without taking the population size into consideration. For example, at 95% confidence, with maximum variance and MOE ±.05, the initial sample size, n', is 384. If the population size, N, is 200, then the adjusted sample size would be $n = 384/[1 + (383/200)] = 132$.

Affordable sample size. Another approach to estimating sample size is to specify the sample size that available resources may support, and then assess whether either the corresponding margin of error or confidence level is acceptable. In the first instance, a confidence level may be specified, and then the corresponding margin of error may be determined, where MOE = ±$z(\sigma/\sqrt{n})$. For example, at the 95% confidence level, with maximum variance, MOE = ±1.96(.5/$\sqrt{n}$). If resources are sufficient to select a sample of 225 elements, then MOE = ±1.96(.5/$\sqrt{225}$) = ±.065. The other approach involves specifying a margin of error and then determining the corresponding confidence level. Rewriting the basic sample size formula, the confidence level (z) may be calculated as z = MOE/($\sigma/\sqrt{n}$). For example, with a margin of error set at ±.05, z = .05/(.5/$\sqrt{n}$). If resources are sufficient to select a sample of 300 elements, then z = .05/(.5/$\sqrt{300}$) = 1.73, which corresponds to a 92% confidence level.

Sample size for a mean. When calculating the sample size for estimating a mean, it often is not possible to specify the maximum variance. Variances for means may vary substantially. The variance for key interval-/ratio-level variables must be estimated from a pilot study, previous studies, or records. Moreover, studies typically also measure other key variables as proportions. Therefore, most often an overall sample size for a study is calculated using the conservative strategy for estimating a proportion, for which variance may be set at maximum. Nevertheless, when the main purpose is to estimate the mean for one key variable, it is best to calculate the sample size based on an estimate of that variable's variance.

Difference between proportions

The sample size for estimating a difference in proportions ($p_1 - p_2$) is derived from the formula for the standard score (z) for a difference between proportions: $z = p_1 - p_2/\sqrt{[(p_1q_1/n_1) + (p_2q_2/n_2)]}$, where $\sqrt{[(p_1q_1/n_1) + (p_2q_2/n_2)]}$ is the standard error of the difference between proportions. When n is set to be equal in both groups, which minimizes the standard error of the difference, the formula may be simplified to $z = p_1 - p_2/\sqrt{[(p_1q_1) + (p_2q_2)/n]}$, where n is the sample size required for *each* group. Solving for the sample size: $n = z^2(p_1q_1 + p_2q_2)/(p_1 - q_2)^2$.

For example, this formula might be applied to estimate the sample size to detect a difference of 10% (.10) in the prevalence of mammography screening during the past two years for two groups of women. If prevalence is estimated at 30% (.30) in group one and 20% (.20) in group two, then at the 95% confidence level, $n = 1.96^2[(.3 \times .7) + (.2 \times .8)]/.10^2 = 142$ per group, and the total sample size would be 284. With the most conservative approach, whereby the group variances are assumed to be equal and maximum, the sample size formula may be simplified to $n = z^2(2pq)/(p_1 - q_2)^2$. At the 95% confidence level, $n = 1.96^2[2(.5 \times .5)]/.10^2 = 192$ per group and a total sample size of 384. Alternatively, for a given specific sample size per group, and assuming group variances are equal and maximum, the size of a difference between proportions may be estimated as $p_1 - q_2 = z\sqrt{2pq/n}$. For example, if a sample of 100 will be collected per group (total $n = 200$), a difference between proportions of about .14 (14%) may be detected with 95% confidence.

Statistical power analysis

Statistical power is the probability that when a statistical test for differences is applied (e.g., a *t* test for differences between proportions or means), the **null hypothesis (H_0)** of no difference will be rejected when it is false (Chapter 15). A statistical power analysis is beyond the scope of this book. It is recommended to seek consultation from a statistician. Cohen (1988) generally is regarded as the definitive treatment of statistical power analysis. A useful summary of statistical power analysis is available in Cohen (1992). Power analysis software may be accessed free online at http://powerandsamplesize.com/ (accessed September 7, 2018). Also, G*Power software may be downloaded free at https://download.cnet.com/G-Power/3000-2054_4-10647044.html (accessed September 7, 2018).

Field sample size

The sample size calculations presented in the preceding sections assume 100% contact, eligibility, and cooperation rates. Such conditions virtually never are encountered in practice. A **field sample size (FSS)** should be calculated to account for such contingencies by increasing the sample size so the number of subjects from whom data are analyzed is approximately equal to the number intended. Contact, eligibility, and cooperation rates may be estimated based on previous studies, a pilot study, and/or records. The field sample size is calculated by dividing the intended sample size (n) by the product of the contact rate, eligibility, and cooperation rates: FSS = n/(Contact Rate × Eligibility Rate × Cooperation Rate). Other contingencies, such as sampling frame duplicates, may be included in the denominator as appropriate. For example, suppose the following rates are expected: contact = 85%, eligibility = 90%, and cooperation = 70%. If the intended sample size is 300, then the field sample size would be FSS = 300/(.85 × .90 × .70) = 560. The expectation is that 476 individuals will be contacted (560 × .85), 428 of those will be eligible (476 × .90), and 300 of those will cooperate (428 × .70). The best practice when estimating contact, eligibility, and cooperation rates is to be conservative by assuming rates somewhat lower than expected. Also, inasmuch as sample sizes are estimates, a conservative approach is to round up. For instance, it is not necessary to select a sample of exactly 383 elements. Instead, such an estimate typically is rounded to 400. These strategies ensure the field sample size will be large enough to provide the sample size intended for analysis.

Logistical aspects

Typically, sample size assessment is a two-step process, whereby after considering statistical aspects, adjustments are made based on logistical considerations, such as

- importance,
- data quality,
- target population, and
- resources.

Importance. The more potential for a study to make an important contribution to the current state of knowledge, theory, and/or practice, the stronger the justification for selecting a large sample for which the confidence level will be high and the margin of error will be low. For example, a large sample size may be justified if there is a potential for harm from inferential errors (i.e., caused by a low confidence level and/or a large margin of error) that might have an adverse impact on practice guidelines.

Data quality. Another consideration is data quality standards/expectations among the audience(s) to whom results will be reported. For instance, a 95% confidence level might be regarded as too low, or a .05 margin of error might be regarded as too large.

Target population. A concern about the target population is whether it is feasible to gain access to the intended number of sites, groups, and/or individuals that will be included in a sample. A smaller sample size may enable employing more intensive and effective contact strategies by reducing the points of access to be negotiated. Also, a smaller sample size may be justified if there is a substantial potential risk to study participants and/or data collection staff.

Resources. The sample size must be supportable by available and/or obtainable financial and staff resources. In particular, data collection travel time and costs typically increase when a large sample is distributed widely over a large geographic area. When resources are not adequate to support an intended sample size, the sample size that is feasible should be estimated. Then the corresponding confidence level and margin of error should be calculated and assessed in view of the study's importance. Also, consideration should be given to the time required to collect data, especially if collecting data from a large sample might expose a study to a time-related interval validity threat (Chapter 5).

> **CHECK YOUR UNDERSTANDING 7.5**
>
> - Explain how sample size is related to each of the following:
>   - Confidence level
>   - Population variance
>   - Margin of error
> - Identify the four logistical aspects that should be taken into consideration when determining sample size, and explain why each one is important.

Random Assignment

Random assignment, also called **randomization**, is the most effective strategy for addressing nonequivalence as an internal validity threat (Chapter 5) to a research design that includes two or more groups (e.g., treatment and control groups). There is no relationship between selection and assignment methods:

- Participants who are selected by random sampling may be assigned either randomly or nonrandomly.
- Random assignment does not enhance the representativeness of a nonrandom sample.
- For a nonrandom sample, random assignment still will yield statistically equivalent groups.

Randomly assigning study groups to conditions may be done simply by a coin toss for two groups or a lottery drawing for three or more groups. The most common strategies for randomly assigning individuals or multiple intact groups (e.g., eighth-grade classrooms) to conditions are as follows:

- *Separate random samples:* Separate random samples are selected corresponding to the number of study conditions and randomly assigned to conditions.
- *Simple random assignment:* A determination is made randomly for each participant.
- *Stratified random assignment:* Equal numbers of participants from each stratum are assigned to each study condition.
- *Block randomization:* Participants are assigned within subgroups, called blocks, as they are recruited.
- *Matching:* This version of stratified random assignment may enhance comparability across conditions when participants are very diverse and their number is small.

When a research design includes one or more pretest observations, random assignment typically is indicated as the first component in a diagram (Chapter 4). However, if that sequence is implemented in practice, nonequivalence may result owing to a differential loss of participants between random assignment and treatment implementation. In particular, the burden of pretest participation may lead participants to drop out. That is especially likely for those who already have been assigned to a control condition and expect to derive no benefit from further participation. Therefore, the best practice is to implement random assignment *after* all pretest observations are complete to eliminate differential loss of participants prior to treatment implementation.

Separate Random Samples

When individuals are selected by random sampling, an efficient strategy is to select *k* separate random samples, corresponding to the number of conditions. Then randomly assign the *k* samples to conditions using a coin toss or lottery drawing. In addition to selecting separate random samples from a large population, this method may be employed to randomly assign an entire population or a nonrandom sample, such as a pool of volunteers. In such situations, if the research design includes only two conditions, only one random sample must be selected; the remaining subjects constitute a separate random sample.

Simple Random Assignment

Although it is less efficient than separate random samples, **simple random assignment** may be employed for each individual, such as by tossing a coin or rolling a die. However, it is most efficient to use software to generate a random series of numbers between 1 and *k*, corresponding to the number of study conditions. Unfortunately, simple random assignment does not necessarily assign equal numbers of participants across conditions. The solution is to stop assigning participants to a condition when the condition's designated number is assigned. Then assign the remaining participants to the other condition for a two-group design, or continue random assignment to the other conditions for a design with three or more groups. When the designated number of participants is assigned to one condition, assigning the remaining participants to the other condition is a result of a random process that does not introduce bias.

Stratified Random Assignment

Stratification may enhance comparability of participants across conditions by ensuring equal numbers with a particular characteristic are assigned to each condition. For example, volunteers might be stratified by age and sex; then simple random assignment may be implemented within each age × sex stratum. **Stratified random assignment** requires advance information about participants and requires additional time and resources. It is most appropriate when a study's main focus is on comparing participants who are as similar as possible regarding the stratification variable(s). Otherwise, it is important to recognize that selecting separate random samples or using simple random assignment generally will yield groups with similar frequency distributions on *all* variables.

Block Randomization

Sometimes all participants cannot be selected and assigned at once, such as when a *rolling recruitment* strategy is employed as participants become eligible (e.g., with a particular diagnosis) and/or available (e.g., seek particular services). Moreover, it may be necessary to expose participants to study conditions, such as counseling strategies for posttraumatic stress disorder, shortly after they are recruited. Therefore, it may not be feasible to conduct random assignment after all participants are enrolled in a study.

Block randomization assigns participants within series, called *blocks*, as they are recruited. The block size corresponds to the number of study conditions (k). The number of blocks (b) is determined by dividing the number of participants by the number of study conditions: $b = n/k$. For example, if 300 participants are recruited and randomly assigned to three conditions, there will be 100 blocks, each containing three randomly assigned participants. Individuals may be assigned within blocks by simple random assignment. When block randomization is applied across a large number of blocks, on average, it will assign participants equitably in all possible orderings of conditions, called *permutations*. Table 7.8 illustrates block randomization to three conditions.

Matching

When participants are diverse and their number is small, random variation may yield assignments that deviate in ways that might confound interpreting outcome differences. Matching is a version of stratified random assignment that may enhance comparability across conditions in such a situation. Although it may be implemented regarding more than one matching variable, recruiting and identifying matches becomes more difficult as the number of variables increases. Matching is effective to the extent matching variables are potential moderators of a study's outcome, or are correlated with key moderators (Chapter 3). Moreover, accurate measures of matching variables must be available at the time of participant assignment.

Frequency matching is employed to yield groups with similar *frequency distributions*, which means the groups have similar numbers of participants at each value on the matching variable(s). That may be achieved through stratified random assignment with participants stratified on the matching variable(s). Also, block randomization may be used in combination with stratification, as illustrated in Table 7.9 where participants are listed hierarchically by age. The illustration includes all six possible permutations for assigning participants in blocks to three conditions. Although there is only one participant at each age, three participants are randomly assigned within each age block/stratum. The impact of this approach is demonstrated by the fact that the mean age of all participants is 37, which also is the mean age of the participants assigned to each condition.

Pairwise matching

Pairwise matching, which also is called **matched pairs**, is a one-for-one approach that randomly assigns each of two matched participants to alternate conditions. It may be implemented using block randomization. Pairwise matching becomes increasingly challenging the more rigorous the matching criteria. For example, it is more difficult to identify age matches within a narrow interval of ±1 year than within a broader interval of ±2 years.

CHECK YOUR UNDERSTANDING 7.6

- Explain how random sampling and random assignment are
  - related, and
  - not related.

Conducting Health Research

TABLE 7.8 ● Block Randomization of 300 Participants to Three Conditions

	Block 1			Block 2			Block 3			...	Block 100		
Participant	1	2	3	4	5	6	7	8	9	...	298	299	300
Condition	2	3	1	3	1	2	1	2	3	...	2	1	3

TABLE 7.9 ● Block Randomization With Participants in Ascending Order by Age

Block	Participant	Age	Condition
1	1	20	1
	2	22	2
	3	24	3
2	4	26	1
	5	28	3
	6	30	2
3	7	32	2
	8	34	1
	9	36	3
4	10	38	2
	11	40	3
	12	42	1
5	13	44	3
	14	46	1
	15	48	2
6	16	50	3
	17	52	2
	18	54	1

Key Points

Reasons for Sampling

The primary reasons for studying a sample are to
- minimize costs,
- minimize time,

- improve access to subjects,
- improve data quality, and
- minimize population exposure.

Random Sampling Concepts

- Each population element has an independent chance to be selected; the selection probability for each element is known, or may be calculated.
- Simple random sampling is the foundational random sampling design.
- A sampling design for which each element has the same selection probability is called an EPSEM design (Equal Probability Selection Method).
- Simple random sampling with replacement returns a selected element to the population before making the next selection.
- Simple random sampling without replacement does not return a selected element to the population.
- A sampling distribution is the distribution of a sample statistic for all possible random samples of size n from a population of size N.
- According to the central limit theorem, the sampling distribution will approach a normal distribution, regardless of the shape of the population distribution.
- Sampling error is the difference between a random sample statistic and its corresponding population parameter.
- Sampling error is taken into account by calculating a confidence interval around a point estimate.

Random Sampling Procedures

- A sampling frame is a source that identifies population elements and is a vehicle from which a sample may be selected.
- Random number selection is the most often employed basic random selection method.
- Systematic random selection uses a fixed interval from a random starting point in a sampling frame.

Stratified Random Sampling

- Divides a population into subgroups, called strata; a random sample is selected from each stratum.
- Reduces sampling error.

Cluster Random Sampling

- Selects elements within a sample of preexisting subgroups, called clusters.
- The number of individuals within clusters, called the cluster size, is taken into account by selecting clusters with probabilities proportionate to size.
- Within-cluster homogeneity reduces the number of independent observations in a sample, which is called the design effect.

Sample Size

- A larger sample size is required the higher the desired confidence level, the larger the population variance, and/or the smaller the desired margin of error.
- The field sample size accounts for contingencies such as the cooperation rate.
- Logistical aspects of sample size include a study's potential importance, data quality, the target population, and resources.

Random Assignment

- Best practice is to implement random assignment after a pretest observation.
- The most common random assignment strategies are
    - separate random samples,
    - simple random assignment,
    - stratified random assignment,
    - block randomization, and
    - matching.

BOX 7.4: KEY RANDOM SAMPLING FORMULAS

Sampling fraction (f)	n/N
Standard error (SE)	σ^2/n or $\sigma/\sqrt{n}$
Standard error sample estimate	$s/\sqrt{n}$
Confidence interval for a sample mean	$\bar{x} \pm z\, SE_{\bar{x}} = \bar{x} \pm z(s/\sqrt{n})$
95% confidence interval for a sample mean	$\bar{x} \pm 1.96(s/\sqrt{n})$
Systematic random selection interval (k)	N/n
Proportionate allocation among strata (n_h)	$N_h(n/N)$ or $n \times P_h$
Equal allocation among strata (n_h)	n/L
Stratum weight (w_h)	P_h/p_h or f/f_h
Cluster systematic random selection interval (s)	N/m
PPS cluster sample overall selection probability (P_0)	$m(MOS/N) \times n_c/MOS$
Cluster sample size adjusted for design effect	$n \times \text{deff}$
Cluster sample effective sample size	n/deff
Sample size for a point estimate	$z^2\sigma^2/MOE^2$ or $(z\sigma/MOE)^2$
Sample size for a proportion with maximum variance	$z^2(.25)/MOE^2$
Sample size adjusted for population size	$n'/[1 + (n' - 1/N)]$
Margin of error (MOE)	$\pm z(\sigma/\sqrt{n})$
Confidence level (z)	$MOE/(\sigma/\sqrt{n})$
Sample size (per group) for a difference between proportions	$z^2(p_1 q_1 + p_2 q_2)/(p_1 - q_2)^2$

Review and Apply

1. Review the research plan you developed in the "Review and Apply" section of Chapter 1 or 3. If you did not do that previously, either do it now or identify a health-related problem that interests you.

   a. What do you estimate to be the **population size**, N?

   b. Identify the **sampling frame** you would use to select a random sample of the population, assess how well it covers the population, and identify any potential noncoverage bias.

   c. Identify the **sample design** you would employ and explain why it is appropriate for your study.

   d. Using the methods described in this chapter, calculate the **sample size**, n, for estimating a population proportion. Specify the confidence level, variance estimate, and margin of error. Adjust your sample size estimate for the population size, if appropriate.

   e. Specify assumptions for contact, eligibility, cooperation rates, and any other contingencies that should be taken into account and calculate the **field sample size** (FSS).

2. Perform the following calculations related to sample size:

   a. The sample size to estimate a population proportion at the 95% level of confidence, assuming variance is maximum, and a margin of error of ±3% (.03).

   b. The sample size to estimate a population proportion at the 99% level of confidence, assuming variance is maximum, and a margin of error of ±3% (.03).

   c. The margin of error for an estimate of a population proportion at the 99% confidence level, assuming variance is maximum and the sample size is 200.

   d. The confidence level for an estimate of a population proportion assuming maximum variance, a margin of error of ±8% (.08), and the sample size is 200.

   e. The sample size to estimate a population proportion at the 95% level of confidence, assuming variance is maximum, and a margin of error of ±3% (.03) where the population size is 300.

   f. The **total** sample size to estimate a difference between population proportions at the 99% level of confidence, assuming variance is maximum, and a margin of error of ±5% (.05). Be sure to calculate the sample size for two population subgroups combined, not for a single group.

3. Select a published journal article of interest to you that used random sampling and write an evaluation of the following aspects of the sampling design and procedures:

   a. Identify the **target population** and assess its appropriateness for addressing the study's purpose.

   b. Describe the **sampling frame** and assess its appropriateness for the study population and any potential bias.

   c. Describe the **sampling design** and **selection procedures** used for selecting the sample (in your own words, using appropriate sampling terminology—do not simply quote the article) and assess any potential sources of bias.

   d. Identify the **strengths** and **weaknesses** of the sampling design and procedures, and assess the study's external validity.

   e. Suggest ways the sampling design and/or selection procedures might be improved.

4. Choose a state comprising 50 or more counties (called *parishes* in Louisiana) and obtain a list of all counties and population sizes at www.cubitplanning.com/data/quick-reports (accessed November 1, 2018) or at www.census.gov/data/datasets/2017/demo/popest/counties-total.html (accessed November 1, 2018).

   a. Calculate the mean (μ) population size for all N counties in the state.

   b. Select the following samples, each with a sample size (n) of 20 counties, and for each sample calculate the mean population size ($\bar{x}$), the standard error (SE) of the sample mean, and the 95% confidence interval about the sample mean. Then compare your results and identify which sample provides the best estimate of the population mean.

1. A simple random sample without replacement.
2. A systematic random sample.
3. A stratified random sample with proportionate allocation (use your judgment to specify the strata).
4. A stratified random sample with equal allocation (use the same strata you specify for proportionate allocation).
5. Apply stratum weights so the total weighted sample size equals 20 when calculating your estimate of the mean county size.

Study Further

Blair, E., & Blair, J. (2015). *Applied survey sampling*. Thousand Oaks, CA: Sage.

Frankel, M. (2010). Sampling theory. In P. V. Marsden & J. D. Wright (Eds.), *Handbook of survey research* (2nd ed., pp. 83–137). Bingley, UK: Emerald Group.

Khan Academy. (2018). Retrieved from https://www.khanacademy.org/

Levy, P. S., & Lemeshow, S. (1980). *Sampling for health professionals*. Belmont, CA: Lifetime Learning.

Piazza, T. (2010). Fundamentals of applied sampling. In P. V. Marsden & J. D. Wright (Eds.), *Handbook of survey research* (2nd ed., pp. 139–168). Bingley, UK: Emerald Group.

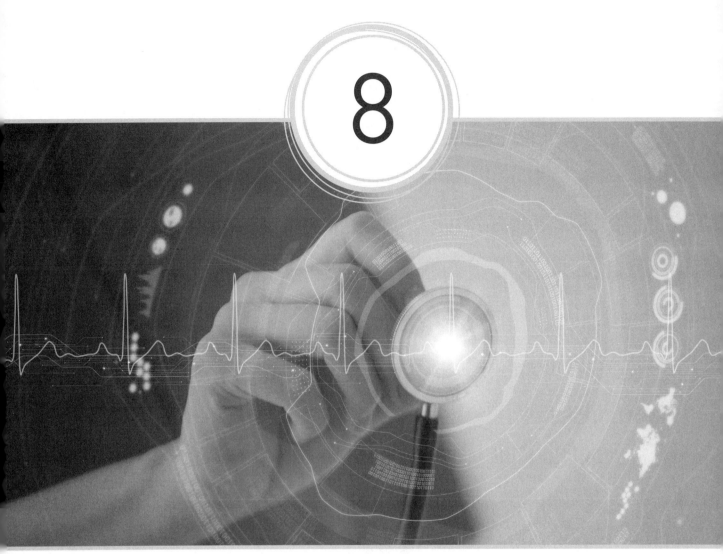

iStock.com/metamorworks

The Measurement Process, Reliability, and Validity

Chapter Outline

Overview
Learning Objectives
From Concepts to Data
    Conceptualization
    Operationalization
    Instrumentation
    An Example
Levels of Measurement
    Nominal Level
    Ordinal Level
    Interval/Ratio Level
    Comparative Summary
Measurement Theory
    Random Error
    Measurement Reliability
    Systematic Error
    Measurement Validity
    The Relationship Between Reliability and Validity
Assessing Measurement Reliability
    Test–Retest Reliability
    Interrater Reliability
    Parallel Forms Reliability
Assessing Measurement Validity
    Judgment-Based Validity
    Performance-Based Validity
Item Response Theory
Key Points

Learning Objectives

After studying Chapter 8, the reader should be able to:

- Implement the measurement process
- Distinguish between levels of measurement
- Apply classical test theory to developing and assessing a measurement
- Apply and interpret methods for assessing measurement reliability
- Apply and interpret methods for assessing measurement validity

Overview

Measurement is familiar from everyday use, such as a person's height or usual travel time from home to workplace. Many measurements already are established, and one needs only to apply them appropriately. However, sometimes it is necessary to modify an existing measurement to improve its fit and performance in a particular situation. Other times, a new measurement device or procedure must be developed for a new concept.

It is essential to understand the full measurement process, from theory-based conceptualization to operationalization of a measurement protocol. Moreover, regardless of whether a measurement already exists or is newly developed, it is essential to be able to assess its reliability and validity.

From Concepts to Data

Measurement is the process of systematically assigning labels and/or numbers to differentiate observations in terms of quality or quantity, across units and/or time. Measurements are empirical indicators of abstract constructs that are not observable directly. For example, although it is not possible to observe directly people's concern about the health effects of smoking cigarettes, it is possible to obtain an indication of their concern by asking them to describe it in their own words, or to rate their concern on a 5-point scale. Although perhaps it is less obvious, the relationship between concepts and indicators applies as well to more familiar measurements. For example, it is not possible to observe temperature directly. Instead, an instrument called a thermometer typically is employed to obtain an indication of temperature.

Figure 8.1 depicts the measurement process. It begins with the **conceptualization** stage, where an abstract construct is defined in theoretical terms. Then, the **operationalization** stage identifies observable *variables* that represent the construct. Finally, the **instrumentation** stage specifies procedures for observing and recording empirical indicators of the variables.

Conceptualization

Constructs are abstract factors that are not observable directly. Examples are social support to get a mammogram and concern about the health effects of smoking cigarettes. Advanced analysis methods, such as structural equation models (SEM), refer to constructs as "latent variables" (Bollen, 1989). The measurement process starts with a **conceptual definition** of a construct derived from a theory or

> **Key Concept**
>
> *A construct is an abstract factor that is not observable directly.*

FIGURE 8.1 ● The Measurement Process

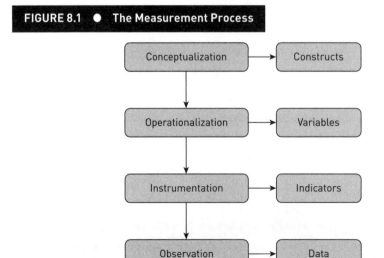

conceptual model (Chapter 1). For example, *perceived susceptibility* is a construct of the Health Belief Model (Janz & Becker, 1984; Rosenstock, Strecher, & Becker, 1988) that describes why individuals do or do not perform health-promotive behaviors. Generally, perceived susceptibility is defined conceptually as individuals' subjective perception of their risk for contracting an adverse health condition. However, to guide a study, such a general definition must be linked to a particular health condition. For example, a study about disparities in mammography screening would specify that perceived susceptibility refers to the risk for getting breast cancer.

Operationalization

An **operational definition** describes how a construct may be observable through collecting information about one or more variables. Operational definitions are based on theory, logic, and prior research. Some constructs are considered to be unidimensional, meaning there is only one facet of their manifestation. The connection between conceptual and operational definitions for such a construct often is direct and easily specified. For example, a person's height is a unidimensional construct for which the following could be applied as both a conceptual and an operational definition: the distance from the bottom of a person's bare feet to the crown of his or her uncovered head. However, many constructs are considered to be multidimensional. For example, a measurement of perceived susceptibility for getting breast cancer might include several risk dimensions, such as

> **Key Concept**
>
> *An operational definition describes how a construct may be observable.*

- overall risk—in lifetime,
- time-conditional risk—within a specific time period, and
- comparative risk—compared to other women of similar age.

Instrumentation

Instrumentation specifies procedures for collecting data about indicators of a study unit's status regarding the variables of interest. In this context, the term *instrument* encompasses a broad spectrum of methods for collecting and recording observations. It is not limited to employing a physical device or to quantitative approaches. For example, instrumentation may include self-administered questionnaires, structured interview questionnaires, unstructured interview guides, focus group moderator guides, nonparticipant observation guides, and records review protocols. Moreover, some variables may be observed through more than one instrumentation approach. For instance, an individual's health status might be measured as a self-assessment and/or a health care provider's clinical assessment. Box 8.1 displays key aspects to consider when developing an instrumentation strategy.

An Example

Table 8.1 presents an example of the measurement process for perceived susceptibility for breast cancer. It starts with a conceptual definition of the construct based on the Health Belief Model. The operational definition postulates three variables representing different dimensions of the construct. Instrumentation specifies that data will be collected using a structured internet questionnaire and presents the question wording and response choices for each indicator.

BOX 8.1: KEY INSTRUMENTATION ASPECTS

- **Mode** (e.g., interview, observation, or records review)
- **Degree of structure** (e.g., structured survey interview questionnaire or unstructured interview guide)
- **Degree of interaction with participants** (e.g., in-person interview vs. online questionnaire)
- **Location** (e.g., clinic or home)
- **Staff** (e.g., professional or volunteer)
- **Timing** (e.g., time of year, day(s) of week, time(s) of day)

TABLE 8.1 Measurement Process for Perceived Susceptibility for Breast Cancer

Conceptual definition: an individual's subjective perception of personal risk for breast cancer			
Operational definition: perceived likelihood of getting breast cancer ...		**Instrumentation: structured internet questionnaire**	
Variable 1	**Overall risk:** in lifetime	Indicator 1	On a scale from 1 to 5, where 1 is *not likely* and 5 is *very likely*, how likely do you think it is that you will get breast cancer in your lifetime?
Variable 2	**Time-conditional risk:** within a specific time period	Indicator 2	On a scale from 1 to 5, where 1 is *not likely* and 5 is *very likely*, how likely do you think it is that you will get breast cancer in the next five years?
Variable 3	**Comparative risk:** compared to other women of similar age	Indicator 3	Compared to other women about your age, would you say the chance that you will get breast cancer is lower, about the same, or higher?

CHECK YOUR UNDERSTANDING 8.1

- Describe each of the following key aspects of the measurement process:
  - Conceptualization
  - Operationalization
  - Instrumentation

Levels of Measurement

The way variables are measured influences the analytic procedures that may be applied to them. Measurements are classified in a series of levels according to the nature and amount of information they capture.

Nominal Level

Nominal-level measurement distinguishes between observations in terms of *kind* or *quality*. Decision rules are developed and applied to group observations judged to be the same, or sufficiently similar, in two or more categories. Nominal measurement does not indicate the quantity of a variable. Therefore, nominal categories may not be interpreted as indicating a hierarchical order among observations or the amount of difference between them. Thus, although the number and percentage of observations in each category may be calculated, mathematical operations and interpretations may not be applied to nominal-level measurements. By their nature, some variables only may be measured at the nominal level. Examples are fresh fruit an individual purchased most recently, marital status, race/ethnicity, and birthplace.

Applying numeric labels to observations does not necessarily indicate differences in quantity. For example, U.S. postal ZIP codes indicate different geographic locations that alternatively could be designated by alphabetic labels. Similarly, although numeric labels may be assigned to nominal categories to facilitate analysis using computer software, such arbitrarily assigned labels do not imply quantity. For example, a list of fruit items individuals purchased recently might be labeled as 1 = *apples*, 2 = *bananas*, and 3 = *oranges*. However, the nature of the information would not differ if numeric labels were assigned as 1 = *oranges*, 2 = *apples*, and 3 = *bananas*.

Strategies

The most simple nominal measurement strategy is **dichotomous classification** according to whether a particular characteristic is present or not. For example, individuals might be classified as HIV-positive or not HIV-positive. Another dichotomous strategy is to classify observations by similarity/difference, grouping together ones that are similar and separating them from ones that are different, such as classifying schools as public or private. **Polychotomous classification** assigns observations to three or more nominal categories. For example, cigarette smoking status may be classified as current smoker, former smoker, or never smoked.

Ordinal Level

Ordinal-level measurement distinguishes between observations in terms of *relative amount*, such as whether one observation contains more, less, or about the same quantity as another. Thus, observations may be placed in hierarchical order, such as from lowest to highest. For example, a woman's risk for breast cancer might be classified as low, medium, or high. Numeric labels may be assigned to ordinal categories to indicate their relative position on a continuum. For example, if breast cancer risk is labeled as 1 = *low*, 2 = *medium*, and 3 = *high*, then a higher value indicates a higher risk. However, mathematical operations may not be applied to numeric labels for ordinal categories because ordinal measurement does not employ standard quantitative units, such as pounds or inches. Differences between ordinal categories indicate *relative* positions on a continuum, but the distances between them are not necessarily consistent across all categories. Thus, if individual A rates her breast cancer risk as high and individual B rates her risk as medium, the measurement does not indicate *how much* higher the perceived risk is for individual A than for individual B.

Moreover, intervals between ordinal-level categories may be perceived differently by different individuals. For example, Table 8.2 displays two individuals' ratings of five fruits using an ordinal scale, where 1 = *do not like* and 10 = *like very much*. They rated each fruit using the same numeric label. That is, they both rated bananas = 1, grapes = 2, and so on.

TABLE 8.2 ● Two Ratings of Five Fruits	
Individual A	**Individual B**
1 Bananas	1 Bananas
	2 Grapes
2 Grapes	3
3	
4	4
	5 Pears
5 Pears	
6	6
7	7
8	8
	9 Oranges
9 Oranges	
10 Apples	10 Apples

Therefore, the apparent differences between their ratings are the same, such as 1 for grapes and bananas, and also 1 for apples and oranges. However, as illustrated in the table, those differences are not necessarily equal. Individual A perceives a greater difference between grapes and bananas than individual B, while individual B perceives a greater difference between apples and oranges.

Ordinal-level measurement is employed extensively because it generally is quick and easy to apply, especially when asking individuals to provide self-reports about attitudes, or behaviors they perform infrequently. Moreover, often it is not possible to measure a variable using standard quantitative units. For instance, there are no standard units to measure how much an individual likes various kinds of fruit. Even when it is possible to employ a standard measurement unit, it may not be reasonable or necessary to do so. For example, suppose individuals are asked to report the time it takes to travel from home to the nearest hospital. Unless they made the trip frequently or recently, they might not be able to provide an accurate response. Furthermore, the analysis plan might not require measurement with a high degree of precision, such as the exact number of minutes. Instead, it might be sufficient and more efficient to measure travel time in terms of ordinal categories, such as less than one hour, about one hour, and more than one hour.

Strategies

Ordinal-level measurement may be performed using several strategies, the most basic of which is *direct comparison*. For example, the relative height of students in a particular classroom might be measured by asking them to stand back-to-back and placing them in order from shortest to tallest. Another strategy is *reference category comparison*, for which several approaches are possible. One is the *usual or typical state*. For example, in a study about nutrition behavior, participants might be asked to describe the portion size of a dinner meal by comparing it with the usual size of their dinner meal as smaller, about the same, or larger. Another type of reference category is *other people*. For example, women might be asked to describe their breast cancer risk compared with other women about their age as lower, about the same, or higher. Still another type of reference category is *other times*, such that participants might be asked to describe their current physical health status compared with the past; for example, compared to one year ago, are they less healthy now, about the same, or more healthy now?

A third strategy classifies observations by assigning them a **rating** along a continuum, which often is used to measure attitudes or beliefs. For example, participants might be asked to rate their experience with their current source of health care overall on a 5-point scale, ranging from 1 = *not satisfied* to 5 = *very satisfied*. A fourth strategy is **ranking** instances of a variable in a hierarchical order. For example, participants in a smoking cessation study might be asked to rank a list of reasons why a smoker might decide to stop smoking from least to most important.

Interval/Ratio Level

Interval-level measurement and ratio-level measurement share the same characteristics, with one exception that rarely is encountered in practice. Interval-/ratio-level measurement uses *standard units*, such as inches or years, to indicate the amount within categories and differences between them. For example, using a standard U.S. ruler, all objects that have the same length, such as 5 inches, have the same measurement outcome of 5 inches. Also, differences between units are equal. For instance, the distance between 2 and 3 inches, 1 inch, is the same as the distance between 3 and 4 inches. Moreover, the numeric labels that designate each measurement outcome have mathematical meaning. Thus, mathematical operations and interpretations may be applied. For example, an object measuring 8 inches in length is 4 inches longer than one that is 4 inches. It also may be stated that an object measuring 8 inches in length is twice as long as one measuring 4 inches.

The only difference between interval- and ratio-level measurement is that the zero point for interval-level measurement is set arbitrarily, while the zero point in ratio-level measurement is absolute. The most common example for illustrating this distinction is temperature measurement systems. The Fahrenheit (F) and Celsius (C) temperature scales are interval-level measurements, but not ratio level. Their zero points are set arbitrarily, according to different principles, and they do not represent the same amount of heat. For instance, 0°C = 32°F, and both indicate the point at which water freezes. Moreover, neither scale has an absolute zero point that represents the absence of heat. Thus, negative values are possible with both scales. In contrast, the Kelvin (K) temperature scale is a ratio-level measurement because its zero point represents the absence of heat, defined as the temperature at which thermal motion ceases. In the absence of an absolute zero point, it is not possible to compute ratios between measurements. For example, although a temperature of 90°F is twice as high above 0°F as is 45°F, 90°F may not be interpreted as being twice as warm as 45°F because temperatures below 0°F are possible.

However, virtually all interval-level measurements also are ratio measurements. The example of temperature scales with arbitrary zero points is unique. Examples of common interval-/ratio-level measurements are weight, height, age, annual income, and number of physician visits during the past 12 months. Although such measurements have absolute zero points, in practice it is not possible to observe a zero value for some interval/ratio measurements. Although it is possible for a person's annual income or number of physician visits to be zero, it is not possible for a person's weight, height, or age to be zero.

Strategies

There are two interval-/ratio-level measurement strategies, both of which are familiar from everyday practice. One strategy employs an instrument with a standard metric, such as a ruler (inches or centimeters), weight scale (pounds or kilograms), or calendar (days and months). It often is possible to make such measurements with various degrees of precision. For example, distance may be measured in terms of inches, feet, yards, or miles; time may be measured in terms of seconds, minutes, hours, days, weeks, months, or years. Therefore, it is essential to decide the degree of precision that is appropriate for the purpose of a particular study. For instance, most often it is sufficient to measure an adult's age in years, rather than days, or years plus days. However, it would be appropriate to measure the age of a newborn in weeks and/or days. An important distinction is that measurement *precision* is not the same as measurement *accuracy*. **Measurement precision** is the degree of detail at which a measurement is made. **Measurement accuracy** is the degree to which a measurement is free of error or bias.

The second strategy is counting. Examples of a count variable are the number of children age 17 or younger living in a household, and the number of visits to a health care provider an individual made during the past 12 months. Count measurements employ a counting rule that specifies what to count and how to count it. Sometimes a rule is simple, such as the number of students currently enrolled in the sixth grade at a particular school. Other times, a rule might be complex, such as when asking participants to report the number of alcoholic beverage drinks they consumed during a particular time period. That measurement requires specifying what is meant by both an alcoholic beverage and a drink so participants will know what drinks to count. For example, to ask participants to report the number of drinks of alcohol they consumed during the past 30 days, the Behavioral Risk Factor Surveillance System (Centers for Disease Control and Prevention, 2016) questionnaire defines what counts as an *alcoholic beverage* as "beer, wine, a malt beverage or liquor" and defines *one drink* as "equivalent to a 12-ounce beer, a 5-ounce glass of wine, or a drink with one shot of liquor."

Comparative Summary

Table 8.3 presents a comparative summary of levels of measurement, illustrating their hierarchical relationship from the nominal through interval/ratio levels. Each successive level includes all the information from the preceding level(s) plus additional information that distinguishes more effectively between observations and enables applying more powerful analytical methods.

For convenience of interpretation and presentation, sometimes it is helpful to transform a measurement from a higher level to a lower one. Most often, that is done by transforming an interval-/ratio-level measurement to the ordinal level by grouping measurements into more broad categories. For example, annual household income might be grouped into intervals such as $40,000 or less, $40,001–$80,000, $80,001–$120,000, $120,001–$200,000, and more than $200,000. However, such transformations sacrifice precision and analytic power.

It is not possible to transform a measurement from a lower level to a higher one. For instance, suppose undergraduate college students are asked to indicate on a self-administered questionnaire whether their class status is freshman, sophomore, junior, or senior. Class

TABLE 8.3 ● Comparative Summary of Levels of Measurement

Feature	Nominal	Ordinal	Interval	Ratio
Differences in kind/quality	Yes	Yes	Yes	Yes
Relative amount		Yes	Yes	Yes
Amount within and between categories			Yes	Yes
Absolute zero point				Yes

status cannot be transformed to the interval/ratio level, such as the exact number of credit hours each student has completed. Therefore, in general, the best practice is to measure a variable at the highest level possible and reasonable, which provides the option to transform measurements to a lower level as appropriate. For example, undergraduate college students might be asked to report the number of credit hours they have completed, which may be analyzed in terms of credit hours completed or transformed into the four traditional ordinal categories.

CHECK YOUR UNDERSTANDING 8.2

- Describe the following three levels of measurement:
  - Nominal
  - Ordinal
  - Interval/ratio
- Explain how the three levels of measurement are related to each other.

Measurement Theory

The predominant theoretical measurement model, called **classical test theory (CTT)**, assumes there is a **true value** for every observation. If a measurement is perfectly accurate, then the **observed value** will equal the true value; observed values will differ only owing to variation in true values across observation units and/or time. However, it is not realistic to expect any measurement to be perfect. The goal of the measurement process is to obtain measurements that are as error-free as possible to reduce the chance of drawing incorrect conclusions. Although errors may occur at any level of measurement, for simplicity of presentation the interval/ratio level is assumed. The following equation represents the relationship between an observed value, a true value, and two basic types of measurement error, systematic error and random error (Zeller & Carmines, 1980):

$$Observed\ Value = True\ Value + Systematic\ Error + Random\ Error$$

Random Error

Random error is an *unsystematic* deviation of an observed value from its true value. Using a concept from everyday experience, random errors are inadvertent "mistakes" that occur by chance; thus there is no pattern to them. For example, when completing a self-administered questionnaire, random errors might occur if nearby activities distract participants from focusing on the questions and response choices, they are fatigued and not able to concentrate, or they are not motivated to read questions and record responses carefully. Random errors also might be introduced by observers who collect measurements, such as interviewers being fatigued or careless when asking questions and recording responses. Random errors are not correlated with the variable being measured. That is, they are just as likely to occur for one variable as for another one. Also, random errors are not correlated with other variables. For example, the accuracy of participants' report about the number of times they saw a health care provider during the last 12 months will not vary according to their age, such that owing to differences in recall ability older participants are more likely than younger ones to underreport that information.

The true and observed values of a measurement vary across observation units. For example, the number of times participants saw a health care provider during the last 12 months is likely to vary across individuals. Figure 8.2 depicts random error distributions for two sets of observed values (O) relative to their true values (TV). The location of each observed value indicates the amount and direction of its deviation from its own true value. The true value along the horizontal axis in Figure 8.2 is a *relative* reference point that may be different for each individual that is observed. It is *not* necessarily the same value for every individual.

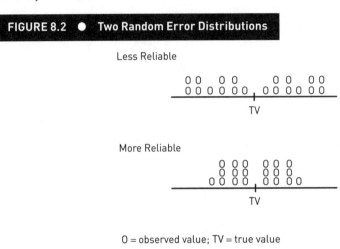

FIGURE 8.2 • Two Random Error Distributions

O = observed value; TV = true value

Owing to random error, some observed values are lower than the true value, while others are higher. Over the course of *many* observations, there will be an equal number of observed values lower (negative) and higher (positive) than the true value. Overall, the sum of random errors will equal zero. Because random errors are unsystematic and cancel each other over repeated measurements, they do not cause measurement bias, such that observed values consistently are lower or higher than the true value. However, that does not mean the observed value for any *individual* observation is error-free.

Measurement Reliability

Measurement reliability is the extent to which a measurement is free of random error and thus obtains consistent outcomes when the true value is constant. If only the absolute values (ignoring negatives and positives) of random errors are considered, the closer observed values are to their true value *overall*, the less total random error and the more reliable the measurement. Accordingly, the measurement depicted in the second distribution in Figure 8.2 is more reliable than the one in the first distribution.

Systematic Error

Systematic error is a consistent deviation of an observed value from its true value that results in **measurement bias**, whereby the observed value always is lower or higher than its true value. For example, systematic errors might occur owing to *social desirability bias*, whereby interview participants respond in ways they expect are socially acceptable. Accordingly, they might underreport performing a negative behavior, such as drinking an alcoholic beverage to the point of being intoxicated. Conversely, they might overreport performing a positive behavior, such as engaging in physical activity for exercise. Figure 8.3 depicts systematic error distributions for two sets of observed values that have the same degree of random error, and therefore are similarly reliable. However, owing to systematic error, the sum of the measurement errors in both distributions will not equal zero. The observed values in the first distribution are negatively biased, consistently underestimating their true values; those in the second distribution are positively biased, consistently overestimating their true values. The second distribution is more biased than the first one because, on average, the distances between its observed and true values are greater.

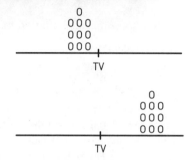

FIGURE 8.3 • Two Systematic Error Distributions

O = observed value; TV = true value

Measurement Validity

Measurement validity is the extent to which a measurement accurately measures the construct it is intended to measure. As illustrated in Figure 8.4, a valid measurement is free of both random and systematic error. Thus, all observed values equal their true values. Unfortunately, virtually all measurements have some degree of both random and systematic error. The general measurement goal is to minimize them to the extent it is feasible.

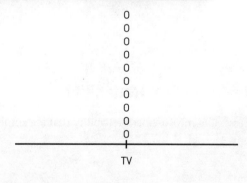

FIGURE 8.4 • Observed Values for a Valid Measurement

O = observed value; TV = true value

TABLE 8.4 ● Measurement Error, Reliability, and Validity

Aspect	Random Error	Systematic Error
Reliability	Yes	No
Validity	Yes	Yes

The Relationship Between Reliability and Validity

Table 8.4 summarizes the relationship between random and systematic measurement error, and measurement reliability and validity. Reliability is influenced *only* by random error, while validity is influenced by *both* random and systematic error. Thus,

- reliability is a necessary but not sufficient condition for validity, and
- a valid measurement also is reliable.

Measurement reliability is influenced most directly by instrumentation and the observation protocol. Validity is influenced directly by all aspects of the measurement process, from conceptualization through observation.

Evidence supporting a measurement's reliability indicates that it also *might* be valid, but it does not provide assurance of validity. Assessing validity requires assessing systematic error *and* random error. As illustrated in Figure 8.5, a reliable measurement might not be valid. However, as illustrated in Figure 8.4, a valid measurement also is reliable because it is relatively free of random error as well as systematic error.

Virtually all measurements have some degree of both random and systematic error. Figure 8.6 depicts examples of measurement error distributions for two sets of observed values. On average, the measurements have the same amount of systematic error in the sense that their mean values are the same distance below their true values. However, owing to less random error, the measurement in the second distribution is more reliable than the measurement in the first. Therefore, the second measurement also is more valid.

> **CHECK YOUR UNDERSTANDING 8.3**
>
> - Describe the following measurement theory concepts and explain how they are related to each other.
>   - Random error
>   - Systematic error
>   - Reliability
>   - Validity

Assessing Measurement Reliability

Three methods for assessing measurement reliability that are employed frequently are

- test–retest,
- interrater, and
- parallel forms.

FIGURE 8.5 ● **Observed Values for a Reliable but Not Valid Measurement**

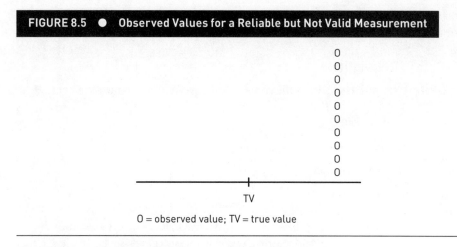

FIGURE 8.6 ● **Two Measurement Error Distributions**

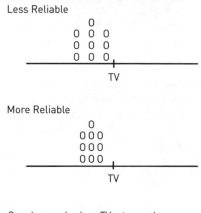

As illustrated in Figure 8.5, reliability may be high even when there is substantial systematic error. Whereas reliability is a function only of random error, each reliability method assumes that any systematic error is constant, although it is not necessarily zero. Therefore, any measurement inconsistency should be attributable to random error. Each method assesses only one potential source of random error. Therefore, the best practice is to employ more than one reliability assessment method whenever feasible.

Measurement reliability is assessed on a continuum, where reliability coefficients range from 0 to 1.00, indicating no reliability to perfect reliability, respectively. Although some sources present guidelines for interpreting reliability assessment results, there are no generally accepted standards for deciding whether reliability is acceptable (McDowell & Newell, 1996). Reliability should be considered within the context in which a measurement will be applied (Morera & Stokes, 2016). An important factor to take into consideration is the current state of the art regarding measuring a particular construct. When employing a new measurement, a lower degree of reliability might be acceptable as indicating a measurement has potential to be refined in future studies. When using a well-established measurement, reliability should be comparable to that reported in other studies in which it was used. Also, a study's potential importance should be considered. The greater the potential contribution to knowledge, theory, and/or practice, the higher should be the reliability of key measurements.

Test–Retest Reliability

Test–retest reliability assesses the correlation between repeated measurements of

- the *same* individual(s),
- under the *same* conditions,
- by the *same* observer, and
- using the *same* procedure.

If the true value does not change between test and retest measurements, then the same or a very similar result should be obtained when a reliable measurement is repeated. The terms *test* and *retest* are derived from educational testing. However, in this context, they may refer to any type of measurement. Test–retest reliability is assessed by computing the Kappa coefficient (described in the "Interrater Reliability" section) or the McNemar test for nominal-level measurement, Spearman's rank-order coefficient (rho, ρ) for ordinal-level measurement, or Pearson's product moment correlation coefficient (r) for interval-/ratio-level measurement.

Limitations

The main challenge to interpreting test–retest reliability is whether the true value, which is not known, is the same at the test and retest measurement. If the true value changes, a low test–retest correlation might indicate one of two possible interpretations:

- The measurement is not reliable.
- The measurement is reliable, and it detected the true value's change.

The likelihood of the true value changing varies with the nature of the construct being measured and the length of the test–retest interval. Test–retest reliability may be employed with greater confidence when measuring a construct that is not likely to change during the test–retest interval. Examples are measuring a person's body weight twice within a few minutes and extracting patient demographic information from the same record. Test–retest reliability is less trustworthy when measuring constructs such as an individual's knowledge, attitude, or behavior that may change even over a brief interval, and is increasingly likely to change as the test–retest interval is lengthened.

Test–retest change in a true value might be caused by history or maturation, similar to how those factors may threaten internal validity for a pretest–posttest research design (Chapter 5). The chance for a true value change may be minimized by specifying as brief a test–retest interval as is feasible. However, when measuring factors such as knowledge, attitudes, or behaviors, the shorter the interval, the greater the chance that participants might recall and repeat their initial performance at the retest. That would inflate a measurement's apparent reliability. Thus, depending on the nature of the construct being measured, specifying a test–retest interval may involve a compromise between being too short and being too long. Another potential threat to interpreting test–retest reliability is the test might cause the true value to change similar to the way a testing threat to internal validity might cause a change in the dependent variable among a control group (Chapter 5). For example, asking participants about their knowledge regarding signs of a heart attack might motivate them to seek information to improve their knowledge during the test–retest interval.

It may not be feasible to perform test–retest reliability assessment if the additional financial and time resources are not available to repeat a measurement. In such situations, consideration should be given to selecting a random subsample of observation units with which the test–retest method may be employed. Another situation in which test–retest may not be feasible is when a measurement is applied to a onetime event for which an audio–video recording is not available. An example of such a situation is conducting in-person interviews with anonymous injecting drug users. Finally, participants might not be willing to repeat a measurement activity after a relatively brief interval, such as responding to the same questions in an interview or self-administered questionnaire.

Interrater Reliability

Interrater reliability (also called **"interobserver"** or **"intercoder" reliability**) assesses agreement between independent *concurrent* observations of the same individual(s) using the same procedure. Independent measurement by more than one observer (typically two) at the same time ensures that the true value has not changed. Therefore, if a measurement is reliable, then each observer will obtain the same or a very similar result. Concurrent measurement does not necessarily mean simultaneous observation. Some data sources are fixed in time, such as patient or student records, photographs, videos, and interview transcripts. Nevertheless, the timing of independent observations from such sources should be as close as possible to eliminate potential influences from extraneous factors. Interrater reliability is assessed by computing the Kappa coefficient for nominal-level measurement, Spearman's rank-order coefficient (rho, ρ) for ordinal-level measurement, or Pearson's product moment correlation coefficient (r) for interval-/ratio-level measurement.

Kappa coefficient

The most frequent application of interrater reliability is to assess the consistency of coding data from records and interview/focus group transcripts into nominal-level categories. The procedure for computing the **Kappa coefficient**, also called "Cohen's Kappa" (Cohen, 1960), assumes two independent observers assign each observation to one of two mutually exclusive categories. A common approach is to assess whether a characteristic is present or absent, such as whether a clinic record indicates a patient has been diagnosed with breast cancer, or whether an interview transcript includes a participant mentioning gang activity as a concern about raising children in his or her community.

Although it might appear reasonable to assess interrater reliability by computing the percent of agreement between observers, that approach is misleading because some agreement may occur by chance. Table 8.5 depicts outcomes for 200 observations for which each of two independent observers assigned each observation to one of two categories randomly.

TABLE 8.5 ● Percent of Agreement by Chance

Observer A	Observer B		
	Absent	Present	Total
Absent	50	50	100
Present	50	50	100
Total	100	100	200

Percent of agreement: [(50 + 50)/200] × 100 = 50%

For example, they might have tossed a coin to determine which category to assign each observation. Common sense would suggest that is not a reliable measurement procedure. However, as indicated by the highlighted cells, on average, two independent observers will agree 50% [(50 + 50)/200] of the time by chance.

Kappa adjusts for chance agreements by computing the ratio of the proportion of agreements above and beyond what may be attributable to chance $(P_o - P_e)$ and the proportion of agreements that are not attributable to chance $(1 - P_e)$. Thus, the formula for computing Kappa is $\kappa = (P_o - P_e)/(1 - P_e)$, where P_o is the proportion of *observed* agreements and P_e is the proportion of agreements *expected* by chance. Kappa's values range from 0, indicating no agreement other than what is possible by chance, to 1.00, indicating complete agreement among observers. Notably, if all agreement is owing to chance, then Kappa will be 0, whereas the unadjusted percent of agreement will be 50%, or .50 in decimals.

In practice, it is not expected that observers will assign all observations randomly as in Table 8.5. Instead, the proportion of chance agreements depends on the marginal distributions of observers' assignments. Table 8.6 depicts an example where the observed proportion of agreements (P_o) is .90 [(70 + 110)/200]. The expected proportion of agreements is computed using a method that might be familiar from computing the chi-square statistic, where the value expected by chance in any cell of a cross-classification table is the cell's (row total × column total)/grand total. For Table 8.6, the expected agreements by chance are $(P_e) = [(75 \times 85)/200] + [(125 \times 115)/200] + (32 + 72)/200 = 104/200 = .52$. Thus, $\kappa = (.90 - .52)/(1 - .52) = .79$.

TABLE 8.6 ● Kappa Computation

Observer A	Observer B		
	Absent	Present	Total
Absent	70	5	75
Present	15	110	125
Total	85	115	200

$P_o = [(70 + 110)/200] = .90$

$P_e = [(75 \times 85)/200] + [(125 \times 115)/200] = .52$

$\kappa = (.90 - .52)/(1 - .52) = .79$

Limitations

Employing more than one observer requires additional financial and time resources that might not be available. In such situations, consideration should be given to selecting a random subsample of observation units for which the interrater reliability method may be applied.

Parallel Forms Reliability

Parallel forms reliability (also called **alternate forms reliability**) assesses the correlation between equivalent, concurrent measurements of the same construct, with the same individual(s). Concurrent measurement ensures that the true value has not changed. Therefore, if *both* measurements are reliable, then they will obtain the same or a very similar result. Also, as for interrater reliability, concurrent measurement does not necessarily mean simultaneous observation. However, the timing of independent observations should be as close as possible to eliminate potential influences from extraneous factors. Parallel forms reliability is used most often to assess the reliability of multiple-item measures of knowledge, attitude, or behavior. For example, to assess the reliability of an assessment of patients' knowledge about cancer risk factors, they might be asked to respond to two sets of the same number of questions.

Limitations

Administering parallel form requires additional financial and time resources. A measurement may appear to be unreliable if the alternate form is not reliable. Thus, their correlation appropriately would be low. Moreover, parallel forms reliability cannot be employed if an equivalent measure is not available. In particular, often there is only one form of a **multiple-item scale** or test. The following sections present strategies for addressing such situations. Also, the strategies enable estimating reliability without requiring additional financial and time resources, and without increasing the participation burden. A key assumption of the strategies is that a multiple-item measure is unidimensional, such that each item measures the same construct.

Split-half reliability

Split-half reliability is the correlation between parallel forms created by randomly dividing a multiple-item measure, such as a test or scale, into halves (Chapter 7). Although sometimes it is suggested that a multiple-item measure may be divided conveniently by selecting alternate items, such as an odd–even split, or by a first-half/second-half split, those strategies are not random. For example, if every other item is "true" or "false," then selecting alternate items is likely to result in a nonequivalent split. If items increase in difficulty, then a first-half/second-half split will divide the least and most difficult items.

However, the reliability of a multiple-item measure is proportional to the number of items (Streiner & Norman, 1995). Therefore, even with a random split, dividing a measure reduces the reliability of each half, which underestimates the full measure's reliability. The reliability of the full measure (r), adjusted for the full number of items, may be estimated by the Spearman-Brown prophesy formula: $r = 2r_{AB}/1 + r_{AB}$, where r_{AB} is the correlation between Form A and Form B after a random split. For example, if the observed correlation (r_{AB}) is .70, the estimated reliability of the full measure is .82.

Split-half reliability may be used to assess the reliability of alternate forms when dividing a multiple-item measure to address a potential testing threat to internal validity, where one half (Form A) is administered at the pretest and the other half (Form B) is administered at the posttest. A stronger version of that method is to randomly assign participants to receive Form A or B at the pretest and receive the other form at the posttest. Thus, each form would be administered to a random half of the participants at pretest and posttest. A limitation of split-half reliability is it assesses only one random split out of all possible random splits. Thus, the reliability coefficient may vary depending on which random split is assessed.

Cronbach's coefficient alpha

Cronbach's coefficient alpha is the most frequently used measure of reliability for multiple-item measures. There are many possible random splits of a multiple-item measure. For example, there are 126 possible random splits for 10 items, 92,378 for 20 items, and 77,558,760 for 30 items. Although it is not feasible to create and assess so many random splits in practice, Cronbach's coefficient alpha estimates the average split-half correlation for all possible random splits of items. The formula is

$$\alpha = \frac{k}{k-1}\left[1 - \left(\frac{\sum_{1}^{k} s_i^2}{s_T^2}\right)\right]$$

where k is the total number of items, s_i^2 is the variance of each item, and s_T^2 is the variance of the total multiple-item measure. An alternate formula for coefficient alpha is

$$\alpha = \frac{k\bar{r}}{1 + (k-1)\bar{r}}$$

where $\bar{r}$ is the mean of the interitem correlations, that is, the arithmetic average of each item correlated with each other item. Although the formulas may appear somewhat daunting, the information to compute coefficient alpha typically is readily available from most analysis software. Moreover, it may be computed by software, such as the reliability procedure in IBM SPSS Statistics.

Sometimes it is suggested that coefficient alpha should be applied only to items that are continuous measures. This perspective also recommends assessing the reliability of dichotomous measures, such as yes/no items, by the Kuder–Richardson Formula 20, which typically is referred to as KR-20. However, that is not necessary because coefficient alpha actually is an extension of KR-20 to accommodate continuous measures. If coefficient alpha is computed for dichotomous items, the result will be identical to KR-20 (Zeller & Carmines, 1980).

Limitations. Coefficient alpha typically is interpreted as an indicator of the "internal consistency" of a multiple-item measure. However, that interpretation rests on the assumption that a composite measure is unidimensional (Morera & Stokes, 2016). That is, if the items measure the same construct, then they should be highly correlated with each other. However, sometimes a construct is relatively heterogeneous in nature. For example, a multiple-item measure of knowledge about HIV risk factors or a measure of physical activity will comprise items that are not necessarily correlated with each other. Knowledge about one HIV risk factor may be independent of knowledge about another one. Performing one physical activity may be independent of performing another one. Therefore, assessing the reliability of such measures using coefficient alpha should be done with caution, and consideration should be given to employing another reliability method in addition to or instead of coefficient alpha.

When a composite measure comprises more than one dimension, coefficient alpha should be computed separately for the items that measure each dimension. For example, the Health Belief Model construct of perceived threat comprises two dimensions, perceived susceptibility and perceived seriousness/severity. If multiple items are used to measure those two dimensions, then their reliability should be assessed separately.

CHECK YOUR UNDERSTANDING 8.4

- Describe the following methods for assessing a measurement's reliability.
    - Test–retest
    - Interrater
    - Parallel forms

Assessing Measurement Validity

The ultimate measurement goal is to obtain a valid measurement of a construct. Whereas reliability is influenced only by random error, validity is influenced by *both* random and systematic error. Thus, while a reliable measurement is not necessarily valid, a valid measurement is also reliable, as illustrated in Figure 8.4. Ideally, validity assessment would compare measurement outcomes with a construct's true values. However, in measurement theory, true values, especially for abstract constructs such as health knowledge and beliefs, are not known. Moreover, there are no "standard" validity coefficients. Instead, validity is assessed in terms of whether a measurement is acceptable for its intended application.

> **Key Concept**
>
> *A valid measurement is also reliable.*

There are two basic validity assessment approaches:

- **Judgment-based validity** assesses whether a measurement appears to measure the construct it is intended to measure.

- **Performance-based validity** compares empirical outcomes for a measurement with those of other measures with which it is or is not expected to be correlated.

The most frequently employed methods for assessing measurement validity are summarized in Table 8.7. Measurement validity may vary with factors such as a study's time, place, population characteristics, and data collection mode. Therefore, the best practice is to employ as many validity assessment methods, in as many different contexts, as are feasible.

In general, validity assessment of a new measurement proceeds from the top through the bottom of Table 8.7. When employing an existing measurement, although it is appropriate to consider evidence from previous studies, the validity of key measurements should be assessed within each study's specific context. Assuming an existing measurement has been previously "validated" may result in misinterpreting a study's findings. Moreover, sometimes it is necessary to modify an existing measurement to make it appropriate for a particular context. For example, it might be translated into another language, or the protocol might be changed depending on participants' characteristics (e.g., age, gender, race/ethnicity, or education). It is essential to assess the impact of such modifications on a measurement's validity.

Judgment-Based Validity

Face validity

Face validity is the most basic measurement validation method, whereby a measurement is assessed in terms of whether it appears to represent a particular construct. The fundamental question addressed by face validity is "Does it make sense to measure this construct this way?" Unfortunately, face validity tends to be overlooked because it is so basic and subjective. There is no formal method for assessing the degree of face validity a measurement demonstrates. As it is a subjective assessment, there may be disagreements about a measurement's face validity, which are especially likely to arise regarding measures of abstract constructs. Nevertheless, without face validity, it is not logical to assess measurement validity by any other method. Table 8.8 presents three examples of face validity.

TABLE 8.7 ● Measurement Validity Assessment Methods

Approach	Method	Description
Judgment-Based	Face Validity	A measurement appears to represent a particular construct.
	Content Validity	A measurement appears to represent a construct's content domain.
Performance-Based	Concurrent Criterion Validity	A measurement agrees with a criterion measurement of the same construct at the same time.
	Predictive Criterion Validity	A measurement agrees with a future measurement with which it is expected to be correlated.
	Convergent Validity	Measures of the same construct correlate with each other.
	Discriminant Validity	Measures of different constructs are not correlated or are weakly correlated.
	Construct Validity	Relationships with measurements of other constructs are consistent with theoretical expectations.

TABLE 8.8 ● Face Validity Examples

Construct	Measurement
Body weight	Mechanical scale
Perceived health status	Self-report using an ordinal scale
Use of health services	Review of clinic records

Three face validity strategies, which typically are employed in the following order, are

- theoretical guidance about the nature of the construct,
- logic and common sense, and
- input from independent experts.

First, theoretical guidance should be sought about the nature of the construct to be measured. In particular, it is important to determine if it is unidimensional or multidimensional. For example, a physiological construct such as body weight appears to be unidimensional, whereas abstract concepts, such as social support, typically appear to be multidimensional (perceived sources of support, support actually received, type of support, etc.).

Second, logic and common sense provide insight into whether a measurement is reasonable or feasible, or whether one measurement appears to be more or less valid than another measurement of the same construct. For example, although it is possible to measure height by placing individuals back-to-back and observing who is taller than whom, it appears more precise and efficient to employ a device called a ruler, which is marked in standard units. Finally, input may be solicited from independent experts who have no vested interest in a particular study and have relevant theoretical and/or practical expertise.

Content validity

Content validity assesses whether a measurement appears to represent a construct's content domain. Typically, content validity methods are employed to assess a multiple-item measurement, such as a series of questions asking patients to rate their satisfaction with their usual source of health care. Figure 8.7 presents two examples of content validity for the same construct. The large circles represent the construct's content domain; the small circles represent three items, such as ratings of different aspects of patient satisfaction. The shaded area within a small circle represents part of the construct's content that the item covers. The unshaded area within a small circle and outside a large circle represents aspects of the item that are not relevant to the construct. The unshaded area within a large circle represents the part of the construct's content the three items do not cover.

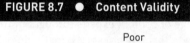

FIGURE 8.7 ● Content Validity

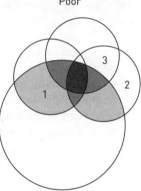
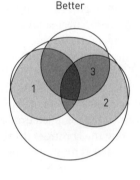

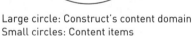

Large circle: Construct's content domain
Small circles: Content items

Content validity is poor in the first example, where the three items cover only a small portion of the construct's content domain. Moreover, while it is expected and desirable that items in a multiple-item measurement such as a patient satisfaction scale will be correlated with each other, the overlap among the items is substantial. Thus, each item contributes little additional information about the construct beyond using any one of them alone. Indeed, the item represented by circle 3 does not contribute any additional information because its content is completely redundant with the two other items. Content validity is better in the second example, where the three items cover most of the construct's content domain. While there is some overlap among them, each item contributes a substantial amount of additional information about the construct.

The general content validity process and strategies are

- identify the nature and scope of the construct,
- develop an initial content list that is as comprehensive as possible, and
- trim the initial content list to include items that are most relevant and feasible to administer.

Although content validity assessment involves a more systematic process than assessing face validity, it still is a judgment-based approach to measurement validity. Thus, there may be disagreements about a construct's scope of content as well as whether a measurement adequately covers its content.

First, the nature and scope of the construct must be identified. Typically, this involves seeking theoretical guidance, examining existing measures of related constructs, and brainstorming with content experts who have relevant theoretical and/or practical expertise. Second, an initial list of the construct's content that is as comprehensive as possible is developed. Sometimes the content may be organized within subdomains. For example, the most recent revision of the Patient Satisfaction Questionnaire (PSQ-III) (RAND Health, n.d.) includes seven subscales and 50 items that measure global satisfaction with medical care plus satisfaction with six specific aspects of care: technical quality, interpersonal manner, communication, financial aspects of care, time spent with doctor, and accessibility of care.

Although an initial content list should be as comprehensive as possible, it often is not feasible to administer a measurement that includes 100% of a construct's content. In such situations, the measurement goal is to include a representative (nonrandom) sample of a construct's content universe. Therefore, the content may be trimmed to include items that content and methodological experts deem to be most relevant and feasible.

The best practice is to seek input from a broad range of content experts throughout the content validity process. Content experts may include theoretical experts, methodological experts, researchers studying the same or related constructs, practitioners, and target population members. Expert input may be obtained by individual interviews, focus groups, or panel discussions. In particular, an often used strategy called a Delphi panel (Hsu & Sandford, 2007; Thangaratinam & Redman, 2005) is useful, whereby content experts participate in an iterative process that typically comprises three rounds. In the first round, they independently nominate potential content items. In the second round, they review an initial content list compiled from their nominations and rate each content item's relevance for measuring the construct. In the final round, they review a list of items compiled from those they rated as most relevant and confirm including those items.

Performance-Based Validity

Concurrent criterion validity

Concurrent criterion validity assesses agreement with another measurement of the same construct, the *criterion*, at the same time. The criterion measurement, sometimes called the "gold standard," is generally regarded as providing results as close as possible to a construct's true value. For example, patients' self-reported body weight may be compared with their clinically measured weight as the criterion. In most situations, the reason for employing this method is to assess a more feasible alternative to the criterion measurement, which may be expensive, invasive, or time-consuming, or require special equipment and expertise. For instance, the validity of a patient's self-report about cigarette smoking may be assessed by comparing it with a biomarker criterion (Rebagliato, 2002; Vartiainen, Seppälä, Lillsunde, & Puska, 2002). When resources are not sufficient to assess concurrent criterion validity for all observation units, consideration should be given to assessing a random subsample.

Selecting a criterion measurement is a critical aspect of concurrent criterion validity. If the criterion does not adequately represent a construct's true value, then an incorrect conclusion about measurement validity may result. Unfortunately, a criterion is not available for most abstract constructs, such as social support, perceived barriers to getting a mammogram, or intention to engage in physical activity for exercise. When measuring such constructs, a common application of concurrent criterion validity is to assess a shortened version of an existing long version of a multiple-item scale to reduce administration cost, time, and burden for staff and/or participants. For example, Marshall and Hays (1994) employed that approach to develop a short form (PSQ-18) of the PSQ-III (RAND Health, n.d.), to reduce the number of items from 50 to 18. The validity of a short version of a longer instrument may be assessed by administering the two versions independently to randomly selected subgroups of the same population. If a short version appropriately represents the original long version, there should not be a statistically significant difference (Chapter 15) between their results.

Predictive criterion validity

Predictive criterion validity assesses agreement with a future measurement with which a measurement is expected to be correlated. For example, if a self-report of intention to stop smoking cigarettes within the next six months is valid, then it may be expected that smokers who report a strong intention will be more likely than others to have stopped smoking six months later. As for concurrent criterion validity, selecting a criterion measurement is a critical aspect of predictive criterion validity. If the criterion is not a valid measure of a construct that is correlated with the measurement being assessed, then an incorrect conclusion about validity may result. For example, even if records about purchasing an automobile during the next six months are valid, they would not be an appropriate predictive validity criterion if they are not correlated with intention to stop smoking cigarettes.

Convergent and discriminant validity

Convergent and discriminant validity are used to assess items in multiple-item measurements.

- **Convergent validity** assesses whether measures of the same construct are correlated with each other.
- **Discriminant validity** assesses whether measures of different constructs are *not* correlated or are weakly correlated.

Convergent validity is based on the concept that items intended to measure the *same* construct are expected to be correlated with each other. That is, the items should *converge* on the construct they are intended to measure. Discriminant validity is based on the concept that items intended to measure *different* constructs are expected not to be correlated with each other. Thus, a *divergence* should be observable among them.

Figure 8.8 depicts convergent and discriminant validity for two Health Belief Model constructs, perceived susceptibility to breast cancer and perceived seriousness of breast cancer (Janz & Becker, 1984; Rosenstock, Strecher, & Becker, 1988). Measurement items are linked to their respective constructs by straight, single-headed arrows, which indicate the items are functions of the constructs. A two-headed, curved arrow between items indicates they are correlated. Both sets of items demonstrate convergent validity. The perceived susceptibility items are correlated with each other, as are the perceived seriousness items. They demonstrate discriminant validity by not being correlated with items intended to measure the other construct.

Convergent validity does not require high correlation levels, such as .70 or higher. From a content validity perspective, high correlations indicate redundancy. Instead, moderate correlations, such as between .20 and .50, typically are considered to indicate convergence while each item contributes some unique information about the construct. Moreover, interitem correlations may be positive or negative. For example, a negative correlation would exist if participants report they believe (correctly) a woman is more likely to get breast

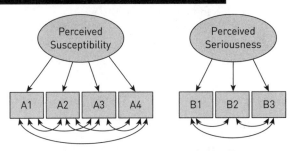

FIGURE 8.8 • Convergent and Discriminant Validity

cancer if she has a family history of breast cancer and is less likely to get breast cancer if she exercises four or more hours a week (National Cancer Institute, 2018).

There are two critical aspects to selecting a discriminant construct. First, its measurement must be valid. Second, it must be relevant to the target construct. For example, it is relevant to assess discrimination between items intended to measure physical health and mental health. An artificially high degree of discriminant validity may be observed by selecting a discriminant construct that is not relevant to the target construct. For example, demonstrating that items measuring perceived susceptibility to breast cancer are not correlated with items measuring beliefs about factors contributing to teenage pregnancy would not be convincing evidence of discriminant validity. It would be more convincing to demonstrate discrimination between items measuring perceived susceptibility to breast cancer and items measuring perceived severity of breast cancer.

In the interest of simplifying the presentation, Figure 8.8 does not display potential correlations between items measuring susceptibility and severity. However, the Health Belief Model treats those constructs as subdomains of perceived threat: The higher the perceived susceptibility and the higher the perceived severity, the higher the perceived threat. Therefore, it is likely that items measuring susceptibility and severity will be correlated to some degree. For example, women with a female blood relative who was diagnosed with breast cancer may be more likely to believe they are susceptible to getting breast cancer and that breast cancer is a serious disease. Nevertheless, valid items measuring susceptibility and severity are expected to be correlated more strongly with other items measuring the same construct (convergent validity) than with items measuring the other construct (discriminant validity).

Construct validity

Construct validity assesses whether a measurement relates to measurements of other constructs in a way that is consistent with theoretical expectations. Accordingly, a valid measurement should be correlated with measurements of certain other constructs, and it should *not* be correlated with measurements of certain other constructs. For example, as depicted in Figure 8.9, according to the Health Belief Model, the more a woman perceives she is susceptible to breast cancer and the fewer her perceived barriers to getting a mammogram, the more likely she is to get a mammogram. Thus, a valid measurement of perceived susceptibility should be related to the likelihood of getting a mammogram. Also, it should not be related to perceived barriers because neither construct causes the other, nor are they dependent variables of a common cause (Chapter 3).

Construct validity is assessed after data are collected. The strongest evidence is derived from a consistent pattern of relationships found by independent researchers, in multiple studies, in diverse settings, with diverse populations, and across a substantial period of

FIGURE 8.9 ● Construct Validity for Perceived Susceptibility to Breast Cancer

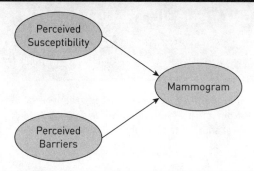

time (Zeller & Carmines, 1980). The main analytic construct validity methods are multiple regression and structural equation models. When appropriate, known groups analysis (also called "extreme groups" or "discriminant groups") assesses a measurement's ability to distinguish between participants with different characteristics. For example, in theory, women with a family history of breast cancer should score higher on perceived susceptibility to breast cancer than women without a family history of breast cancer.

Construct validity is founded on guidance from an existing well-developed theory, which McDowell and Newell (1996, p. 33) observed is "a requirement that is not easily met." Moreover, construct validity assessment must be independent of any analysis from which the guiding theory is developed because using the same data for both purposes would result in a false positive validity outcome. In addition to a well-developed theory, measurements of other constructs must be acceptably valid. Construct validity results may be misinterpreted if the guiding theory is flawed or measurements of other constructs are not valid.

Box 8.2 presents an example of a study that assessed the reliability and validity of a new instrument.

Item Response Theory

Item response theory (IRT) is an approach to measurement that was developed for educational achievement testing, but also has been applied to scales measuring attitudes and behaviors (Baker, 2001). Whereas classical test theory (CTT) treats a multiple-item measurement as comprising parallel or equivalent measures of the same construct, IRT treats items as assessing levels of difficulty, such as ability to solve different types of mathematical problems. IRT also has been applied to measurements of characteristics such as physical functioning, where it may be assumed participants who are able to perform a high-difficulty task, such as running, also are able to perform a less difficult task, such as walking (Vasudevan et al., 2015; Velozo, Forsyth, & Kielhofner, 2006). For achievement testing, IRT scores are assigned in terms of whether a response is correct or incorrect. Scores for a characteristic such as physical functioning may be assigned in terms of whether a participant is able or not able to perform a task.

Although IRT may be applied to multiple-choice items, such as a 5-point attitude scale, a dichotomous scoring method must be imposed to simulate treating responses as "correct" or "incorrect." However, applying such coding to items measuring abstract constructs, such as attitudes, is arbitrary because there is no general criterion for determining whether an individual's attitude is "correct." The methods for developing and assessing multiple-item measurements presented in this chapter and Chapter 9 assume items are parallel/equivalent

> **BOX 8.2: EXAMPLE OF ASSESSING MEASUREMENT RELIABILITY AND VALIDITY**
>
> DEVELOPMENT OF THE BARRIERS TO PHYSICAL ACTIVITY QUESTIONNAIRE FOR PEOPLE WITH MOBILITY IMPAIRMENTS
>
> Vasudevan, Rimmer, and Kviz (2015) assessed the reliability and validity of a new measure, the Barriers to Physical Activity Questionnaire for People With Mobility Impairments (BPAQ-MI). A summary of some of the methods employed is presented below.
>
> **Content Validity**
>
> First, an extensive review of previous studies was conducted to develop an initial item bank comprising 112 items. Second, a Delphi panel of 11 experts made recommendations for deleting and adding items. The final instrument comprised 63 items in eight subscales.
>
> **Concurrent Criterion Validity**
>
> The instrument was administered to 150 participants, and results were compared with those from a preexisting instrument that previously demonstrated good reliability and validity with a similar population of participants.
>
> **Test–Retest Reliability**
>
> A randomly selected subsample of 30 participants completed the instrument a second time within approximately 7 to 14 days of their initial assessment.
>
> **Internal Consistency**
>
> Cronbach's coefficient alpha was computed for each of the eight subscales.

> **CHECK YOUR UNDERSTANDING 8.5**
>
> Describe the following methods for assessing a measurement's validity.
>
> - Judgment-based
>   - Face validity
>   - Content validity
> - Performance-based
>   - Concurrent criterion validity
>   - Predictive criterion validity
>   - Convergent validity
>   - Discriminant validity
>   - Construct validity

measures for which CTT-based methods are appropriate. As Streiner and Norman (1995, p. 186) observed, CTT-based methods "generally yield satisfactory scales," and "a substantial majority of the well-known and highly regarded scales used in social science research were developed using such procedures." Nevertheless, IRT methods should be considered when assessing a multiple-item measurement comprising items that indicate levels on a hierarchy of difficulty.

Key Points

From Concepts to Data

Measurement is the process of systematically assigning labels and/or numbers to differentiate observations in terms of quality or quantity, across units and/or time.

- **Conceptualization**: defines an abstract construct in theoretical terms.
- **Operationalization**: identifies observable variables that represent the construct.
- **Instrumentation**: specifies procedures for observing and recording empirical indicators of the variables.

Levels of Measurement

Measurements are classified in a series of levels according to the nature and amount of information they capture.

- **Nominal**: distinguishes between observations in terms of kind or quality.
- **Ordinal**: distinguishes between observations in terms of relative amount.
- **Interval/ratio**: distinguishes between observations in terms of the amount in terms of standard units.

Measurement Theory

Classical test theory, the predominant theoretical measurement model, posits that an observed value is equal to the sum of an observation's true value, systematic error, and random error.

- **Random error**: unsystematic deviation of an observed value from its true value.
- **Reliability**: the extent to which a measurement is free of random error and thus obtains consistent outcomes when the true value is constant.
- **Systematic error**: a consistent deviation of an observed value from its true value that results in measurement bias, whereby the observed value always is lower or higher than its true value.
- **Validity**: the extent to which a measurement accurately measures the construct it is intended to measure; a valid measurement is free from both random and systematic error.

Assessing Measurement Reliability

- **Test–retest reliability**: correlation between repeated measurements of the same individual(s), under the same conditions, by the same observer, and using the same procedure.
- **Interrater reliability**: agreement between independent concurrent observations of the same individual(s) using the same procedure. Cohen's Kappa adjusts for chance agreement.
- **Parallel forms reliability**: correlation between independent, concurrent measurements of the same individual(s) using similar procedures.

- **Split-half reliability**: correlation between random splits of a multiple-item measure.
- **Cronbach's coefficient alpha**: average split-half correlation for all possible random splits of a multiple-item measure.

Assessing Measurement Validity

- **Judgment-based**: assesses whether a measurement appears to measure the construct it is intended to measure.
  - **Face validity**: A measurement appears to represent a particular construct.
  - **Content validity**: A measurement appears to represent a construct's content domain.
- **Performance-based**: compares empirical outcomes for a measurement with those of other measures with which it is or is not expected to be correlated.
  - **Concurrent criterion validity**: A measurement agrees with a criterion measurement of the same construct at the same time.
  - **Predictive criterion validity**: A measurement agrees with a future measurement with which it is expected to be correlated.
  - **Convergent validity**: Measures of the same construct are correlated.
  - **Discriminant validity**: Measures of different constructs are not correlated.
  - **Construct validity**: Relationships with measurements of other constructs are consistent with theoretical expectations.

Item Response Theory (IRT)

- IRT treats a multiple-item measurement as comprising items that indicate levels on a hierarchy of difficulty.
- Scores are assigned in terms of whether a response is correct or incorrect.
- When measuring abstract constructs such as attitudes, there is no general criterion for whether a participant's attitude is "correct."

Review and Apply

1. Review the research plan you developed in the "Review and Apply" section of Chapter 1 or 3. If you did not do that previously, either do it now or identify a health-related problem that interests you.
2. Choose one key independent or dependent variable related to the problem.
   a. What theoretical guidance is available for measuring the variable?
   b. Brainstorm, by yourself and/or with others, about ways to measure the variable and select the measurement strategy you consider to be most appropriate.
      1. Identify the challenges to implementing the measurement in a *research setting* and recommend strategies for addressing those challenges.
      2. Identify the challenges to implementing the measurement in a *practice setting* and recommend strategies for addressing those challenges.

c. Identify method(s) appropriate to assess the *reliability* of the measurement.

d. Identify method(s) appropriate to assess the *validity* of the measurement.

3. Search the research literature to discover if and how the variable has been measured in previous studies.

4. If the variable has been measured differently in previous studies, select the measurement you consider to be the most reliable and valid.

    a. Identify evidence supporting the measurement's reliability, and explain why you consider the evidence to be supportive.

    b. Identify evidence that does *not* support the measurement's reliability, and explain why you consider the evidence not to be supportive.

    c. Identify evidence supporting the measurement's validity, and explain why you consider the evidence to be supportive.

    d. Identify evidence that does *not* support the measurement's validity, and explain why you consider the evidence not to be supportive.

    e. What recommendations do you propose to improve the measurement?

Study Further

DeVellis, R. F. (2017). *Scale development: Theory and applications.* Thousand Oaks, CA: Sage.

Streiner, D. L., Norman, G. R., & Cairney, J. (2015). *Health measurement scales: A practical guide to their development and use* (5th ed.). Oxford, UK: Oxford University Press.

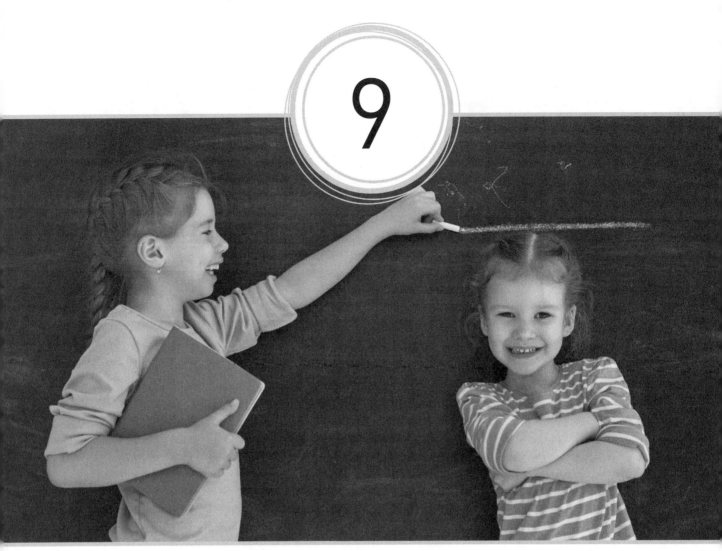

9

Developing a Measurement Instrument

Chapter Outline

Overview
Learning Objectives
The Instrument Development Process
    Specifying Variables
    Specifying Format
    Drafting and Revising
    Field Pretesting
Using Existing Instruments
    Advantages
    Disadvantages
    Modifications
Developing a Rating Scale
    Single-Item Scales
    Multiple-Item Scales
Key Points

Learning Objectives

After studying Chapter 9, the reader should be able to:

- Implement the instrument development process
- Assess the advantages and disadvantages of using an existing instrument
- Develop a single-item rating scale
- Decide when to use a bipolar versus a unipolar rating scale
- Combine single-item scales to form a multiple-item scale

Overview

Some measurement instruments used in research are familiar from everyday applications, such as a clock to measure travel time and a ruler to measure a person's height. In the research context, a measurement **instrument** is a method for collecting and recording observations. It is not necessarily a physical device, and it may take many forms, such as a thermometer, photographs of public park conditions, self-ratings of health status, or notes about observations of parent–child interactions. Moreover, there may be more than one method for measuring the same variable. For example, an individual's body weight might be assessed using a physical weight scale in a clinical setting or by obtaining a self-report in a questionnaire. When an appropriate measurement instrument is not already available, one must be developed, or an existing instrument must be modified. In addition to the construct to be measured, instrumentation must take into consideration factors such as the nature of the target population, the research setting, and the administration mode. It is essential to understand the instrument development process to develop effective new instruments, and assess and modify existing ones as appropriate.

The Instrument Development Process

As described in Chapter 8, some variables may be measured in multiple ways. Moreover, virtually all research involves measuring more than one variable, and some instruments may measure several variables. For example, a questionnaire for a mammography screening study might ask women about their health history, knowledge about breast cancer risk factors, health behaviors, attitudes toward screening, access to health care resources, and demographic characteristics. In view of the broad range of potential measurement instruments, for convenience of presentation, the discussion of the instrument development process assumes collecting data through interviews and/or questionnaires, which are employed extensively to measure a wide variety of variables. However, the basic principles for developing such instruments generally may be extended to other types of instruments. Figure 9.1 depicts the instrument development process, which is described further in the following sections.

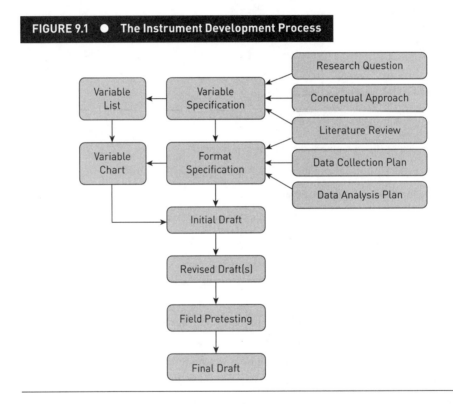

FIGURE 9.1 ● The Instrument Development Process

Specifying Variables

The research question and the conceptual approach are the primary guides for specifying the variables to be measured. Also, reviewing relevant research literature may indicate variables to consider. A **variable list** specifies the independent, dependent, moderator, and mediator variables, as appropriate (Chapter 3). Table 9.1 presents an example of a variable list for a study of the effectiveness of a program to enhance perceived benefits of mammography and reduce perceived barriers to getting a mammogram among married women by promoting spousal support for mammography screening. For convenience of presentation, the list does not include all the variables that might be measured for such a study.

TABLE 9.1 ● Variable List for a Mammography Screening Intervention

Variable Type	Variable Name
Independent	Program participation
Dependent	Spousal support for mammography screening
Mediator	Perceived benefits of mammography
	Perceived barriers to getting a mammogram
Moderator	Number of years married
	Family history of breast cancer

Specifying Format

Next, the measurement format must be specified. It is helpful to develop a **variable chart** that extends the variable list by specifying the mode, timing, and measurement protocol for each variable. The variable chart in Table 9.2 assumes a pretest–posttest research design to evaluate the effectiveness of a mammography screening intervention to enhance spousal support to increase perceived benefits and reduce perceived barriers for obtaining a mammogram. Depending on factors such as the nature of the variables, participants, and measurement context, some measurements might be collected by different modes and at different times, as illustrated in the table.

The study illustrated in Table 9.2 will employ three measurement instruments: a program participation record, a pretest self-administered questionnaire, and a posttest telephone interview questionnaire. As appropriate, a variable chart may include additional columns, such as data analysis file labels (e.g., "ATTREC" for *attendance record*), theories from which variables are derived, sources of existing measurements (a summary of reliability and validity evidence also may be included), and whether existing measurements will be used as is or modified. For variables that will be measured by multiple items, usually it is sufficient to include only one or two representative items.

Drafting and Revising

The path from an initial draft to a final draft typically involves several rounds of review and revision. It is essential to take this aspect into consideration when developing a study time schedule. Drafting, revising, and finalizing an instrument may take several weeks or months depending on factors such as the nature of the key variable(s), the innovativeness of the measurement strategy, and an instrument's length and complexity. Regardless of whether a measurement instrument will be entirely original or adapted from an existing one, each draft should be reviewed independently by experts regarding theoretical content, data collection feasibility, data processing and analysis, and relevance to professional practice. Such reviews may be obtained from individual consultations, focus groups, and/or panel reviews.

Field Pretesting

Whenever feasible, an instrument should be assessed by conducting a **field pretest** (Chapter 10), which is a small-scale trial run to assess an instrument under study conditions. Box 9.1 presents key instrumentation factors that a field pretest may assess. Primary methods for evaluating a field pretest, as appropriate, include real-time observation by a

TABLE 9.2 Variable Chart for Mammography Screening Intervention

Variable Type	Variable Name	Measurement Mode	Timing	Measurement
Independent	Program participation	Attendance record	Intervention	Number of sessions attended
Dependent	Spousal support for mammography screening	Self-administered questionnaire	Pretest	"On a scale from 1 to 5, where 1 is *not supportive* and 5 is *very supportive*, how would you describe your husband's support for you to get a mammogram?"
		Telephone interview	3 months postintervention	"During the time since you attended the Women's Health Program three months ago until now, on a scale from 1 to 5, where 1 is *not supportive* and 5 is *very supportive*, how would you describe your husband's support for you to get a mammogram?"
Mediator	Perceived benefits	Self-administered questionnaire	Pretest	"On a scale from 1 to 5, where 1 is *no benefits* and 5 is *many benefits*, how would you describe the benefits of getting a mammogram within the next two years?"
		Telephone interview	3 months postintervention	
	Perceived barriers	Self-administered questionnaire	Pretest	"On a scale from 1 to 5, where 1 is *no barriers* and 5 is *many barriers*, how would you describe the barriers for you to get a mammogram within the next two years?"
		Telephone interview	3 months postintervention	
Moderator	Number of years married	Self-administered questionnaire	Pretest	"In what month and year were you and your husband married?"
	Breast cancer history	Self-administered questionnaire	Pretest	"Has anyone who is a blood relative to you ever been diagnosed with breast cancer?"

BOX 9.1: KEY FIELD PRETEST INSTRUMENTATION FACTORS

- Ease of administration
- Clarity of instructions
- Clarity of key terms
- Participants' willingness and ability to provide information
- Procedure for recording measurements
- Appropriateness of the measurement setting (e.g., location, time of day, or day of week)

staff trainer, reviewing audio or video recordings of instrument administration, and debriefing participants and staff about their experience with the measurement protocol. Because the number of field pretest participants typically is small, about 15 to 30, assessments of an instrument's reliability and validity should be interpreted with caution.

CHECK YOUR UNDERSTANDING 9.1

- Describe a variable list and a variable chart, and explain the role of each one for developing a measurement instrument.

Using Existing Instruments

Before starting the process of developing an instrument, a search should be made to determine if an appropriate existing instrument is available that may be used as is or with modifications. For instance, an instrument might be included in, or referenced by, a research report when reviewing literature related to the research problem. Box 9.2 lists resources for locating an existing instrument. A citation to an existing instrument's source must be included in any report of research in which it is used. If an instrument is modified to accommodate a study's purpose or context, then the reason(s) for and nature of the modification(s) should be described. In general, it is not necessary to obtain permission to use an instrument that is published in a research journal or available at a federal government website. However, some instruments are proprietary, and require permission and perhaps a fee to use them. When there is any doubt about permission to use an instrument, the author should be contacted to ensure no copyrights are infringed.

BOX 9.2: RESOURCES FOR LOCATING AN EXISTING INSTRUMENT

- Journals that publish reports related to the research problem
- Consultation with a reference librarian
- Instrument compendia
  - Online (e.g., Health and Psychosocial Instruments [HaPI] and Measurement Instrument Database for the Social Sciences [MIDSS])
  - Published (e.g., McDowell, 2006)
- Federal government (e.g., Behavioral Risk Factor Surveillance System, health-related quality of life measures, National Health Interview Survey)
- Academic and nonprofit research centers
- Google Scholar search

Advantages

There are three major advantages to using an existing instrument:

- Save time
- Save costs
- Facilitate comparison with other studies

As described in the "Drafting and Revising" section, developing a new instrument often requires a substantial investment of time, money, and other resources. Using an existing instrument reduces that investment and enables initiating data collection sooner than if a new instrument is developed. Also, using an existing instrument facilitates comparing results across studies that use the same instrument. For example, results may be compared with a *benchmark*, such as binge drinking prevalence measured in a community survey versus Behavioral Risk Factor Surveillance System data for the state (Centers for Disease Control and Prevention, 2018b, 2018c).

Disadvantages

Potential disadvantages to using an existing instrument are that it might not

- adequately cover a construct's content,
- be up to date,
- be appropriate for the target population, and
- be appropriate for the data collection mode.

First, an existing instrument might not adequately cover the content required for a study's purpose. For example, Champion's (1999) barriers scale for mammography screening comprises 11 items that measure attitudes about obtaining a mammogram. While the items cover attitudinal content, such as fear ("I am afraid to have a mammogram because I might find out something is wrong") and embarrassment ("Having a mammogram is too embarrassing"), the scale does not include items that measure other barriers, such as availability of services, transportation, and insurance coverage. A related issue is that an existing instrument might not be up to date. For example, terms referring to sexual orientation, sexual behavior, and gender identification have changed substantially over recent decades (Federal Interagency Working Group on Improving Measurement of Sexual Orientation and Gender Identity in Federal Surveys, 2016).

Another potential disadvantage is an existing instrument might not be appropriate for the target population. For example, Cranford, McCable, and Boyd (2006, p. 1902) found that a revised binge drinking definition incorporating the duration of a drinking episode, and extending the time frame from the past two weeks to the past year, "captures a dimension of risky alcohol involvement in college students that is not fully assessed by the standard measure" (National Institute on Alcohol Abuse and Alcoholism, 2004).

In other situations, the operational definition of a construct may differ according to a population's culture. For example, in western cultures such as the United States, a person's age is described as the number of years he or she has lived, typically rounded to the last whole year. Accordingly, a parent would report the age of a child who has lived four years and three months as four years. However, in many Asian cultures, a person's age is described in terms of the year of life he or she is living. Thus, the age of a child who has lived four years and three months would be reported as five years because the child is in his or her fifth year of life. Such reporting differences will have a trivial effect for most studies of the general adult population. However, they could have a substantial effect on results for studies about young children, such as immunizations, in a multicultural population or for cross-cultural comparisons.

A fourth potential disadvantage is an existing instrument's format might not be appropriate for the data collection mode. For example, visual aids such as photographs or graphic representations of response scales cannot be employed in a telephone interview (Lavrakas, 2010).

Modifications

Potential reasons for modifying an existing instrument are to

- enhance coverage of content;
- reduce administration time, cost, and/or participant burden;
- adapt it for a different administration mode; and
- adapt it for a different population.

An instrument's content might be expanded or modified in other ways to enhance its coverage of a multidimensional construct. For example, Champion's (1999) barriers scale for mammography screening might be supplemented to include items that measure barriers such as availability of services, transportation, and insurance coverage. In other situations, an instrument might be shortened to reduce administration time, cost, and/or participant burden. For example, as described in Chapter 8, Marshall and Hays (1994) developed a short form (PSQ-18) of the Patient Satisfaction Questionnaire (PSQ-III) (RAND Health, n.d.), to reduce the number of items from 50 to 18.

Perhaps the most frequent reason for modifying an existing instrument is to adapt it for a different administration mode or population. For example, an instrument initially designed for a self-administered mode might be adapted for an interview by making the tone of instructions conversational and adding transitional phrases to facilitate changes in topics or response formats. An instrument also might be adapted for administration with a population that is substantially different from the one for which it was developed initially. For example, Wiklander et al. (2013) adapted the HIV Stigma Scale (HSS-40), which was developed for adults, to be administered to children and youth aged 8–18.

To reduce excluding participants according to linguistic proficiency, typically in English, and to enhance cross-cultural comparisons, an existing instrument may be translated for administration in multiple languages (Edwards, 2015). In the past, translation validity was assessed by **back-translation**, whereby an instrument is translated from the source language into a second language, and then is independently translated from the second language back into the source language. That practice predominantly has been replaced by **committee translation**, of which there are several variations. The typical committee translation process employs a team of three or more translators who work both independently and collaboratively to determine the most appropriate terminology, grammar, and syntax (Harkness et al., 2010; Harkness, Pennell, & Schoua-Glusberg, 2004).

CHECK YOUR UNDERSTANDING 9.2

- What are the advantages and disadvantages of using an existing instrument?

Developing a Rating Scale

Using a self-administered or interview questionnaire, a **rating scale** asks participants to locate themselves along an ordered continuum representing the range of possible values for a continuous variable (Chapter 3). Rating scales commonly are used to measure subjective phenomena that are not directly observable, such as attitudes, beliefs, expectations, and intentions. They enable ordinal comparisons across participants, such as whether their attitude is more or less strong than that of others. Also, ratings by the same participant may be compared over time. Scale points may be indicated by verbal and/or numeric labels. Typically, scales are analyzed in terms of numbers assigned to verbal labels.

Single-Item Scales

The simplest rating scale is a **single-item scale**, which may be employed for three purposes. One is to assess a participant's status regarding a unidimensional construct, such as the degree of abdominal pain he or she is experiencing at the time of measurement. Another is to assess a participant's status overall regarding a multidimensional construct, such as satisfaction with his or her usual source of health care. Third, several single-item scales measuring different facets of a multidimensional construct may be combined to form a multiple-item scale.

Bipolar scale

A **bipolar scale** measures ordinal levels in opposite directions, such as degree of satisfaction or dissatisfaction. Most bipolar scales are modeled after Likert's (1932) technique and often are referred to as a **Likert scale** (although frequently pronounced as "LY-kert," the correct pronunciation is "LIK-ert"). Participants are asked to respond to a statement about a topic by choosing among ordinal options ranging from the most negative to the most positive. A typical Likert scale presents five ordered points indicating degrees of agreement or disagreement, as illustrated in Box 9.3.

There are several potential problems with the typical Likert scale format. First, the focus of the scale is a *directional* statement, which might bias results in that direction. For instance, the statement in Box 9.3 might lead participants who are eager to please others to be more likely to choose a positive response, a problem called **acquiescence bias**. Second, the risk of a positive bias is compounded by presenting the positive end of the scale first, which participants might interpret as an expectation for them to have positive opinions about the topic, a problem called **social desirability bias**. Moreover, perceiving such an expectation may be especially likely if clinic staff administer the scale.

Neither of these issues may be resolved by presenting the statement in a negative direction. Both acquiescence and social desirability bias may lead some participants even to agree with negative statements that do not reflect their true opinion. Furthermore, participants

---

BOX 9.3: BIPOLAR SCALE

How much do you agree or disagree with the following statement?

In general, I am very satisfied with the services I receive at my usual source of health care.

1. Strongly agree
2. Somewhat agree
3. Neither agree nor disagree
4. Somewhat disagree
5. Strongly disagree

Note: Sometimes unmodified *agree* and *disagree* are used instead of *somewhat*.

with a positive opinion must respond negatively by *disagreeing* with a negative statement such as "In general, I am very dissatisfied with the services I receive at my usual source of health care." Such double-negative situations may confuse participants and result in responses that may be opposite their true opinions.

Third, presenting scale points in a vertical format might imply that the first responses are most acceptable. Finally, presenting scale points from positive to negative requires recoding them so higher ratings indicate more positive positions (Chapter 15). That is, scale points would be recoded as *strongly agree* = 5, *somewhat agree* = 4, *neither agree nor disagree* = 3, *somewhat disagree* = 2, and *strongly disagree* = 1.

Box 9.4 presents two revised versions of the scale. In the first revision, although the statement still is in a positive direction, the format provides several improvements. Presenting the negative end of the scale first indicates negative ratings are acceptable, which may reduce the risk of acquiescence and social desirability bias (Bradburn, Sudman, & Wansink, 2004; Liu & Keusch, 2017). Also, it is not necessary to recode responses for the analysis. Moreover, a horizontal format better represents the concept of a continuum and implies that all scale points are equally acceptable. The second revision replaces the directional statement with a neutral request for participants to rate services at their usual source of health care. Accordingly, instead of degrees of agreement/disagreement, the scale measures degrees of satisfaction/dissatisfaction, and addresses the goal of rating health care services equitably.

BOX 9.4: REVISED BIPOLAR SCALES

How much do you agree or disagree with the following statement?
In general, I am very satisfied with the services I receive at my usual source of health care.

Strongly Disagree	Somewhat Disagree	Neither Agree nor Disagree	Somewhat Agree	Strongly Agree
1	2	3	4	5

In general, how would you rate the services you receive at your usual source of health care?

Very Dissatisfied	Somewhat Dissatisfied	Neither Satisfied nor Dissatisfied	Somewhat Satisfied	Very Satisfied
1	2	3	4	5

Unipolar scale

A **unipolar scale** measures ordinal levels in one direction, from a null or zero point to a maximum end point. Typically, the scale direction is positive, such as *not satisfied* to *very satisfied*, and the negative end of the scale is presented first to reduce the risk of acquiescence and social desirability bias (Bradburn et al., 2004; Liu & Keusch, 2017), as displayed in Box 9.5. If satisfaction were measured in the negative direction, *not dissatisfied* to *very dissatisfied*, the null end label (*not dissatisfied*) probably would strike most participants as odd. Worse, it would present a double-negative condition that is almost certain to be confusing.

> **BOX 9.5: UNIPOLAR SCALE**
>
> In general, how would you rate the services you receive at your usual source of health care?
>
> | Not Satisfied | Slightly Satisfied | Somewhat Satisfied | Mostly Satisfied | Very Satisfied |
> |---|---|---|---|---|
> | 1 | 2 | 3 | 4 | 5 |

Bipolar or unipolar? Some variables inherently are bipolar, such as a rating in comparison with a reference standard, which typically is located at the scale midpoint. Box 9.6 presents an example where participants are asked to rate their current health status in comparison with others of a similar age. Other variables inherently are unipolar, such as those measured in terms of quantity or frequency, where negative ratings are not possible. Box 9.7 presents an example of using a unipolar scale to measure a quantity. Other continuous variables may be measured using either a bipolar or unipolar scale, as illustrated for satisfaction with services in Box 9.4 and Box 9.5. Nevertheless, unipolar scales generally are preferable because they more clearly focus on a single dimension and tend to be less cognitively difficult than bipolar scales (Schaeffer & Presser, 2003; Dillman, Smyth, & Christian, 2014).

> **Key Concept**
>
> *Unipolar scales generally are preferable.*

> **BOX 9.6: INHERENTLY BIPOLAR SCALE**
>
> In general, compared to other people about your age, how would you describe your health at this time?
>
> | Much Worse | Somewhat Worse | About the Same | Somewhat Better | Much Better |
> |---|---|---|---|---|
> | 1 | 2 | 3 | 4 | 5 |

> **BOX 9.7: INHERENTLY UNIPOLAR SCALE**
>
> During the past 12 months, how much did your husband encourage you to get a mammogram?
>
> | Not at all | A Little | Somewhat | Very Much |
> |---|---|---|---|
> | 1 | 2 | 3 | 4 |

Branching

"Branching," sometimes called "unfolding," is a strategy for simplifying a participant's burden when responding to a bipolar scale (Malhotra, Krosnick, & Thomas, 2009; Schaeffer & Presser, 2003). It should be considered when there are three or more positive and negative scale points. Branching combines features of bipolar and unipolar scales. First, a simple bipolar scale is used to assess *direction* by asking participants if their opinion about a topic generally is positive, negative, or neutral. For example, they might be asked if in general they are satisfied, dissatisfied, or neither satisfied nor dissatisfied with services they receive at their usual source of health care. Second, depending on the direction, a unipolar scale is used to assess the *intensity* of participants' opinion by asking them to rate how positive or negative (e.g., satisfied or dissatisfied) they feel. While branching may be used effectively for single-item scales, it is not recommended for multiple-item scales where participant burden and administration time would be increased by presenting each item using a two-step format.

Item-specific scale

An **item-specific scale** format (also called **construct-specific**) has been shown to effectively address concerns about acquiescence bias and participant burden associated with the agree/disagree bipolar scale format, and improve reliability and validity (Hanson, 2015; Saris, Revilla, Krosnick, & Shaeffer, 2010). Some researchers (e.g., Dillman et al., 2014, p. 155) recommend against using the agree/disagree format almost entirely and "strongly advocate the use of construct-specific scales." Saris et al. (2010, p. 76) recommend that if the agree/disagree format is used, "great care should be taken in interpreting the results, always keeping in mind the drawbacks of such scales." Nevertheless, the agree/disagree format persists because it is

- familiar to researchers and participants,
- easy to construct,
- versatile and may be used to measure a wide variety of constructs,
- comparable with results from earlier studies that used that format, and
- efficient for presenting multiple-item scales that may be introduced by a simple common question, such as "How much do you agree or disagree with each of the following statements?"

The item-specific format uses a unipolar scale focused directly on the underlying construct to be measured. For example, a bipolar scale might ask cigarette smokers how much they agree or disagree with the statement "I am very concerned about the effects of smoking cigarettes on my health." Specifying the underlying construct as *concern* about the health effects of smoking cigarettes, an item-specific format may be used instead and ask,

How concerned are you about the effects of smoking cigarettes on your health?
Are you

- not concerned at all,
- slightly concerned,
- somewhat concerned, or
- very concerned?

In most situations, the item-specific format requires presenting a different scale dimension for each item (concern, importance, effectiveness, etc.), which increases participation burden and administration time. A more efficient method is to ask participants to rate how much each statement in a series applies to them, such as

Using a scale from 1 to 5, where 1 is *not at all* and 5 is *very much*, please rate how each of the following statements applies to you.

Number of points

Reviews of scale construction methods have concluded that there is no apparent standard practice regarding the number of points that should be included in a rating scale (Cox, 1980; Krosnick & Presser, 2010). Nevertheless, substantial research evidence suggests the optimal number of scale points generally is between four and seven (Bollen & Barb, 1981; Bradburn et al., 2004; Cox, 1980; Dillman et al., 2014; Krosnick & Fabrigar, 1997; Krosnick & Presser, 2010; Miller, 1956; Revilla, Saris, & Krosnick, 2014; Schaeffer & Presser, 2003).

Key Concept

The optimal number of scale points generally ranges between four and seven.

Deciding the number of scale points involves a balance between providing enough options so participants may appropriately indicate their position, and not providing so many that they are unable to discern meaningful differences among them. In general, the more scale points, the more opportunity for participants to indicate their appropriate scale level, and the more variance a scale may capture. For example, with a 3-point bipolar scale (e.g., *dissatisfied*, *neither satisfied nor dissatisfied*, and *satisfied*), participants may express only the direction but not the strength of their opinion. Also, it may capture variance only across three levels.

Although a scale measures a continuous variable, the feasible number of points is limited. As the number of points increases, eventually a participant's ability to distinguish meaning between adjacent points decreases (Bradburn et al., 2004). For example, on a scale from 1 to 100, most participants are not likely to discern a meaningful difference between ratings of 76 and 77. As the number of scale points becomes large, participants tend to round at familiar points such as 10, 25, 50, 75, 90, and 100 (Tourangeau, Rips, & Rasinski, 2000). Consequently, a 100-point scale actually might distinguish only among a few levels that are familiar and manageable.

The foremost consideration about the number of scale points is the goal of the analysis. For example, if ratings from a unipolar scale will be collapsed into three categories (e.g., *low*, *medium*, and *high*), it would be more efficient to present only those three points on the scale. Generally, more points may be considered when participants' knowledge about a topic is substantial and they are motivated to provide information that is as precise as possible. The number of points should be kept at a minimum for a telephone interview because it is cognitively difficult for participants to consider a large number of points if they are not presented a visual scale representation. Also, presenting long scales in a telephone interview increases administration time and an interviewer's burden. In an in-person interview, an interviewer may present a scale on a card, commonly called a "show card."

Including a midpoint

Whether to include a midpoint is an issue that must be addressed primarily for a bipolar scale. Including a midpoint provides an appropriate option for participants who are not inclined in either a positive or negative direction. However, participants might choose the midpoint when it is not their true position (Krosnick & Fabrigar, 1997; Schuman & Presser,

1981). Some might choose the midpoint to avoid expressing what they perceive as an unpopular opinion, a form of social desirability bias. Others might choose the midpoint to reduce their cognitive burden, called **satisficing** (Krosnick, 1991), whereby they satisfy a request to choose a scale point in the easiest way available.

Although these problems may be avoided by not including a midpoint, called a **forced-choice** method, there is no appropriate option for participants who truly are not inclined in either a positive or negative direction. Typically, when presented with a bipolar scale without a midpoint, participants must choose a position that does not apply to them, or they might choose not to respond at all. Moreover, as Krosnick and Fabrigar (1997, p. 148) observed, a midpoint sometimes is "conceptually demanded," as when a scale involves a comparison with a reference standard, such as rating one's current health status in comparison with others of a similar age (Box 9.6). The preponderance of evidence from experimental studies indicates that in most situations providing a midpoint does not reduce a scale's reliability and validity (Bradburn et al., 2004; Dillman et al., 2014; Krosnick & Fabrigar, 1997; Krosnick & Presser, 2010). In general, including a midpoint in a bipolar scale is recommended except when there is a compelling reason to not include one, such as to force participants to commit to one side or another of an issue.

> **Key Concept**
>
> In general, including a midpoint in a bipolar scale is recommended.

Although most attention to including a midpoint understandably has focused on bipolar scales, a midpoint also may be included in a unipolar scale. Unlike a bipolar scale, where the midpoint represents a position between opposite directions, the midpoint of a unipolar scale represents the middle of the range of values from the null or zero point to the maximum end point. For example, the midpoint for a rating of satisfaction with one's usual source of health care on a five-point unipolar scale might be specified as *somewhat satisfied*, as illustrated in Box 9.5. To include a midpoint in a unipolar scale, it is essential to use an odd number of scale points. For example, using a scale from 1 to 10 as illustrated in Box 9.8, some participants might interpret 5 as the midpoint. However, it actually is in the lower half of the scale.

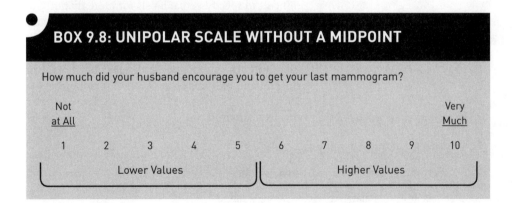

Labeling

Scale point labels may be numeric, verbal, or a combination, as illustrated in Box 9.9. *Numeric labels* alone present a greater cognitive burden than when they are combined with verbal labels because they require participants to ascribe meaning to them (Krosnick & Presser, 2010; Schaeffer & Presser, 2003). Moreover, there may be substantial variation in how they interpret numeric labels (Schwarz, Knauper, Hippler, Noelle-Neumann, &

> **BOX 9.9: SCALE LABELING EXAMPLES**
>
> "In general, how would you rate the services you receive at your usual source of health care?"
>
> Bipolar: Fully Labeled
>
> | Very Dissatisfied | Somewhat Dissatisfied | Neither Satisfied nor Dissatisfied | Somewhat Satisfied | Very Satisfied |
> |---|---|---|---|---|
> | 1 | 2 | 3 | 4 | 5 |
>
> Unipolar: Fully Labeled
>
> | Not Satisfied | Slightly Satisfied | Somewhat Satisfied | Mostly Satisfied | Very Satisfied |
> |---|---|---|---|---|
> | 1 | 2 | 3 | 4 | 5 |
>
> Unipolar: End Points Only Labeled
>
> | Not Satisfied | | | | | | | | | Very Satisfied |
> |---|---|---|---|---|---|---|---|---|---|
> | 1 | 2 | 3 | 4 | 5 | 6 | 7 | 8 | 9 | 10 |

Clark, 1991). *Verbal labels* help establish a common meaning for scale points. Regardless of whether numeric labels are used, scale reliability and validity generally are enhanced when a verbal label is assigned to every point (Krosnick, 1999; Krosnick & Fabrigar, 1997; Krosnick & Presser, 2010; Schaeffer & Presser, 2003). Unfortunately, it is difficult to specify verbal labels for more than five or seven points such that they represent approximately equal-appearing intervals (Krosnick & Presser, 2010). Therefore, when the number of points is large, typically only the end points (also called "anchors"), or the end and midpoints, are labeled (Bradburn et al., 2004).

Key Concept

Scale reliability and validity generally are enhanced when a verbal label is assigned to every point.

The following are guidelines for verbal scale point labels.

- Verbal labels must be unidimensional.
- Labels should indicate approximately equal intervals.
- Labels must be balanced across the scale range.

Verbal labels must refer to a single dimension. For example, for a scale to rate satisfaction with services at one's usual source of health care, all labels must refer to levels of satisfaction. They must not mix dimensions, such as *not satisfied*, *acceptable*, and *very good*. Also, labels should indicate approximately equal intervals and be balanced across the scale range. In Box 9.9, the labels for the "Bipolar: Fully Labeled" scale are approximately equidistant because the same modifiers, *somewhat* and *very*, are used to indicate levels of both satisfaction and dissatisfaction.

The scale in Box 9.9 also is balanced because it includes the same number of points for satisfaction and dissatisfaction. A bipolar scale would be unbalanced if labels on opposite sides of the midpoint were more or less extreme than on the other side, such as the following:

Dissatisfied	Slightly Dissatisfied	Neither Satisfied nor Dissatisfied	Very Satisfied	Completely Satisfied
1	2	3	4	5

In this example, the labels for the positive (*satisfied*) end of the scale are more extreme (*very* and *completely*) than for the negative (*dissatisfied*) end. A bipolar scale also would be unbalanced if there were different numbers of points on opposite sides of the midpoint, such as the following:

Very Dissatisfied	Somewhat Dissatisfied	Somewhat Satisfied	Very Satisfied	Completely Satisfied
1	2	3	4	5

In this example, there are only two negative (*dissatisfied*) scale points while there are three positive (*satisfied*) ones.

It is more challenging to specify verbal labels at approximately equal intervals for a unipolar scale than for a bipolar one because it is not possible to start with a foundational concept (e.g., satisfaction/dissatisfaction) and apply the same modifiers to both sides of the midpoint. The "Unipolar: Fully Labeled" scale in Box 9.9 would be unbalanced, favoring high satisfaction levels, if instead the scale labels were as follows:

Not Satisfied	Somewhat Satisfied	Mostly Satisfied	Very Satisfied	Completely Satisfied
1	2	3	4	5

The verbal label for a bipolar midpoint should indicate a position of neutrality between opposite sides of the scale. It should not indicate an inability or unwillingness to commit to a position regarding the topic, such as "don't know," "uncertain," "not sure," "undecided," or "no opinion." Such response choices are not aspects of the construct a scale measures. Therefore, if they are offered, they should be separated from the scale (Dillman et al., 2014) as illustrated in Box 9.10.

Key Concept

The verbal label for a bipolar midpoint should indicate a position of neutrality.

There is no consensus about when it is appropriate to present such response choices. The major concern about offering such response choices is some participants might choose them instead of an appropriate scale point, a form of satisficing (Krosnick, 1991). However, if such response choices are not offered, then some participants who are not familiar with the topic and/or have not formed an opinion about it might choose the middle category. In general, offering a response choice such as "don't know" is recommended

> **BOX 9.10: BIPOLAR SCALE WITH A "DON'T KNOW" OPTION**
>
> In general, how would you rate the services you receive at your usual source of health care?
>
> | Very Dissatisfied | Somewhat Dissatisfied | Neither Satisfied nor Dissatisfied | Somewhat Satisfied | Very Satisfied | Don't Know |
> |---|---|---|---|---|---|
> | 1 | 2 | 3 | 4 | 5 | 8 |

for a bipolar scale except when there is a compelling reason not to do so (Blair, Czaja, & Blair, 2014, p. 202).

Multiple-Item Scales

A single-item scale, such as to measure overall satisfaction with usual source of health care, is appealing because it is simple and convenient. However, such a global measure does not indicate what facets of a multidimensional construct a participant takes into consideration when responding. For instance, some may consider a wide array of facets of their usual source of care and conceptually calculate an "average" rating. Others may consider only one or two facets, which may differ across participants. The validity and reliability of a measurement of a multidimensional construct generally may be improved by using a multiple-item scale, which combines several single-item scales measuring different facets of the construct. This strategy helps to ensure both that participants consider all relevant facets and that they all consider the same set of facets.

Although not essential, it is most efficient to administer and combine results when a set of single-item scales uses the same format, such as all are bipolar or unipolar, and all use the same labels. However, sometimes it is necessary to use different labels for different facets. For example, a series of 5-point unipolar scales might label some points in terms of satisfaction, others in terms of importance, and so forth. Whatever the single-item format(s), it is best to use the same number of scale points to avoid transforming scores to a common base, such as transforming 4- or 7-point items to a 5-point scale base.

When single-item scales are unipolar, it is best for them all to be oriented in the same direction to reduce a participant's cognitive burden and avoid having to reverse coding items. For example, in Box 9.11, two single-item scales assess different facets of perceiving cigarette smoking as a lung cancer risk factor, the effects of continuing to smoke and stopping smoking. A *higher* score for the first item (continuing to smoke) indicates participants who smoke cigarettes are more likely to perceive smoking is a lung cancer risk factor. However, a *lower* score for the second item indicates participants are more likely to perceive smoking is a lung cancer risk factor. That is, smoking is perceived as a lung cancer risk factor because getting lung cancer is *not likely* if one stops smoking. This problem may be resolved by presenting the second item in a positive direction, such as "How likely do you think it is that you can prevent getting lung cancer if you stop smoking within the next 30 days?" Now a *higher* score related to stopping smoking indicates smoking is a lung cancer risk factor. Participants are less likely to be confused when responding to the items, and it will be straightforward to combine scores for the two items.

Box 9.12 presents an example of a multiple-item scale comprising seven items measuring various facets of a usual source of health care. As described in Chapter 8, the pool of single-item scales is best identified by seeking input from a broad range of content

BOX 9.11: REVERSE CODED SINGLE-ITEM UNIPOLAR SCALES

1. How likely do you think it is that you ever will get lung cancer if you continue to smoke cigarettes?

Not Likely	Slightly Likely	Somewhat Likely	Most Likely	Very Likely
1	2	3	4	5

2. How likely do you think it is that you ever will get lung cancer if you stop smoking cigarettes within the next 30 days?

Not Likely	Slightly Likely	Somewhat Likely	Most Likely	Very Likely
1	2	3	4	5

BOX 9.12: MULTIPLE-ITEM SCALE

Please rate your usual source of health care in terms of each of the following aspects.

	Very Dissatisfied	Somewhat Dissatisfied	Neither Satisfied nor Dissatisfied	Somewhat Satisfied	Very Satisfied
a. Convenience of location	1	2	3	4	5
b. Convenience of hours	1	2	3	4	5
c. Ability to get an appointment	1	2	3	4	5
d. Out-of-pocket costs	1	2	3	4	5
e. Waiting time at the clinic	1	2	3	4	5
f. Explanations about your health	1	2	3	4	5
g. Explanations about treatment	1	2	3	4	5

experts to establish support for the face and content validity of the multiple-item scale. There is no standard number of items that should be included in a multiple-item scale, which may be as few as two, such as to measure perceptions of smoking cigarettes as a lung cancer risk factor. Although the reliability of a multiple-item scale generally tends to increase as the number of items increases, increasing the number of items is counterproductive if the additional items are redundant or are not relevant to the underlying construct. Moreover, a large number of items is inefficient in terms of participant burden and administration costs.

Typically, individual items are weighted equally, and the summary score for a multiple-item scale is computed as the mean (arithmetic average) across the items. Computing the mean yields a score within the range of possible scores for the individual items, such as from 1 to 5. Thus, it may be interpreted in terms of the individual item metric. For example, the circles in Box 9.13 indicate a participant's ratings for the seven items, for which the sum is 26 and the mean is 3.7. Interpreting the sum of 26 is difficult because that value's meaning depends on the number of items. For instance, the maximum sum for the seven items is 35. A sum of 26 would be a relatively higher score if there were only six items, for which the maximum sum would be 30. However, regardless of the number of items, the mean of 3.7 may readily be interpreted as being on the positive end of the scale.

BOX 9.13: MULTIPLE-ITEM SCALE: SUM = 26, MEAN = 3.7

Please rate your usual source of health care in terms of each of the following aspects.

	Very Dissatisfied	Somewhat Dissatisfied	Neither Satisfied nor Dissatisfied	Somewhat Satisfied	Very Satisfied
a. Convenience of location	1	2	3	④	⑤
b. Convenience of hours	1	2	3	④	5
c. Ability to get an appointment	1	2	③	4	5
d. Out-of-pocket costs	1	2	3	4	5
e. Waiting time at the clinic	1	②	3	4	5
f. Explanations about your health	1	2	3	④	5
g. Explanations about treatment	1	2	3	④	5

Chapter 9 • Developing a Measurement Instrument   **239**

> ### CHECK YOUR UNDERSTANDING 9.3
>
> - What are the guidelines for deciding whether to employ a bipolar or unipolar rating scale?
> - Describe an item-specific rating scale and explain how it might enhance results instead of using a bipolar rating scale.
> - When developing a rating scale, present guidelines for determining
>   - the number of scale points, and
>   - whether to include a scale midpoint.

Key Points

The Instrument Development Process

- Specifying variables
- Specifying format
- Drafting and revising
- Field pretesting

Using Existing Instruments

- **Advantages**
  - Save time
  - Save costs
  - Facilitate comparisons with other studies

- **Disadvantages**
  - Might not adequately cover a construct's content
  - Might not be up to date
  - Might not be appropriate for the target population
  - Might not be appropriate for the data collection mode

- **Modifications**
  - Enhance coverage of content
  - Reduce administration time, cost, and/or participant burden
  - Adapt for a different administration mode
  - Adapt for a different population

Developing a Rating Scale

- A rating scale
  - asks participants to locate themselves along an ordered continuum,
  - is commonly used to measure subjective phenomena (e.g., attitudes, beliefs, expectations, and intentions),

- enables ordinal comparisons across participants, and
- enables comparisons for the same participant over time.

Single-Item Scales

- Single-item scales assess a participant's status regarding a unidimensional construct.
- They also assess a participant's status overall regarding a multidimensional construct.
- A **bipolar scale** measures ordinal levels in opposite directions.
- A **unipolar scale** measures ordinal levels in one direction.
- **Branching** may simplify a participant's burden for a bipolar scale by assessing first direction and then intensity of the participant's opinion.
- An **item-specific** format is a unipolar scale focused directly on the underlying construct.
- The optimal **number of points** generally is between four and seven.
- Include a **midpoint** in a bipolar scale unless there is a compelling reason to not include one.
- Scale reliability and validity generally are enhanced when a **verbal label** is assigned to every point.

Multiple-Item Scales

- Multiple-item scales combine several single-item scales measuring different facets of multidimensional construct.
- They ensure that participants consider all relevant facets and that they all consider the same set of facets.
- Using multiple-item scales generally improves the validity and reliability of a measurement of a multidimensional construct.
- There is no standard number of items that should be included.
- Increasing the number of items is counterproductive if items are redundant or not relevant to the construct.
- A large number of items is inefficient in terms of participant burden and administration costs.

Review and Apply

1. Make a variable list of the key variables you would measure to conduct your individual study. As appropriate, include independent and dependent variables, and mediator and moderator variables (Chapter 3). Limit your list of variables only to include key variables that are essential to conduct an appropriate analysis of your study's results.

2. For each key variable in your list, specify the most appropriate mode for measuring it (records review, interview, etc.) and the format for recording each measurement (a count of number of clinic visits, presence/absence of a characteristic, expressing an opinion using a 5-point scale, etc.).

3. Search for existing instruments you might use or adapt to measure at least one each of your key independent and dependent variables. Then select an instrument and
   a. assess its fit for your study population, setting, and data collection mode; and
   b. describe why and how you might modify it to be more appropriate for your study.

4. Select one variable in your study that may be measured using a single-item rating scale.
    a. Develop a bipolar version of the scale; explain why you did or did not decide to include a middle point.
    b. Develop a unipolar version of the scale.
    c. Identify which version of the scale you think would be most effective for your study, and explain why.

Study Further

Colton, D., & Covert, R. W. (2007). *Designing and constructing instruments for social research and evaluation.* San Francisco, CA: Jossey-Bass.

DeVellis, R. F. (2017). *Scale development: Theory and applications.* Thousand Oaks, CA: Sage.

McDowell, I., & Newell, C. (2006). *Measuring health: A guide to rating scales and questionnaires.* New York, NY: Oxford University Press.

Streiner, D. L., Norman, G. R., & Cairney, J. (2015). *Health measurement scales: A practical guide to their development and use* (5th ed.). Oxford, UK: Oxford University Press.

Zeller, R. A., & Carmines, E. G. (1980). *Measurement in the social sciences: The link between theory and data.* Cambridge, UK: Cambridge University Press.

10

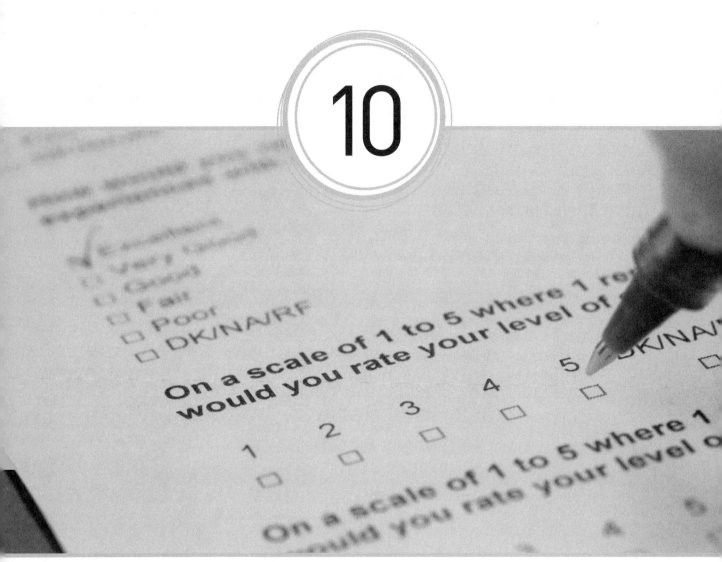

Developing a Structured Questionnaire

Chapter Outline

Overview
Learning Objectives
Key Concepts
    Standardization
    The Response Process
    Satisficing
Questionnaire Development Process
    Outline
    Drafting
    Cognitive Interviewing
    Field Pretesting
Questionnaire Design and Data Collection Mode
    Data Collection Modes Overview
    Understanding Questions
    Question Order Control
    Response Situation Control
    Recorded Response Quality
    Question Complexity
    Questionnaire Complexity
    Questionnaire Length
    Visual Aids
    Records Referral
    Sensitive Topics
    Open Questions
    Summary
Questionnaire Format
    Type
    Layout
    Instructions
    Web Questionnaires
Questionnaire Structure
    Question Order Overall
    Question Order Within a Topic
    Navigation
Key Points

Learning Objectives

After studying Chapter 10, the reader should be able to:

- Decide when to employ a structured questionnaire
- Employ strategies to minimize response satisficing
- Employ cognitive interviewing to develop and assess a questionnaire draft
- Conduct field pretesting to evaluate a questionnaire draft
- Design a questionnaire that is appropriate for the data collection mode
- Format and organize a questionnaire to collect reliable responses

Overview

A structured questionnaire is the measurement instrument used primarily to conduct a survey, where participants, called "respondents," are asked to respond to prepared questions, typically by choosing among a predetermined set of response choices. Such instruments also may be used in combination with nonsurvey research methods. For example, they may be used to collect background information about focus group participants, record on-site observations of clinic or community conditions, or extract information from records. Given that a survey always uses a structured questionnaire, and in view of the high prevalence of employing survey methods to study a wide variety of research problems, this chapter focuses on concepts and strategies for developing a structured questionnaire in the survey research context.

Key Concepts

Standardization

A **structured questionnaire**, hereafter referred to as a **questionnaire**, is used to collect comparable data about the research question from each participant, called a **respondent**. Most questions use a **closed-response format** that presents a predetermined set of response choices. Research has shown that responses may vary substantially depending on question wording, response choices, the order in which questions and/or response choices are presented, and the mode and protocol for administering a questionnaire (Bradburn, Sudman, & Wansink, 2004; Dillman, Smyth, & Christian, 2014; Krosnick & Presser, 2010; Schaeffer & Presser, 2003; Schwarz, 1999; Tourangeau, Rips, & Rasinski, 2000). Accordingly, a questionnaire is designed using a *standardized approach* whereby for each respondent the following aspects are the *same*:

- *Wording* of each question
- *Response choices* for each question
- *Order* in which questions are presented
- *Mode* of administration
- *Protocol* for implementing the data collection mode

Key Concept

Questionnaire design uses a standardized approach.

The underlying assumption is that by holding these factors constant, differences or similarities in responses across respondents, or within respondents across time, are most likely to be valid and reliable rather than measurement artifacts.

The Response Process

A questionnaire collects information by means of *self-report*. Therefore, the primary design focus is on the respondent. It is essential to write questions and response choices that

- are easy to understand,
- address topics familiar to the respondent,
- minimize the response burden, and
- request information respondents are able and willing to provide in the designated format.

As formulated by Tourangeau et al. (2000) and illustrated in Figure 10.1, responding to a question typically requires respondents to perform a series of four cognitive tasks. First, they must understand the question and decide what information is being requested. There are two major questionnaire design concerns at this stage: whether each respondent will understand what information the question is intended to solicit, and whether all respondents will understand the question in the same way. Second, respondents must search their memory to retrieve relevant information. Next, they must assess the retrieved information to formulate a summary judgment. Finally, they must decide which response choice most appropriately represents their judgment. They might edit their response, such as to be more or less precise, or to be more socially acceptable. Moreover, they might consider whether to respond at all, such as for a question with a heavy response burden or one that addresses a highly sensitive topic.

> **Key Concept**
>
> *Responding to a question typically requires performing a series of four cognitive tasks.*

FIGURE 10.1 • Cognitive Model of Survey Response

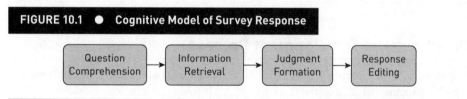

Source: Based on Tourangeau, Rips, & Rasinski (2000).

This model of the **response process** is a useful guide to considering questionnaire design factors that may enhance a respondent's ability to provide a valid and reliable response to each question. Although Figure 10.1 depicts it as linear, respondents may move back and forth in the response process. For example, they might reconsider their understanding of a question while retrieving information or forming a judgment.

Satisficing

The goal of questionnaire design is to facilitate each respondent in carefully and completely performing each cognitive task for every question. Such respondent behavior is called **optimizing**, according to **satisficing theory** (Krosnick, 1991), which addresses how respondents go through the response process. Satisficing refers to respondents not performing every task carefully and completely, which may result in an inaccurate or biased response. For example, they might give minimal thought to a question's meaning, not search their memory for all relevant information, not carefully assess retrieved information, and/or not take care to select the most appropriate response choice. A respondent's performance may vary across questions and topics in the same questionnaire. The likelihood of satisficing is greatest when task difficulty is high, a topic is unfamiliar, a topic is sensitive/threatening, and/or a respondent is not motivated to contribute to the goal of the study. Examples of satisficing behavior are as follows:

- Selecting the first reasonable response choice
- Arbitrarily selecting a response choice
- Selecting a socially desirable response (e.g., the scale midpoint, endorsing the status quo)
- Selecting the same scale point for each item in a multiple-item rating scale (called **nondifferentiation bias**)
- Retrieving only the most recent information from memory
- Avoiding a judgment by responding "don't know" or "undecided," or providing another nonresponse

CHECK YOUR UNDERSTANDING 10.1

- In what ways is a structured questionnaire "standardized"?
- Describe the four cognitive tasks that responding to a question typically requires.
- Identify at least three types of response behaviors that might result from satisficing.

Questionnaire Development Process

The process for developing a questionnaire, depicted in Figure 10.2, starts with reviewing the variable list and variable chart, which should be developed as described in Chapter 9. Typically, developing a valid and reliable questionnaire is hard work and time-consuming. Throughout the process, it is important to collaborate with content experts, questionnaire design experts, and staff who will administer the questionnaire and process responses.

Outline

Drawing on the variable list and variable chart, an outline should be developed that specifies the order for the topics and how a respondent should be routed to the next appropriate question. Box 10.1 presents an abridged outline for a questionnaire about mammography screening for an interview with women who are age 40 or older and have not been diagnosed with breast cancer.

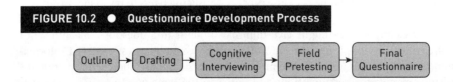

FIGURE 10.2 ● Questionnaire Development Process

> **BOX 10.1: MAMMOGRAPHY SCREENING QUESTIONNAIRE OUTLINE**
>
> I. Self-rated health status
> II. Access to health care services
>   A. Usual source of care—if "none," go to IIB
>   1. Type of place
>   2. Type of provider
>   B. Seen a provider in the past two years?
> III. Family history of cancer
>   A. Breast cancer
>   B. Other cancer
> IV. Knowledge about breast cancer risk factors
> V. Mammography history
>   A. Ever had a mammogram—if "no," go to VI
>   B. Time of last mammogram
> VI. Perceptions about mammography
>   A. Benefits
>   B. Barriers
> VII. Background characteristics
>   A. Age
>   B. Education
>   C. Ethnicity/race

Drafting

Virtually always, developing a valid and reliable questionnaire involves an iterative process of multiple drafts and evaluation. Each draft should be reviewed by content experts, questionnaire design experts, and staff who will administer the questionnaire and process responses. When a reasonable draft is developed, it is helpful to conduct cognitive interviewing to detect and address any previously unidentified problems with instructions, question wording, response choices, and question order.

Cognitive Interviewing

Cognitive interviews are conducted with individual respondents to gain insight into how they understand key questions, search their memory for relevant information, form judgments, and edit their responses (Beatty & Willis, 2007; Willis, 2005). They may be employed to evaluate self-administered questionnaires as well as ones intended for interview administration. The three basic cognitive interview techniques are as follows:

- *Thinking aloud:* Respondents are asked to verbalize aloud their thoughts while responding to a question.

- *Paraphrasing:* Respondents are asked to restate a question in their own words.
- *Probing:* Respondents are asked follow-up questions about how they arrived at their response.

More than one technique may be employed with the same questionnaire and with an individual question. Administering a questionnaire during a cognitive interview requires more time than during the normal course of conducting an interview. Therefore, it is important to minimize the respondent's burden by focusing on aspects that merit special attention, such as questions about a new topic or that use an innovative approach.

Implementation

Cognitive interview respondents are not selected by random sampling because the goal is not to draw inferences about the target population's characteristics. Respondents are selected to assess the appropriateness of a questionnaire with all major target population subgroups (e.g., age and education). Typically, the number of respondents is small, about 10 to 20. They are recruited by advertising strategies and provided a cash or gift incentive. After an initial round of cognitive interviews, the revised questionnaire should be assessed in a second round of cognitive interviews conducted with a new group of respondents. Whenever possible, cognitive interviews should be conducted in-person by experienced interviewers to avoid confounding interviewer errors with questionnaire design issues. Also, experienced interviewers are more likely to detect problems that should be addressed.

Assessment

Box 10.2 lists aspects of the four cognitive tasks of the response model that may be assessed by cognitive interviews. The assessment typically is qualitative in nature, based on interviewer notes and audio recording transcriptions. When an issue is raised by only one or a few respondents, it is challenging to determine whether it merits revising the questionnaire. If the issue is deemed most likely to be unique to that individual, then no revision may be required. However, with a small sample, even a single incidence might turn out to be more prevalent when the main study is conducted. Such an issue should be assessed by **probing** during a second round of cognitive interviewing. Also, if the questionnaire ultimately will be self-administered, consideration should be given to the possibility that an issue might be an artifact of administering it as an interview.

Field Pretesting

When a questionnaire draft is developed about which there are no major concerns identified by cognitive interviews or expert review, it should be assessed further by field pretesting using the same protocol and in conditions as similar as possible to those for the main study. Field pretesting provides information about practical issues of administering a questionnaire and may identify unforeseen problems before conducting the main study.

Field pretesting is especially important if a questionnaire measures a new topic, it will be administered using an innovative method, or there is little prior experience studying the target population. Even a small field pretest may reveal issues that should be addressed before committing resources to administering a questionnaire that otherwise might collect unreliable and invalid information. Whenever feasible, if substantial revisions are made following an initial field pretest, a subsequent field pretest should be conducted to assess them.

BOX 10.2: ASPECTS THAT MAY BE ASSESSED BY COGNITIVE INTERVIEWS

Question Comprehension

- What do respondents think the question is asking?
- Does the way respondents understand the question differ from what is intended?
- Do different respondents understand the question differently?
- What do key words and phrases in the question and response choices mean to respondents?

Information Retrieval

- Do respondents have access to information relevant to the question?
- What type(s) of information are respondents able to retrieve?
- How do respondents retrieve relevant information?
  - Forward or reverse chronology
  - Cues from significant events, times, persons, or places
  - Conceptual domains (e.g., types of health problems)

Judgment Formation

- Are respondents able to formulate a relevant response?
- How do respondents formulate a response?
- How accurate and complete are responses?

Response Editing

- Are respondents able to select a response choice that is relevant to their judgment?
- Are respondents willing to provide an accurate/honest response?

Sample

The field pretest sample should be selected from the target population using procedures similar to those that will be employed for the main study. However, the field pretest sample design may deviate somewhat from the main study sampling design. Typically, that involves oversampling one or more key population subgroups to be as confident as possible that the questionnaire is appropriate for them.

Field pretest respondents should not be included in the main study because they will have been influenced by their exposure to an earlier draft of the questionnaire. Moreover, the best practice is not to combine field pretest and main study data because virtually always there will be differences in the questionnaire and/or administration protocol. If the target population is small, pretest respondents might be selected from a similar population (e.g., another clinic) to avoid depleting the target population respondent pool.

The number of participants in an initial round of field pretesting typically is about 10 to 20. A larger sample may be selected, such as to assess an innovative measurement strategy or to compare alternative strategies, such as alternate question wording, question order, response choices, or format. Field pretest respondents should be offered a gift or cash incentive only if it will be included in the main study. Otherwise, offering an incentive may cause the field pretest experience to misrepresent how the questionnaire is likely to perform in the main study.

Assessment

Several methods may be employed to assess a field pretest experience. The best practice is to employ as many methods as feasible. Typically, these include the following:

- **Respondent debriefing.** Respondents are asked to discuss their experience responding to the questionnaire.
- **Interviewer/staff debriefing.** Interviewers/staff are asked to discuss their experience administering the questionnaire.
- **Response review.** Responses to all questions are examined to detect potential problems.
- **Behavior coding.** For an interview survey, interactions between respondents and interviewers are observed, coded, and assessed.

Respondent debriefing. Field pretest respondents should be asked to report about their experience in responding to the field pretest questionnaire. Although this may be done by asking respondents to complete a brief self-administered questionnaire, it is best to conduct a *debriefing interview*. That may be done regardless of whether the field pretest questionnaire is administered as an interview or is self-administered. A debriefing interview may be conducted in-person or by telephone, although in-person generally is likely to yield more helpful information. Typically, **respondent debriefing** interviews are conducted individually. However, a group interview may be done when feasible. For example, a group debriefing interview might be done with students who complete a self-administered questionnaire during the same class period. If the field pretest questionnaire is administered as an interview, respondent debriefing interviews should be conducted by staff other than those who conducted the field pretest interview so respondents feel free to report issues that might appear to be critical of their interviewer. Debriefing respondents should be provided a gift or cash incentive. Topics that may be addressed during respondent debriefing are as follows:

- Overall experience responding to the questionnaire (length, difficulty, topic familiarity, topic sensitivity)
- Clarity of instructions (especially important for a self-administered questionnaire)
- Questionnaire format/layout (especially important for a self-administered questionnaire)
- Navigating a self-administered questionnaire
- Pacing of an interview
- Performance of interviewer/staff who administered the questionnaire
- Clarity of question wording
- Clarity and relevance of response choices
- Reason(s) for not answering a question

Interviewer/staff debriefing. Interviewers and staff who administer the field pretest questionnaire should be asked to report about their experience. Whenever feasible, it is best for field pretesting of an interview questionnaire to be conducted by experienced interviewers to reduce mistaking errors from inexperience as indicating questionnaire design problems. Also, experienced interviewers generally are more likely to detect problems and suggest solutions. For an interview questionnaire, after reviewing the overall experience, best practice is to conduct a *question-by-question review* to solicit any comments about each individual question. No question should be passed over assuming it would not be problematic because of its apparent simplicity or prior experience with it. Topics that may be addressed during **interviewer/staff debriefing** are as follows:

- Overall experience administering the questionnaire (gaining and maintaining respondent cooperation, time for completion, topic sensitivity)
- Clarity of instructions
- Questionnaire format/layout
- Navigating the questionnaire
- Problems with reading interview questions and response choices aloud verbatim
- Problems with recording responses
- Respondent difficulty understanding questions and/or response choices
- Reason(s) for a respondent not answering a question
- Appropriateness of the interview setting

Response review. Responses to field pretest questions should be reviewed for indications of potential problems. The **response review** should include considering each of the following:

- Whether questions with small response variance merit keeping
- Deleting response choices that are not used
- Revising or deleting questions with high proportions of nonresponse (e.g., "don't know," "not applicable," refusal, left blank)
- Whether "other—please specify" responses indicate a lack of clarity in response choices or a need to add one or more response choices
- Whether open-response format questions might be converted to a closed-response format

Questions for which there is little, or no, response variance may not merit asking in the main study unless it is important to learn that most or all respondents report the same characteristics (e.g., they do not know a certain behavior is a cancer risk factor). Also, consideration should be given to revising or deleting response choices respondents do not use. Questions for which there are high proportions of *nonresponse* (e.g., "don't know," "refuse to answer," or blank) should be revised or deleted. Responses in "other—please specify" response options should be examined to consider whether an intended appropriate response choice should be revised to clarify the content it includes. Also, responses in "other—please specify" response options should be examined to consider whether a response choice should be added to capture them. Typically, it is not worthwhile to create or retain a response choice unless it is expected to include at least 10% of all responses to a question. Finally, responses to open-response format questions should be examined to consider whether the question should be converted to a closed-response format. That might be done if most of the responses appropriately may be captured by closed-response choices, plus an "other—please specify" response option.

Behavior coding. For an interview questionnaire, respondent and interviewer behavior may be observed to identify instances where respondent and/or interviewer behavior does not conform to the intended protocol, as listed in Table 10.1. Staff may observe interviews in real time by accompanying interviewers during in-person interviews, or by monitoring telephone interviews. Audio recordings of interviews also may be reviewed. Whenever feasible, the best practice is to do both, using recordings to verify and supplement real-time observations. Although systematic **behavior coding** strategies have been developed (Cannell, Fowler, & Marquis, 1968; Ongena & Dijkstra, 2006), unless a questionnaire is very complex and will be used for a large-scale survey, typically behavior coding observations may be reviewed in a less formal manner.

TABLE 10.1 ● Behavior Coding Issues

Respondent	Interviewer
• Asks for clarification of question	• Does not read questions clearly or accurately
• Asks for clarification of a response choice	• Does not read response choices clearly or accurately
• Asks for a definition of a term	• Does not present every question
• Asks for a question to be repeated	• Does not present every response choice
• Asks for response choices to be repeated	• Provides an unauthorized definition of a term
• Responds prematurely	• Does not adequately probe a response
• Has difficulty recalling relevant information	• Suggests an answer to a question
• Has difficulty selecting a response choice	• Expresses approval or disapproval of an appropriate response
• Is reluctant to or does not respond to a question	

CHECK YOUR UNDERSTANDING 10.2

- Describe the role of conducting **cognitive interviewing** in developing and assessing a structured questionnaire.
- Describe the role of conducting **field pretesting** in developing and assessing a structured questionnaire.

Questionnaire Design and Data Collection Mode

Data Collection Modes Overview

The data collection mode may have important implications for key questionnaire design aspects, such as question wording, response choices, the number of questions, and questionnaire format/layout. Briefly, the main survey data collection modes in which a questionnaire may be administered are as follows:

- **Self-administered questionnaire (SAQ):** A respondent completes the questionnaire with no or minimal assistance from staff.
  - *Mailed SAQ:* A paper questionnaire is sent by standard mail to respondents (most often at their residence); respondents complete and return the questionnaire by standard mail.
  - *Monitored SAQ:* A paper questionnaire is distributed by staff to respondents (e.g., at a clinic, workplace, or school); respondents complete and return the questionnaire to staff.
  - *Web SAQ:* Respondents are provided a link to a website to complete and submit the questionnaire online.
- **Telephone interview:** An interviewer reads questions aloud on a telephone and records responses on the questionnaire.
- **In-person interview:** An interviewer reads questions aloud in-person and records responses on the questionnaire (also called "face-to-face" and "personal" interviews).

Table 10.2 summarizes implications of each of the main survey data collection modes for questionnaire design. The following discussion presents guidelines for which there may be exceptions depending on factors such as question topics, the target population, and setting. Competent implementation of each data collection mode and a well-designed questionnaire are assumed.

> **Key Concept**
>
> *The data collection mode may have important implications for questionnaire design.*

Understanding Questions

A respondent's ability to understand questions generally is best when conducting a telephone or in-person interview. An interviewer reads every question and response choice slowly and clearly. If the respondent indicates a lack of understanding, the interviewer may reread the question and/or response choices. However, standard practice is for interviewers not to explain the meaning of a question or response choice. If a respondent asks for an explanation, the standard interviewer reply is "Whatever it means to you." Self-administered modes rely on the respondent to read all questions and response choices, which may be especially difficult for respondents with low literacy skills. That concern is not relevant with an interview mode.

Question Order Control

Interview modes control question order best because an interviewer presents the questions by reading them aloud. A web mode may control question order by requiring a response to a question before navigating to the next one. However, a respondent might enter an inaccurate response to proceed to the next question, or break off from completing the questionnaire out of frustration. Also, forcing an answer might not be approved by an institutional review board. However, requiring a response is justified for a **filter question** that determines how to route a respondent through a branching point. For example, only current cigarette smokers should be asked questions about intentions to stop smoking.

TABLE 10.2 ● Questionnaire Design and Data Collection Mode

Aspect	Mailed/Monitored SAQ	Web SAQ	Telephone Interview	In-Person Interview
Understanding questions	Good	Good	**Very good**	**Very good**
Question order control	Poor	Fair	**Very good**	**Very good**
Response situation control	Poor/**Good**	Poor	Fair	**Good**
Recorded response quality	Fair	Good	**Very good**	**Very good**
Question complexity	Somewhat complex	Somewhat complex	Short and simple	**May be complex**
Questionnaire complexity	Simple	**May be complex**	**May be complex**	**May be complex**
Questionnaire length	Short/medium (~4–12 pages)	Short (≤ 15 min.)	Short/medium (~10–30 min.)	**Long** (~30–60 min.)
Visual aids	Good	**Very good**	Usually N/A	**Very good**
Records referral	**Good**/poor	Fair	Fair	**Good**
Sensitive topics	**Good**/fair	Fair	Fair	Fair
Open questions	Poor	Poor	Good	**Very good**

SAQ = self-administered questionnaire; N/A = not applicable. Bolded items indicate methods with the greatest strength in general for each aspect.

With a mailed or monitored self-administered questionnaire, it is possible for a respondent to look ahead to see questions that appear later in a questionnaire. Bias may be introduced if responses to questions that appear earlier are influenced by such premature exposure to later questions. Also, if respondents do not follow the intended question order, they might not respond to all applicable questions, or they might respond to questions that do not apply to them.

Response Situation Control

It is important to minimize the influence of situational factors on whether and/or how a respondent responds to a questionnaire. The main factors of concern are the presence of other persons and distractions. Especially for a sensitive topic, if others may see responses entered in a self-administered questionnaire or overhear an interview, a respondent might not provide complete and accurate responses. In-person interviews provide the most effective response situation control because the interviewer and respondent are in the same location. For example, if another person attempts to listen in or offer his or her opinion, the interviewer may explain why that is not appropriate and ask the person to refrain from doing so. Also, the interviewer may suggest moving away from or suspending a distracting activity, such as a television program. There is less control for a telephone interview because an interviewer is not able to observe a respondent's environment directly. Potential situational influence generally is even greater when a respondent uses a mobile telephone.

For a monitored self-administered mode, such as in a classroom, staff may ask others (e.g., the teacher) to leave the room, instruct respondents not to communicate while completing the questionnaire, and address any distractions. Mail and web modes provide virtually no control over the response situation. At most, a respondent may be encouraged to complete the questionnaire in a quiet, comfortable location, with no one else nearby.

In the worst-case scenario, it is possible someone other than the intended respondent might complete part or even the entire questionnaire.

Recorded Response Quality

An advantage of interviews is the interviewer is trained to record responses clearly, and in the appropriate location and format. For a web mode, response format and clarity are controlled by software. However, a respondent might record an "acceptable" response in the wrong location. For example, a list of fruit items an individual purchased recently might be labeled as 1 = *apples*, 2 = *bananas*, and 3 = *oranges*. If a respondent purchased bananas but erroneously enters a 3 or clicks on the response field for oranges, his or her error is not likely to be detected (Chapter 15).

The risk of an acceptable response being recorded in the wrong location also is present when employing mailed and monitored paper questionnaires, which depend on respondents' ability and care in recording their responses. In addition, with those modes, it is more likely for a response not to be recorded. For example, respondents might neglect to record a response if they are distracted or anxious to move on to the next question. Not recording a response is less likely with a trained interviewer. A web questionnaire may be programmed to remind respondents that they have not recorded their response to a question before proceeding to the next one. Also, with mailed and monitored modes, it is more likely for a response to be recorded in the wrong format or illegibly.

Question Complexity

The complexity of an individual question is a function of several factors:

- Question length
- Question format
- Length of response choices
- Number of response choices
- Response format

An in-person interview is most effective for presenting complex questions. If an interviewer detects it would be helpful, he or she may reread the question and/or response choices without requiring a request by the respondent. Also, the interviewer may present a card with the question and/or response choices on it so the respondent may read along and review them. Questions may be somewhat complex for mailed, monitored, or web modes because the respondent may reread the question and response choices, as necessary. Nevertheless, care must be taken not to include so many complex questions that a high response burden leads the respondent to skip them or not complete the questionnaire. For a telephone interview, questions should be as short and simple as possible because the respondent relies entirely on listening to the interviewer. Also, the respondent may be reluctant to ask for a question to be reread to avoid appearing inattentive or unintelligent.

Questionnaire Complexity

The best practice is for a questionnaire to be as simple to navigate as possible. The main factor that determines a questionnaire's complexity is how difficult it is to navigate. The most common challenge is when a respondent is routed through a branching sequence called a **skip pattern**, where the next appropriate question does not follow immediately after the current one. Instead, the next appropriate question is determined by a response to a filter question. Another questionnaire complexity aspect, called **rostering**, asks respondents to identify by first name or relationship certain other individuals, such as household members or coworkers. Then they are asked to answer a series of questions about each individual on that roster.

Web questionnaires and computer-assisted interviews (Chapter 12) are the most effective modes for administering a complex questionnaire. Even without a computer-assisted format, an interview questionnaire may be rather complex because the interviewer is trained to navigate it. However, a very complex questionnaire still is vulnerable to interviewer errors. Moreover, navigating one may cause an interviewer to appear clumsy. With web questionnaires and computer-assisted interviews, navigation is controlled by software, which may make a complex structure appear simple both to a respondent and to an interviewer. Nevertheless, navigation accuracy depends on accurately programming the software, taking into consideration all possible contingencies when dealing with skip patterns and rosters.

The structure of mailed and monitored self-administered questionnaires must be as simple as possible. Appropriately navigating a mailed self-administered questionnaire depends entirely on a respondent's ability and willingness to follow instructions. A questionnaire may be slightly more complex for a monitored self-administered questionnaire because staff may be present to lend assistance.

Questionnaire Length

The longest questionnaires typically may be employed with interviews, for which interviewer–respondent rapport may be established, and the respondent is not required to perform reading and writing tasks. The longest questionnaires may be administered by in-person interviews, which may take about 30 to 60 minutes to complete. In-person interviews maximize rapport, enable employing the widest variety of question types to engage the respondent's interest, and typically provide the respondent a cash or gift (e.g., a gift card) incentive. A questionnaire must be shorter for telephone than for in-person interviews, taking no more than 20 to 30 minutes to complete. However, a telephone interview generally should be at least 10 minutes, allowing time to introduce the study, obtain informed consent, and administer the questionnaire.

Mailed and monitored paper questionnaires should be short, generally between about four and twelve pages, and require no more than about 20 minutes to complete. A monitored questionnaire may be somewhat longer than a mailed one because staff can provide encouragement and instruction. Web users expect most online activities to be quick. Therefore, a web questionnaire virtually always must be short, requiring no more than about 10 minutes to complete. However, an entire web questionnaire may be longer than what individual respondents see because the software presents only questions that apply to them.

Visual Aids

The most effective modes for presenting visual aids are in-person interviews and web questionnaires. In-person interviews are very effective for presenting visual aids because the interviewer distributes them, provides instructions, answers questions, and retrieves them to avoid distracting the respondent. Videos may be presented on a laptop computer or tablet device. Web questionnaires also generally are very effective for presenting all types of visual aids. However, unless the questionnaire is completed in a monitored setting, no staff is available to provide assistance. Also, depending on the respondent's equipment and service, long download times may lead to frustration, skipping questions, or breaking off from completing a questionnaire.

Mailed and monitored questionnaires are effective for presenting most visual aids. Materials such as photographs, drawings, and maps may be enclosed with a mailed questionnaire. However, whether a respondent uses them appropriately depends on his or her attention to the instructions. For a monitored questionnaire, staff may control when a visual aid is distributed, provide instructions, answer questions, and retrieve it to avoid distracting the respondent while answering other questions. Also, videos may be presented in a monitored situation.

Presenting visual aids directly to a respondent during a telephone interview generally is not possible. When names and addresses are available, visual aid materials may be mailed to respondents in advance of the interview. However, when the interviewer calls, a respondent might have misplaced the material, not have it readily at hand, or have discarded it.

Records Referral

Mailed questionnaires are effective for asking respondents to refer to records (personal, household, or organizational) because they may retrieve the information at a convenient time instead of immediately. In-person interviews also are effective for retrieving information from records because they may be conducted at the site where the records are located, the respondent may be asked in advance to have the records available, interviewer–respondent rapport may put the respondent at ease about retrieving records, and the respondent typically is provided a cash or gift incentive.

A monitored questionnaire typically is not administered in a setting where respondents are likely to have ready access to records. A web mode is not effective for retrieving records because instead of accessing records and returning to complete the questionnaire online, respondents tend to skip those questions. Telephone interview respondents tend to be reluctant to leave an interviewer waiting while they retrieve records unless they are readily accessible. Although web and telephone interview respondents may be asked in advance to have records available, that strategy is not reliable.

Sensitive Topics

Respondents generally tend not to provide complete and accurate responses to questions about sensitive topics (e.g., drug use, sexual behavior, and racial attitudes), and they are likely to skip or refuse to answer them. Self-administered questionnaires generally are most effective for collecting information about sensitive topics because a respondent does not respond directly to another person. Mailed questionnaires may be administered anonymously, with no respondent identifiers on the questionnaire or return mailing envelope. For a monitored questionnaire without identifiers, respondents might not trust assurances of anonymity. Respondents also tend not to trust anonymity of web questionnaires, which may be subject to security breaches. Also, concerns about anonymity are likely to be high if a web questionnaire is accessed using a workplace computer and/or through a link on an employer's website. Respondents are most reluctant to respond to sensitive questions in an interview. Telephone interviews offer an advantage over in-person interviews because they are not conducted face-to-face.

Open Questions

An open question asks respondents to provide an answer in their own words. Interviews are most effective for asking open questions. The interviewer undertakes the recording task, which reduces respondents' burden and allows them to focus on their response. The interviewer records open responses legibly and verbatim, which may be supplemented by audio recording. Also, the interviewer is trained to employ probes to obtain a clear, relevant, and complete response (Chapter 12). Telephone responses tend to be shorter and less complete than for in-person interviews (Groves et al., 2009, pp. 169–170).

Self-administered questionnaires are not effective for presenting open questions mainly because they often are not answered at all. Moreover, responses might not be focused on the point of the question, they might be fragmented, or they might contain serious spelling or grammatical errors. In addition, handwritten responses on mailed and monitored paper questionnaires may not be legible.

Summary

Overall, compared to the other modes, mailed questionnaires are effective for retrieving information from records and asking questions about sensitive topics. Monitored questionnaires are effective for controlling the response situation. Web questionnaires are effective for presenting a complex questionnaire and visual aids. Both telephone and in-person interview modes are effective regarding understanding questions, controlling question order, recorded response quality, and presenting a complex questionnaire. In addition, in-person interviews are effective for controlling the response situation, asking complex questions, presenting a long questionnaire, employing visual aids, retrieving information from records, and asking open questions. However, the advantages of interviews, especially in-person, require a substantially higher commitment of resources compared to self-administered modes.

CHECK YOUR UNDERSTANDING 10.3

- What are the main advantages and disadvantages regarding questionnaire design for each of the following data collection modes?
    - Mailed self-administered questionnaire
    - Monitored self-administered questionnaire
    - Web self-administered questionnaire
    - Telephone interview
    - In-person interview

Questionnaire Format

A well-formatted self-administered questionnaire is a key factor for whether a respondent completes it at all, responds to all applicable questions, and records responses appropriately. It should have a professional appearance to bolster the study's validity and importance, and imply it is easy to complete. The format for an interview questionnaire must facilitate reading questions and response choices aloud, recording responses, and navigating to the next appropriate question. For every administration mode, the format should facilitate processing responses for analysis. Developing a paper questionnaire requires proficiency with word processing format functions. Web questionnaire design software typically provides preset format options, which sometimes may be customized.

The following guidelines apply to all questionnaire administration modes and are based on visual presentation principles that may be applied in various ways. Although the formats illustrated in the examples are recommended, it is not essential to replicate them exactly. However, an essential overall principle is to be consistent within the context of a questionnaire. The same format pattern should be applied throughout a questionnaire so respondents and interviewers may readily recognize the kind of information presented by each element, such as headings, instructions, questions, and response choices.

Type

Box 10.3 presents guidelines for questionnaire type. The typeface family, called a "font," must be easy to read. Examples are Calibri and Cambria. Although it might appear engaging to use a script font that looks handwritten, such special fonts generally are difficult to read. Size should be 11- or 12-point for the general population. For special populations, such as elderly and children, a larger font size, such as 14-point, should be considered. The same font and size should be used for all questions and response choices. Also, instructions, questions, and response choices are presented most effectively in a standard capital and lowercase format. Special styles, such as italics, bold, all capitals, and underlining, may be used to highlight instructions, headings, and key terms. However, long segments of text with such special styles are difficult to read. They should be used sparingly and singly, not in combination.

BOX 10.3: TYPE GUIDELINES

- Choose a font that is easy to read (e.g., Calibri or Cambria).
- Do not use artistic fonts (e.g., script).
- Use 11- or 12-point size for the general population.
- Use 14-point size for a special population (e.g., elderly or children).
- Use the same font and size for all questions and response choices.
- Use capitals and lowercase for questions and response choices.
- Choose special styles (e.g., italics, bold, or underline) for special features (e.g., instructions, headings, and key terms).
- Do not overdo word emphasis so as not to lose its impact.

Layout

Box 10.4 presents guidelines for questionnaire layout. A questionnaire should have a title that appears on the cover page, first page, or first screen. Although allowing a generous amount of "white space" lengthens a paper questionnaire and may seem wasteful, it enhances a questionnaire's readability and lends it a professional appearance. Moreover, for a self-administered questionnaire, respondents recognize a user-friendly layout as being quick and easy to complete. Thus, they are more likely to complete a well-formatted questionnaire.

Box 10.5 illustrates a self-administered paper questionnaire layout that uses little white space in an effort to make it appear short and to save reproduction costs. However, respondents are likely to view it as cluttered, unprofessional, and difficult to read and navigate. Consequently, they are likely to not complete it at all, not answer all questions, and commit recording errors. Data processing errors also are likely because it will be difficult to detect all recorded responses and transcribe them accurately into an analysis file (Chapter 15). Moreover, the layout in the example is not consistent. For example, ordinal scale response choices for question 1 are oriented horizontally,

> **BOX 10.4: LAYOUT GUIDELINES**
>
> - Include a study title on the cover/first page or screen.
> - Make generous use of "white space."
> - Use a vertical flow for questions.
> - Separate questions by line spacing.
> - Single-space questions and instructions that require two or more lines.
> - Separate a question and response choices by line spacing and indentation.
> - Present all parts of a question on the same page/screen.

> **BOX 10.5: POOR LAYOUT**
>
> **Focus Group Participant Background Survey: Current Smokers**
>
> *Please circle ONE number for your answer to each question unless you are given other instructions.*
>
> 1. Compared to other people <u>about your age</u> in general, that is, people who are no more than 5 years younger or older than you, how would you describe your health overall?
>   Much worse...1 Somewhat worse...2 About the same...3 Somewhat better...4 Much better...5
>
> 2. On average, about how many cigarettes <u>per day</u> do you currently smoke?
>   1–10 1   11–20 2   More than 20 3
>
> 3. How concerned are you about the effect of smoking cigarettes on your health?
>   Not concerned at all 1
>   Somewhat concerned 2
>   Very concerned 3
>
> 4. How important do you think the health benefits are for someone <u>your age</u> who stops smoking cigarettes?
>   Not important at all 1
>   Somewhat important 2
>   Very important 3
>
> 5. How much effort do you think it would take for you to stop smoking cigarettes completely?
>   None 1   A little 2   Some 3   Very much 4

but those for questions 3 and 4 are presented vertically. In addition, the close spacing among response choices for question 1 is vulnerable to recording errors. For example, a respondent choosing *about the same* might erroneously record his or her response by circling code 2 instead of 3 because code 2 appears shortly before the *about the same* category label. Instead of following the vertical question flow guideline, questions 3 and 4 are placed side-by-side, a format called *double-banking*, which is vulnerable to recording errors and overlooking a question, such as question 4.

Box 10.6 presents the same questions as in Box 10.5, but it illustrates following the layout guidelines in Box 10.4. Although it uses about twice as much space, it appears professional, well organized, and easy to complete. The questions follow a vertical flow and are separated by extra line spacing. Response choices are indented below each question, making it easy to associate each question with its response choices. Also, response choices are separated by 1.5-line spacing to enhance readability and accurate response recording. As indicated by the general instruction, responses are recorded by circling the code number

BOX 10.6: GOOD LAYOUT

Focus Group Participant Background Survey: Current Smokers

Please circle ONE number for your answer to each question unless you are given other instructions.

1. Compared to other people <u>about your age</u> in general, that is, people who are no more than 5 years younger or older than you, how would you describe your health overall?

   Much worse 1
   Somewhat worse 2
   About the same 3
   Somewhat better 4
   Much better 5

2. On average, about how many cigarettes <u>per day</u> do you currently smoke?

   1–10 1
   11–20 2
   More than 20 3

3. How concerned are you about the effect of smoking cigarettes on your health?

   Not concerned at all 1
   Somewhat concerned 2
   Very concerned 3

4. How important do you think the health benefits are for someone <u>your age</u> who stops smoking cigarettes?

   Not important at all 1
   Somewhat important 2
   Very important 3

5. How much effort do you think it would take for you to stop smoking cigarettes completely?

   None 1
   A little 2
   Some 3
   Very much 4

corresponding to the response. Response codes are aligned at the right margin and connected by a dot leader. On a paper questionnaire, this format facilitates both recording responses and extracting them for data processing.

Placing code numbers before response choices is not recommended. They detract from reading response choices immediately following the question. Moreover, if code numbers appear before response choices, they may influence how a respondent interprets response choices. For example, respondents might perceive a code of 1 as indicating a "preferred" response. Also, if code numbers are placed before numeric response choices, respondents might be confused regarding which value represents their response.

Placing check boxes or lines where responses are to be indicated by entering a mark, such as ✓ or X, before response choices detracts from reading the response choices. Also, not linking responses to numeric codes incurs additional coding time and costs, and increased risk of coding errors (Chapter 15). Although superscript numeric codes may be placed alongside check boxes or lines, such as □[1], they are more difficult to read than non-superscript numbers.

Instructions

Clear instructions for recording responses must be provided, especially on a self-administered questionnaire. In addition to a general instruction, it may be helpful to present an example, as illustrated in Box 10.7. The example question must not be related to the study topic so it does not influence how a respondent might answer the other questions.

Web Questionnaires

Technological aspects make some unique format features available for a web questionnaire. *Radio buttons*, illustrated in Box 10.8, probably is the most often used feature. The software stores a numeric response code assigned to the button a respondent clicks. Other commonly used web features are drop-down lists, slider bars, and text boxes. In addition, web questionnaire software may control navigating to the next appropriate question, which avoids the amount of instructions respondents must read. Couper (2008) and Dillman et al. (2014) provide extensive and detailed guidance for designing a web questionnaire.

BOX 10.7: EXAMPLE OF HOW TO RECORD A RESPONSE

For example, if your answer to the following questions is **red**, then you would draw a circle around the number **5** as shown below.

In general, which of the following colors would you say is your favorite?

Blue	1
Green	2
Orange	3
Purple	4
Red	⑤
Yellow	6

BOX 10.8: WEB QUESTION EXAMPLE

Compared to other people <u>about your age</u> in general, that is, people who are no more than 5 years younger or older than you, how would you describe your health overall?

○ Much worse
○ Somewhat worse
○ About the same
○ Somewhat better
○ Much better

CHECK YOUR UNDERSTANDING 10.4

- Present guidelines for formatting a structured questionnaire.

Questionnaire Structure

Question Order Overall

Box 10.9 presents guidelines for asking *opening questions*, which are the first few questions in a questionnaire. They should be relevant to the study's topic to affirm the study's legitimacy. However, opening questions should not measure a study's key variables, which generally are best asked after respondents are engaged in the general study topic. Opening questions should apply to all respondents so no one feels that their responses are not valued. Also, they should be easy to answer so as to familiarize respondents with the question–response format and assure them of their ability to participate competently. Opening questions should not address sensitive topics, which are best asked after respondents are comfortable in their role and engaged in the general study topic. Unless it is necessary to screen for eligibility (Chapter 1), opening questions should not ask about a respondent's demographic background. Respondents may regard such questions as invasive

BOX 10.9: GUIDELINES FOR OPENING QUESTIONS

Ensure that opening questions

- are relevant to the main topic,
- do not measure key variables,
- apply to all respondents,
- are easy to answer,
- do not ask about sensitive topics, and
- do not ask about demographic background except for screening purposes.

and not relevant to the study's topic. Virtually always, demographic background questions are best placed at the end of a questionnaire.

Following the opening questions, main topics questions should be grouped by topic to maintain a respondent's focus on one topic at a time. For a self-administered questionnaire, it is helpful to include section headings, such as "Perceptions About Mammography," to communicate transitions across topics. An interview questionnaire may include a brief transitional script, such as "Next, I would like to ask some questions about your perceptions about mammography." To engage respondents in a study's purpose, questions asked early in a questionnaire should address topics respondents are likely to regard as important and interesting. It is best to ask questions about sensitive topics after respondents have become comfortable and committed to the study, which generally is about midway in a questionnaire. When appropriate, topics should be presented in chronological order, which respondents are likely to perceive as being logical. More importantly, a chronological order may aid their recall about key events. For example, child-rearing questions might be ordered from their first- through last-born child.

Question Order Within a Topic

Box 10.10 presents guidelines for ordering questions within a topic. Each topic should be introduced with one or more questions that are easy to answer and not sensitive. When appropriate, chronological order may facilitate information retrieval. For example, questions about a health episode might start with experiencing symptoms, then seeking a diagnosis, undergoing treatment, and recovery/rehabilitation. Cognitive interview strategies discussed previously may be used to assess whether a forward or reverse chronological order is most effective for the topic and target population.

Funnel and inverted funnel sequences typically are used when asking for both an overall rating and ratings of components of a complex factor. In general, neither sequence is considered "correct." Their use depends on a study's goal. A **funnel sequence**, illustrated in Box 10.11, first asks for an overall rating, before it might be influenced by the component ratings. An **inverted funnel sequence** first presents the components to ensure a respondent considers them when forming an overall judgment.

A funnel sequence is administered most effectively in an interview or on the web, where greater control over question order is possible. With a self-administered paper questionnaire, an overall rating may be influenced by respondents also seeing the component

BOX 10.10: QUESTION ORDER WITHIN A TOPIC

- Order questions
  - from easiest to most difficult;
  - from least to most sensitive;
  - chronologically, when appropriate;
  - in a funnel sequence—broad to narrow; or
  - in an inverted funnel sequence—narrow to broad.
- Group questions about related topics that use the same stem and response choices.
- Divide long series of questions with the same stem and response choices into subgroups.
- Vary question types and response tasks to maintain interest.
- Avoid long series of questions that are difficult to answer or ask about a sensitive topic.

> **BOX 10.11: FUNNEL SEQUENCE**
>
> 1. Overall, how would you rate the services you receive at your usual source of health care?
>
> | | Not Satisfied | Slightly Satisfied | Somewhat Satisfied | Mostly Satisfied | Very Satisfied |
> |---|---|---|---|---|---|
> | | 1 | 2 | 3 | 4 | 5 |
>
> 2. Please rate your usual source of health care in terms of each of the following aspects.
>
> | | Not Satisfied | Slightly Satisfied | Somewhat Satisfied | Mostly Satisfied | Very Satisfied |
> |---|---|---|---|---|---|
> | a. Convenience of location | 1 | 2 | 3 | 4 | 5 |
> | b. Convenience of hours | 1 | 2 | 3 | 4 | 5 |
> | c. Ability to get an appointment | 1 | 2 | 3 | 4 | 5 |
> | d. Out-of-pocket costs | 1 | 2 | 3 | 4 | 5 |
> | e. Waiting time at the clinic | 1 | 2 | 3 | 4 | 5 |
> | f. Explanations about your health | 1 | 2 | 3 | 4 | 5 |
> | g. Explanations about treatment | 1 | 2 | 3 | 4 | 5 |

questions before providing an overall rating. A general concern about a funnel sequence is that respondents' answer to an earlier question may influence their answer to subsequent ones, which is especially likely when the questions ask about related topics. For example, if respondents' overall rating of their usual source of health care is based primarily on their opinion about their health care provider, they might rate other components of their usual source of health care similarly to be consistent.

Question 2 in Box 10.11 illustrates grouping questions about related topics that use the same *question stem* ("Please rate your usual source of health care . . .") and response choices. For a self-administered questionnaire, that format is more efficient than presenting the seven component questions (2a–g) individually. However, because the rating scales are presented together, it is more vulnerable to satisficing and nondifferentiation bias, whereby a respondent selects the same scale point for each component. That problem may occur with either a funnel or an inverted funnel. The best strategy for avoiding it is to use a web or interview questionnaire, where the respondent does not see all the component ratings at once.

To avoid monotony and fatigue, long series of questions (e.g., more than 10–15) with the same question stem and response choices should be divided into two or more subgroups. In particular, long series of questions that are difficult to answer or that ask about a sensitive topic should be avoided to reduce respondents' burden and potential discomfort. In general, varying question types and response tasks throughout a questionnaire helps to maintain respondents' interest.

Navigation

Question numbering

It is essential to assign a unique number to each question to guide navigation and data processing. Typically, question numbers are not displayed on a web questionnaire because software controls navigation. However, question numbers are embedded in the software. The best practice is to use continuous numbering across topical sections instead of restarting numbering within each section.

For example, suppose fifteen questions are divided into three sections, with five in section A, six in B, and four in C. The five questions in section A would be numbered 1–5, the six questions in section B would be numbered 6–11, and the four questions in section C would be numbered 12–15. If numbering is restarted within each section, there would be more than one version of each of questions "1" through "4." That is, each section would include a question with those numbers. That format is unnecessarily vulnerable to navigation and data processing errors.

Filter questions and skip patterns

As introduced earlier, a filter question determines which of two or more subsequent questions are appropriate for the respondent to answer. A skip pattern is a branching sequence of one or more questions through which respondents are routed depending on their response to a filter question. In such situations, it is essential to provide clear navigation instructions. As illustrated in Box 10.12, if the response to the filter question, 6a, is "Yes," then the respondent or interviewer is instructed to go to the follow-up question, 6b. If the answer to 6a is "No," then 6b should be *skipped*.

Question 7 applies to all respondents. Thus, respondents who follow the branch from 6a to 6b will continue to question 7. Both instructions are positioned so the respondent or interviewer will see them immediately after recording a response to question 6a. Also, the navigation path is reinforced by the "IF YES" flag above question 6b. It is not necessary to present a lengthy and cumbersome statement such as "If your response to question 6a is 'Yes,' then go to question 6b; if your response is 'No,' then go to question 7."

Skip patterns may become quite complex and involve multiple branches within branches. In such situations, it is essential to review every possible branch combination to ensure every respondent is routed appropriately. Questions should be arranged in an order that minimizes the number and complexity of skip patterns, especially for a paper self-administered questionnaire. It is essential to paginate a multiple-page paper questionnaire so the page and question number may be provided when a respondent must skip to a question on another page. Filter questions should be positioned to avoid referring to a response to a previous question, called a **look-back**, which is cumbersome and prone to errors. Although a web questionnaire may be programmed to perform look-backs, it is best to avoid them because they are prone to programming errors as well.

BOX 10.12: FILTER QUESTION AND SKIP PATTERN
(ALL RESPONDENTS ARE CURRENT CIGARETTE SMOKERS)

6a. Have you ever seriously tried to stop smoking cigarettes, that is, when you did not smoke <u>even one puff for at least 24 hours?</u>

    Yes .... 1 → **Go to Q. 6b**
    No .... 2 → **Go to Q. 7**

IF YES

b. When was the <u>last</u> time you tried to quit smoking and you <u>did not smoke even one puff for at least 24 hours?</u>

    Within the last 30 days 1
    1 to 6 months ago 2
    7 to 12 months ago 3
    More than 1 year ago 4

7. Are you seriously thinking about quitting smoking <u>within the next 30 days</u>?

    Yes 1
    No 2

CHECK YOUR UNDERSTANDING 10.5

- Present guidelines for each of the following:
  - Developing opening questions
  - Question order overall
  - Question order within a topic

Key Points

Standardization

For each respondent, the following aspects are the same:

- Wording of each question
- Response choices for each question
- Order in which questions are presented
- Mode of administration
- Protocol for implementing the data collection mode

The Response Process

Responding to a question requires performing a series of four cognitive tasks:

- Understanding the question
- Retrieving information from memory
- Formulating a summary judgment
- Selecting the most appropriate response choice

Satisficing

Optimizing: A respondent carefully and completely performs each cognitive task.

Satisficing: A respondent does not perform each cognitive task carefully and completely, which may result in an inaccurate or biased response.

Questionnaire Development Process

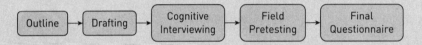

Questionnaire Design and Data Collection Mode

- **Mailed questionnaires** are effective for retrieving information from records and asking questions about sensitive topics.
- **Monitored questionnaires** are effective for controlling the response situation.
- **Web questionnaires** are effective for presenting a complex questionnaire and visual aids.
- **Interview modes (telephone and in-person)** are effective regarding understanding questions, question order control, recorded response quality, and presenting a complex questionnaire.
- **In-person interviews** are effective for controlling the response situation, asking complex questions, presenting a long questionnaire, visual aids, retrieving information from records, and asking open questions.

Questionnaire Format

Key format features include

- type,
- layout, and
- instructions.

Questionnaire Structure

- Opening questions should affirm the study's legitimacy, familiarize respondents with the question–response format, assure them of their ability to participate competently, and engage them in the general study topic.

- Main questions should be grouped by topic, from most to least relevant and interesting, from least to most sensitive, and in chronological order when appropriate.
- Within a topic, questions should flow from easiest to most difficult, from least to most sensitive, and in chronological order when appropriate.
- Question types and response tasks should be varied to maintain interest.
- Questions should be numbered to guide navigation and data processing.
- A filter question determines which of two or more subsequent questions are appropriate for the respondent to answer.
- A skip pattern is a branching sequence of one or more questions through which individual respondents are routed depending on their response to a filter question.

Review and Apply

1. Prepare an outline for a structured questionnaire based on the variable list and variable chart you prepared in the "Review and Apply" section of Chapter 9. See Box 10.1 as an example. Your outline should show
   - the order of topics overall,
   - the order of questions within each topic, and
   - navigation notation.
2. Select a data collection mode using guidance from Table 10.2 and list that mode's advantages and disadvantages for collecting your data from your target population.
3. Review how to use the formatting tools in your preferred word processing software. Reproduce the examples in Box 10.6, Box 10.11, and Box 10.12.
4. Reproduce the examples in Box 10.6, Box 10.11, and Box 10.12 using web survey software. If your school does not provide free access to any web questionnaire software, go to one of the sites listed below or another source of your choice.

   www.qualtrics.com

   www.surveymonkey.com

   www.surveygizmo.com

Study Further

Blair, J., Czaja, R. F., & Blair, E. A. (2014). *Designing surveys: A guide to decisions and procedures*. Los Angeles, CA: Sage.

Bradburn, N. M., Sudman, S., & Wansink, B. (2004). *Asking questions: The definitive guide to questionnaire design—for market research, political polls, and social and health questionnaires*. San Francisco, CA: Jossey-Bass.

Dillman, D. A., Smyth, J. D., & Christian, L. M. (2014). *Internet, phone, mail, and mixed-mode surveys: The tailored design method*. Hoboken, NJ: Wiley.

Presser, S., Rothgeb, J. M., Couper, M. P., Lessler, J. T., Martin, E., Martin, J., & Singer, E. (Eds.). (2004). *Methods for testing and evaluating survey questionnaires*. Hoboken, NJ: Wiley.

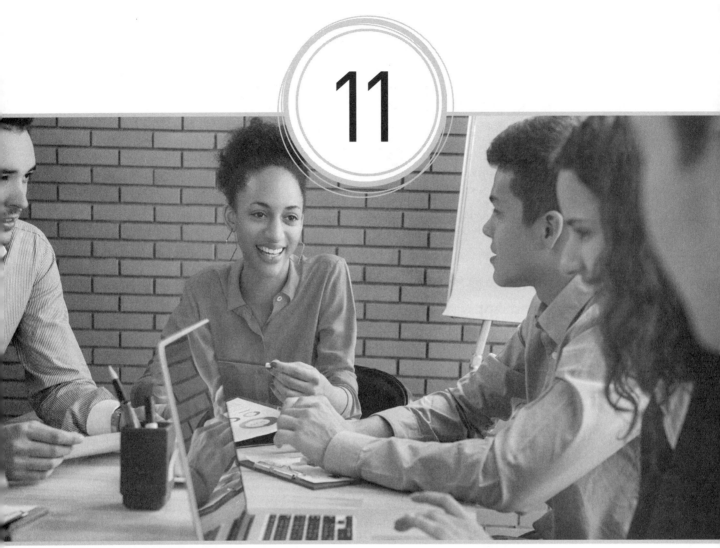

11

Writing Survey Questions

Chapter Outline

Overview
Learning Objectives
Types of Questions
    Closed Questions
    Open Questions
Question Wording
    Vocabulary
    Tone
    Problem Words
Question Structure
    Short and Simple
    Use Complete Sentences
    Ask One Question at a Time
    Do Not Use Double Negatives
    Specify Conditions at the Beginning
    Do Not Ask Biased Questions
    Sensitive Topics
Response Choices
    General Guidelines
    Nominal Level
    Ordinal Level
    Interval/Ratio Level
Key Points

Learning Objectives

After studying Chapter 11, the reader should be able to:

- Identify conditions appropriate for closed and open questions
- Compose questions using appropriate vocabulary and tone
- Avoid using "problem words"
- Compose questions that are clear, specific, and unbiased
- Compose effective questions about sensitive topics
- Compose clear, specific, and unbiased closed-question response choices

Overview

Results from a poorly designed structured questionnaire may not be interpreted with confidence. It is critical to communicate clearly the information that is being requested so it is understood the same way by all respondents. Moreover, questions and response choices must be presented in a neutral manner to avoid potential bias. Writing questions for a structured questionnaire is demanding of time and effort. Key elements of writing questions are wording, structure, and response choices. This chapter presents guidelines and strategies for writing questions to obtain valid and reliable responses to questions in a structured questionnaire.

Types of Questions

There are two basic types of questions, closed and open. Box 11.1 depicts examples of closed and open questions, both of which ask a respondent to report which fresh fruit(s) they ate during the past two weeks. Most questions in a structured questionnaire use a closed-response format (also called "closed-ended") that presents a predetermined set of response choices. Nevertheless, open questions (also called "open-ended"), which ask respondents to answer in their own words, may provide insight into the research problem that is not attainable from closed questions.

BOX 11.1: CLOSED AND OPEN QUESTION EXAMPLES

Closed

During the past 2 weeks, what <u>fresh</u> fruits did you eat?

Did you eat any fresh . . .

	Yes	No
a. Apples?	1	2
b. Bananas?	1	2
c. Grapes?	1	2
d. Oranges?	1	2
e. Pineapple?	1	2
f. Strawberries?	1	2
g. Watermelon?	1	2
h. Other fruit? (*specify*)	1	2
_____	1	2

Open

During the past 2 weeks, what <u>fresh</u> fruits did you eat?

_____

_____

_____

Closed Questions

Advantages

The main advantages of **closed questions** are

- standardization,
- facilitation of data processing and analysis,
- administration, and
- data quality.

The primary advantage of closed questions is standardization (Chapter 10), which ensures responses will reflect the same construct and be expressed in the same unit(s) of measure. A closed question achieves standardization by presenting to each respondent the *same*

- question wording,
- response choice wording,
- response choice format, and
- response choice order.

Standardization enhances comparisons across respondents and time. Closed questions facilitate data processing and analysis by being **precoded**, whereby a numeric code value is assigned to each response choice in advance of administering a questionnaire (Chapter 10). Closed questions typically are quick and easy to administer, which reduces the respondent and interviewer burdens. Also, because respondents are not required to formulate a response in their own words, closed questions reduce the cognitive response burden (Chapter 10), which minimizes the likelihood of item nonresponse. Presenting response choices enhances a respondent's understanding of a question. Response choices also facilitate information retrieval by helping respondents consider responses they might overlook, such as when recalling details about a past event. Also, respondents may be more comfortable answering questions about a sensitive topic when their task is confined to selecting the most appropriate response choice rather than answering in their own words (Tourangeau & Yan, 2007).

Disadvantages

The main disadvantages of closed questions are

- construction,
- vulnerability to satisficing, and
- restriction of spontaneity.

As discussed in Chapter 9 regarding ordinal scales, it is challenging to determine the appropriate number and labeling of response choices. Presenting predetermined response choices is vulnerable to satisficing, whereby a respondent might not take care to select the most appropriate response choice (Chapter 10). Closed questions limit spontaneity and do not capture "colorful" aspects of opinions or experiences, as is possible when respondents answer open questions in their own words.

Open Questions

The most common type of **open question** is *completely* open, as illustrated by question 1 in Box 11.2. Question 2 illustrates a *limited* open question that asks a respondent for a certain number of responses, one in this instance. The intent is to capture the most salient/important factor(s) related to the topic. In other situations, more than one response might be requested. For example, question 2 might ask for the *three* main reasons respondents' families moved into their neighborhood. The number of responses to request depends on a study's purpose, and on the number of responses it is reasonable to expect respondents will be able and willing to provide.

BOX 11.2: OPEN QUESTIONS

1. What signs or symptoms do you think suggest that a person is an alcoholic?
   _____
   _____
   _____

2. What is the <u>one main reason</u> why your family moved into this neighborhood?
   _____
   _____
   _____

An interviewer is trained to probe for clarity and completeness of a response. A key formatting aspect for a paper questionnaire is to provide sufficient space to record an entire response to an open question. Double spacing should be used when more than one line is presented to enhance readability and coding. In a self-administered questionnaire, the length and number of lines communicates an expectation of the extent of a response. This aspect should be assessed during field pretesting. Presenting a single, short line implies a brief response is expected or desired. If the average response is more extensive, respondents might enter abbreviated responses, cram in long responses that might be illegible, or not respond at all. If too much space is provided, to avoid appearing uninformed about the topic respondents might pad their response with extraneous information or not respond at all. An advantage of a web questionnaire is the response space may be expandable to accommodate as much information as a respondent enters.

Advantages

The main advantages of open questions are they

- enhance spontaneity,
- imply that a respondent's true feelings are valued, and
- capture colorful aspects of a respondent's opinion or experience.

Not restricting responses to predetermined choices allows for spontaneity. Also, it implies that a respondent's true feelings are valued. Recording responses in respondents' own words facilitates capturing the full range and nature of their expression about a topic. Moreover, open question responses often may be quoted in reports to illustrate respondents' concerns, reactions, and so on.

Disadvantages

The main disadvantages of open questions are

- heavy administration burden,
- data processing is challenging, and
- data analysis is challenging.

Regardless of the data collection mode, open questions place a heavy burden on respondents, who must recall information without the aid of response choices and formulate responses in their own words. Nonresponse to open questions generally is high because respondents often are not comfortable or able to formulate a response in their own words on demand. Moreover, responses in a self-administered questionnaire may be illegible (paper), incomplete, vague, and not relevant to the question. Although interviews are the most effective mode for asking open questions, they are expensive and time-consuming. Moreover, open questions place a heavy burden on interviewers, who must ask questions, record unstructured responses verbatim, and employ probes to obtain a clear, relevant, and complete response.

Processing responses to open questions is challenging because they must be coded, which is time-consuming and expensive. In addition, it typically is challenging to interpret the meaning of open responses and group them into categories for analysis. Moreover, **multiple responses** might be given when only one is requested. For example, if cigarette smokers are asked for the "one main reason" why they would consider stopping smoking, they might provide several reasons without indicating which one is most salient.

Key Concept

Questionnaire wording is critical for obtaining reliable and valid responses.

CHECK YOUR UNDERSTANDING 11.1

- Describe the main advantages and disadvantages of each of the following:
  - Closed questions
  - Open questions

Question Wording

Question wording is critical for obtaining reliable and valid responses. A question must communicate clearly what information is being requested and do so in a way that its meaning is understood the same way by all respondents.

Vocabulary

Vocabulary guidelines for question wording are to

- use words that are familiar and simple,
- avoid or define technical terms and professional jargon,
- avoid or define abbreviations, and
- use slang cautiously and only when necessary.

To ensure questions are understood similarly by all respondents, they must be written so they are understood by those at the lowest literacy level. In general, that is accomplished by using words that are simple and familiar. For example, the question

"Have you ever been told by a doctor or other health professional that you have *hypertension*?"

may be restated using more universally understood wording as

"Have you ever been told by a doctor or other health professional that you have *high blood pressure*?"

An alternative approach is to define a technical term. For example, the two preceding questions might be combined as

"Have you ever been told by a doctor or other health professional that you have *high blood pressure, also called hypertension*?"

It is best to present a definition *before* introducing the term that is being defined. This is especially important in an interview, where a respondent typically does not see the questions. If an unfamiliar term is presented first, a respondent might engage in thinking about what it could mean instead of listening to the definition that follows. Also, it is best not to place a definition in parentheses, such as

"Have you ever been told by a doctor or other health professional that you have hypertension (high blood pressure)?"

First, this method presents the term before its definition. Second, parenthetical terms might appear unimportant and be ignored on a self-administered questionnaire. Finally, parentheses should not be used in an interview questionnaire because it is awkward for an interviewer to read a parenthetical word or phrase aloud. Consequently, interviewers must develop their own script for presenting a parenthetical term, or they might choose to ignore it. Instead, to maintain standardization of question wording, an otherwise parenthetical term should be incorporated into the question, as described in the hypertension example.

Sometimes it is necessary to define a term that is familiar to respondents, such as *drinking alcohol*, so the term's meaning in a study's context is clear. Moreover, even if a term is familiar to respondents, they might hold different interpretations of its meaning. For example, the National Health Interview Survey adult questionnaire (Centers for Disease Control and Prevention, 2018f) introduces questions about alcohol consumption as follows:

"These next questions are about drinking alcoholic beverages. Included are liquor such as whiskey or gin, beer, wine, wine coolers, and any other type of alcoholic beverage."

This approach ensures that respondents will not restrict the meaning of "drinking alcoholic beverages" to mean drinking only whiskey, beer, or wine. Also, the phrase "any other type of alcoholic beverage" is intended to include alcoholic beverages that the question does not mention specifically, such as brandy and malt liquor.

Abbreviations should be avoided or defined. Although they are efficient, there are two potential problems with abbreviations. First, they are not necessarily unique to a particular referent. For example, depending on one's perspective, "the AMA" may refer to the American Medical Association, the American Marketing Association, or the American Motorcyclist Association. If an abbreviation is used, it should be defined to ensure respondents have a clear and mutual understanding of its referent. As in the hypertension example, the definition should be presented before the abbreviation. For example, a group of related questions might be introduced as follows:

"The next questions are about the human immunodeficiency virus, commonly referred to as HIV."

Then respondents might be asked

"Have you ever been tested for the human immunodeficiency virus, that is, HIV?"

This pattern reinforces the abbreviation's definition. For efficiency, subsequent questions may then use the HIV abbreviation.

It is best not to use slang, or so-called street terms, because terms referring to the same concept may vary across subgroups and within groups over time. Respondents might react to the use of an incorrect or out-of-date term as confusing or even offensive. If deemed necessary, the use of slang should be assessed by methods such as cognitive interviewing and field pretesting.

Tone

Questions should be written using a respectful tone. A question never should sound demanding, especially when it has a substantial response burden. For example, instead of saying

"Rate your usual source of health care . . ."

it is better to say

"Please rate your usual source of health care . . ."

Questions for interviews must use a conversational tone to establish and maintain rapport. However, questions should not be written in a manner that sounds overly familiar, folksy, or streetwise, which may create a condescending or patronizing impression. At the opposite extreme, questions should not be written in an overly sophisticated manner, which unnecessarily increases the respondent's burden, may cause confusion, and may appear elitist. For example, instead of asking

"What is the approximate distance from your residence to the most proximate hospital?"

it is better to ask

"About how far from your home is the nearest hospital?"

Problem Words

Box 11.3 presents a list of problem wording attributes that may introduce confusion and/or bias in a question. Words with ambiguous meanings should be avoided or made specific by adding an appropriate modifier. For example, *government* is a broad term, for which the intended level (city, county, state, or national) should be specified. Also, words that have multiple meanings should be avoided. For example, a rating of *fair* on an ordinal scale may indicate a somewhat low/negative, a moderate/neutral, or a somewhat high/positive position. Even a common preposition, such as *on*, may lead to an unintended interpretation. For example,

"Have you ever attended a class *on* illegal drugs?"

might not be interpreted as intended: to ask if respondents ever attended a class *about* illegal drugs. Alternatively, it might be interpreted as asking if they ever attended a class *about any subject while under the influence of any* illegal drugs. The remedy is to use specific wording, replacing *on* with *about*:

"Have you ever attended a class *about* illegal drugs?"

A related problem may arise with words that are intended figuratively but may be interpreted literally. For example, in response to

"When was the last time you saw your primary care physician?"

respondents might say "Yesterday," referring to having encountered—that is, they "saw"—their primary care physician in a supermarket.

As Payne (1951) observed, some words that appear interchangeable may be nonsynonymous and have different connotations. In particular, he describes differences among *should*, *could*, and *might*. *Should* indicates a *need*, *could* indicates a *possibility*, and *might* indicates a *probability*. Accordingly, the following three questions have different meanings and will obtain different responses.

"Do you think the police *should* do something about gang violence in this community?"

BOX 11.3: BEWARE OF PROBLEM WORDS

- Words with ambiguous meaning
- Words with multiple meanings
- Words with figurative versus literal meanings
- Nonsynonymous words
- Homophones
- Extreme terms
- Emotionally loaded terms/phrases

"Do you think the police *could* do something about gang violence in this community?"

"Do you think the police *might* do something about gang violence in this community?"

For an interview questionnaire, it is important to beware of words, called "homophones," which sound the same as other words but have different meanings. In such situations, either a different word should be used, or a definition should be provided. For example, it would not be obvious whether an interviewer is asking about an *oral* or *aural* examination. Extreme terms, such as *all*, *always*, *completely*, and *never*, should be avoided. Most responses are likely to be "No" to a question such as

"Do you think the police are doing *all* they can to prevent gang violence in this community?"

An example of a better strategy would be to ask for a rating of how effective the police are in preventing gang violence. Finally, emotionally loaded terms such as *tree hugger*, *politicians*, and *patriotic* should be avoided. For example, instead of asking

"Do you think a professional athlete who does not stand while the national anthem is performed is patriotic or not patriotic?"

it is better to ask

"Do you think it is appropriate or not appropriate for a professional athlete not to stand while the national anthem is performed?"

CHECK YOUR UNDERSTANDING 11.2

- Present some guidelines for question wording regarding each of the following aspects:
  - Vocabulary
  - Tone
  - Problem words

Question Structure

Several aspects of a question's structure may influence the reliability and validity of responses. Box 11.4 presents question structure guidelines that are discussed in the following sections.

Short and Simple

Short and simple questions facilitate a respondent's understanding. It is especially important for telephone interview questions to be short and simple because a respondent is not able to see them. For a long or complex question, in-person interview respondents may be presented a card with the question and response choices so they may read silently

BOX 11.4: QUESTION STRUCTURE GUIDELINES

- Ensure questions are short and simple.
- Use complete sentences.
- Ask one question at a time.
- Do not use double negatives.
- Specify conditions at the beginning.
- Do not ask biased questions.

as an interviewer reads it aloud. Nevertheless, for both telephone and in-person interviews, long and complex questions are more difficult for interviewers to read aloud, as well as difficult for respondents to understand. An initially long question often may be rewritten to be more compact and/or broken into parts.

For example, Box 11.5 presents an abbreviated version of a question from an early draft of a self-administered questionnaire to be administered to sixth-grade students for a study about plate waste in a school lunch program (Forrestal, Issel, Kviz, & Chávez, 2008). The question is long and complex. Moreover, it is likely to be confusing for sixth-grade students.

Box 11.6 presents a revised version of the question. The revision still contains all of the components in the early draft. However, it presents each component separately, and they are set off by additional line spacing (1.5 lines). Moreover, the order in which the components are presented is changed to follow a logical progression. The reminder that not all foods are served at every lunch is presented after the initial reference to the food list. Next,

BOX 11.5: DRAFT OF A SCHOOL LUNCH PLATE WASTE QUESTION

15. A list of foods that are served in the school lunch program is below. For foods you eat, please circle the number for how much of your serving you usually throw away. If you do not eat anything from one of the categories, please circle the number for "I Don't Eat This Food." Not all foods are served at every lunch, so please answer based on the days when you are served that item.

	Hardly Any or None	Less Than Half	About Half	More Than Half	All or Almost All	I Don't Eat This Food
a. Fresh fruit	1	2	3	4	5	9
b. Salad or raw vegetables	1	2	3	4	5	9
c. Desserts	1	2	3	4	5	9

BOX 11.6: REVISED SCHOOL LUNCH PLATE WASTE QUESTION

15. A list of foods that are served in the school lunch program is below.

    Not all foods are served at every lunch, so please answer based on the days when you are served that item.

    If you do not eat <u>anything</u> from one of the categories, please circle the number for "I don't eat this food."

    <u>For foods you eat</u>, please circle the number for how much of your serving you <u>usually throw away</u>.

	Hardly Any or <u>None</u>	Less <u>Than Half</u>	About <u>Half</u>	More Than <u>Half</u>	All or Almost <u>All</u>	I Don't Eat <u>This Food</u>
a. Fresh fruit	1	2	3	4	5	9
b. Salad or raw vegetables	1	2	3	4	5	9
c. Desserts	1	2	3	4	5	9

respondents are told what to do if they do not eat anything from one of the food categories. Last, they are instructed how to record their responses about the foods they do eat. In addition, key words and phrases are underlined for emphasis. Response choice labels were made easier to read by capitalizing only the first word for each label instead of capitalizing every word. Finally, the response choice "I don't eat this food" is separated from the others by a vertical line to indicate it is not part of the ordinal response scale.

Use Complete Sentences

A question should be presented as a complete sentence, with correct grammar and spelling. Variable names should not be presented as questions, such as "Age?" "Sex?" or "Race?" Instead, a question should be asked, such as "What is your age?" In a self-administered questionnaire, presenting variable names instead of asking questions creates an appearance of completing a form. In an interview, it sounds demanding and aloof.

Ask One Question at a Time

Only one question should be asked at a time. A **compound question**, also called a "double-barreled" question, which includes more than one concept, is confusing, both for respondents to understand what they are being asked and for researchers to interpret their response. Moreover, a respondent is likely not to answer such a question, especially when it is presented in a self-administered questionnaire.

For example,

"Please rate how clearly your health care provider explained your diagnosis and treatment plan."

asks two questions. It asks respondents to rate (1) the clarity of the diagnosis explanation and (2) the clarity of the treatment plan explanation. The question is confusing, and it is not possible to interpret a response reliably. For example, if respondents provide a rating of 3 on a 5-point ordinal scale, it might indicate they rated both explanations at that level. However, it might indicate their rating for only one explanation, and it is not possible to know which one they rated. Still another possibility is a rating of 3 is an "average," such as respondents might consider one explanation as a 1 and the other as a 5.

Do Not Use Double Negatives

Double-negative terminology, whereby two negative terms indicate a positive condition, never should be used. Double negatives are not necessary, they are confusing, and they compromise a response's reliability. For example, consider the following question:

"Do you think recreational marijuana use should not be illegal?"

The double negative "should not be illegal" is a positive condition, that is, "legal." However, respondents would have to respond negatively, that is, "No," if they think recreational marijuana should be legal. Moreover, some respondents might mistakenly respond "Yes," thinking they are affirming legal recreational marijuana use. Restating the question without the double negative, it would ask

"Do you think recreational marijuana use should be legal?"

Now, the question and responses are clear. If respondents think recreational marijuana use should be legal, they would respond "Yes." If they think recreational marijuana use should not be legal, they would respond "No."

Specify Conditions at the Beginning

A condition for responding to a question should be specified at the beginning. When a condition is specified at or near the end of a question, respondents might formulate their responses prematurely and not take the condition into consideration. A common type of condition is a reference comparison, such as "Compared to other people about your age . . ." or "Compared to a year ago . . ." Inclusions and exclusions also are common types of condition. An example of an inclusion condition is

"Including yourself, how many adults currently live in this household?"

Presenting the inclusion at the question's beginning helps to ensure respondents will include themselves and not report only the number of other adults living in their household. An example of an exclusion condition is

"Not counting special occasions, about how often do you drink red wine at home?"

The condition in this question excludes atypical situations ("special occasions"). Sometimes an exclusion may be expressed indirectly, such as

"If a child has been healthy, how would you rate the importance for that child to get an immunization?"

This question excludes considering a child who has not been healthy.

A time frame is another common type of exclusion. It may be indicated generally, such as "During a typical week . . . ," or specifically, such as "During the past 7 days . . ." Sudman and Bradburn (1982) recommend that specifying a time period should be guided by the salience of the topic and the frequency of the event. A longer time period (e.g., one year) may be referenced for high-salience, less frequent events such as being injured in an automobile collision. A shorter time period should be used for lower-salience, more frequent events such as how often the respondent eats French fries.

Do Not Ask Biased Questions

In addition to bias that may result from wording (e.g., extreme or emotionally loaded terms), various aspects of a question's structure may introduce bias by indicating one or more responses are expected, condoned, or preferred.

Response choices

Just as emotionally loaded terms should not be used in a question, they also should not be used in response choices. For example, a question about causes of substance abuse among high school students should not include a response choice such as "Irresponsible parents." Instead, nonjudgmental wording should be used, such as "The way parents raise their children."

Another way a question may be biased is if not all response choices are presented. For instance, when asking a respondent to provide a rating on an ordinal scale, reference should be made to the entire scale range. The question

"How effective do you think the police have been in addressing gang violence in your community?"

mentions only the positive/highest end of the scale, "effective." A better formulation is

"On a scale from 1 to 5, where 1 is *not effective* and 5 is *very effective*, how would you rate the police in addressing gang violence in your community?"

This question refers to the entire scale range and requests a rating in a neutral manner by not asking "How effective . . ." Both response choices for a dichotomous response question always should be presented. For example,

"Do you favor a national health insurance program?"

mentions only the positive opinion, "favor," and is likely to obtain more "Yes" responses than if the negative response also is presented. Moreover, a response of "No" cannot be interpreted reliably as indicating a respondent opposes national health insurance. "No" could also mean a respondent is undecided, has mixed feelings, or does not care about national health insurance. A better formulation is

"Do you favor or oppose national health insurance?"

This question is balanced by presenting both response options. Also, it explicitly presents "Favor" and "Oppose" as response choices, which is more specific than implying a "Yes" or "No" response.

Interval-/ratio-level response choices may imply certain levels are expected or socially undesirable. For example, consider a question that asks respondents who drink alcoholic beverages how many drinks of alcohol they had during the past seven days. The following response choices imply that a low number is expected:

1 drink

2 drinks

3 drinks

4 drinks

5 drinks

More than 5 drinks

In contrast, the following response choices imply that a high number is expected:

1 to 5 drinks

6 to 10 drinks

11 to 20 drinks

More than 20 drinks

An alternative strategy is to ask two questions, where the first one asks whether during the past seven days respondents had one of the following:

5 drinks or fewer

More than 5 drinks

Then, according to the response, a follow-up question would ask respondents to provide a more detailed response, such as the following:

If 5 drinks or less	If more than 5 drinks
1 drink	6 to 10 drinks
2 drinks	11 to 20 drinks
3 drinks	More than 20 drinks
4 drinks	
5 drinks	

Providing information

A question may be biased by providing information about an issue that a respondent might not previously have known. For example, suppose the following question is asked in a survey of African American women:

"The risk of dying from breast cancer is especially high for African American women. On a scale from 1 to 5, with 1 being *not concerned* and 5 being *very concerned*, how would you rate your concern about getting breast cancer?"

The information about a high risk of dying might lead respondents to rate their concern higher than they might otherwise.

Citing authority

A related problem is introduced by citing an authority regarding an issue. For example,

"Doctors and other health professionals recommend not smoking cigarettes because it increases risks for cancer, heart disease, and other serious health problems. What do you think, is smoking cigarettes harmful to a person's health or not?"

This formulation might pressure respondents to agree with the cited authority. Two alternative strategies are possible. First, respondents may simply be asked whether they think smoking cigarettes is or is not harmful to a person's health. A variation on this strategy is to ask for an ordinal rating of how likely it is that smoking cigarettes is harmful to a person's health.

One-sided

Presenting only one side of an issue may lead a respondent to an unbalanced assessment that does not take other positions into consideration. For example, a question might present an argument in favor of childhood immunizations and ask if respondents favor or oppose childhood immunizations. Instead, arguments both in favor of and against an issue should be presented, such as "Some people say children should be immunized because.... Other people say children should not be immunized because.... What do you think?"

Presenting examples

Presenting examples may influence how respondents answer a question. For instance,

"Do you think vegetables, like broccoli, should be included in your child's diet?"

might focus respondents' attention on the example, excluding other vegetables. In effect, respondents might interpret the question as asking if broccoli specifically should be included in their child's diet. Although the child might like other vegetables, if he or she does not like broccoli, respondents might answer "No." It would not be reliable to conclude respondents do not think any vegetables should be included in their child's diet.

Assumptions

A question may be biased by stating or implying an assumption about respondents' status, attitude, or behavior. For example,

"How long does it usually take to travel from your home to your usual source of health care?"

assumes respondents have a usual health care source. Considering that having one is socially desirable and apparently expected by the researcher, even if respondents do not have a usual health care source, they might respond in terms of traveling to where they might go if they need health care. The solution to this problem is first to ask a filter question to determine if the respondent has a usual source of health care.

Sensitive Topics

Special consideration should be given to questions about sensitive topics, which may make a respondent feel uncomfortable, embarrassed, or threatened. The range of potentially sensitive topics is wide. Some are negative in nature, such as unethical and illegal behavior, and socially undesirable attitudes, such as racial prejudice. Others may be personally upsetting, such as being a victim of or witness to a crime. Some are personal and private, such as sexual behavior, a medical diagnosis, and income. Still others may be positive and socially desirable, such as voting or being a good neighbor. Guidelines for asking questions about sensitive topics are to

- introduce the topic,
- generalize negative conditions,
- make responses acceptable,
- provide an excuse, and
- ask for an opinion.

Introduce the topic

A sensitive topic should be introduced by a transitional statement so a respondent is prepared to address it and does not feel ambushed. For example, a sensitive topic may be introduced simply by a statement such as "The next questions are about . . ." In addition, it is helpful to provide a brief explanation for asking about a sensitive topic, acknowledge that the topic is a sensitive one, and reassure the respondents that their responses will be confidential.

Generalize negative conditions

Respondents' concern about answering truthfully to a question about a sensitive topic may be reduced by generalizing negative responses so they do not feel they are being singled out. For example, a respondent's comfort in responding to a question about a negative condition may be enhanced by beginning a question with a generalization, such as "Many parents find it difficult to keep track of their children's immunization schedule. . . ."

Make responses acceptable

A question about a sensitive topic may be made less threatening by making a negative response acceptable. For example, in a follow-up with smoking cessation program participants 30 days after completing the program, some participants might be reluctant to admit that they did not stop smoking. Instead of asking "Did you stop smoking since the program ended?" the interviewer might ease their discomfort by asking "Have you managed to stop smoking since the program ended?" Using *managed* implies that it is understood that stopping smoking is difficult and not everyone is able to do it.

Provide an excuse

Another strategy to reduce a respondent's response anxiety about a sensitive topic is to build an excuse into a question. For example,

"Sometimes things happen that make it difficult for people to stay on their diet all the time. During the past seven days, was there a time when you were not able to stay on your diet?"

This example refers to not maintaining a diet as an occasional event, attributes it to external causes, and refers to not being able to perform the behavior instead of being disparaging (e.g., "failing"). An excuse should not include an example, such as

"Sometimes it is difficult is to stay on a diet because of attending a special event, such as a birthday party."

If respondents did not participate in such an event recently, they are likely not to regard it as an excuse that applies to them. Consequently, discomfort due to reporting that they did not maintain their diet might be increased because it appears to be inexcusable if the example does not apply to them.

Ask for an opinion

Respondents may be anxious about responding to knowledge questions, especially ones on topics about which they think they should be well informed. They might avoid such anxiety and potential embarrassment by not responding or saying "I don't know." Knowledge questions should not appear as a test and imply there are right and wrong answers, such as

"Which of the following are risk factors for heart disease?"

"True/false" response choices also imply a question is a test for which there are right and wrong answers. Unless the intention is to apply a test, it is better to ask for an opinion, such as

"In your opinion, how likely is drinking alcohol while pregnant to cause health problems for the mother's baby?"

A related strategy is to present opposing views and ask respondents which one most closely describes their view. For example,

"Some people say if a woman drinks alcohol while she is pregnant, it will cause health problems for her baby. Other people say. . . . What do you think?"

> ### CHECK YOUR UNDERSTANDING 11.3
>
> - Other than strategies for questions about sensitive topics, present guidelines for question structure to avoid biasing responses.
> - What are some guidelines for asking questions about sensitive topics?

Response Choices

General Guidelines

There are several aspects of response choices that must be considered when developing a closed-response question. The following are guidelines for developing closed question response choices:

- Be responsive to the question.
- Present one response at a time.

- Ensure response choices are
  - unidimensional,
  - exclusive,
  - exhaustive, and
  - short and simple.
- Use "Don't know" cautiously.

Be responsive to the question

First and foremost, response choices must be responsive to the question. Otherwise, respondents' understanding of the question might be confused, they might not answer it, or their response might not be interpreted reliably. For example, consider the following question.

> When did you have your last mammogram?
>> I was experiencing health problems.
>> It was a regularly scheduled exam.
>> My doctor told me it was time.

The question asks for a *time*, such as the approximate date or how long ago the respondent had her last mammogram. However, the response choices refer to reasons or occasions that prompted her to have her last mammogram.

Present one response at a time

Response choices should not be **double-barreled**, such that responses to more than one question are presented at a time. For example, consider the following question.

> How would you describe your health care provider's explanation of your treatment?
>> Clear and thorough
>> Clear but not thorough
>> Not clear but thorough
>> Not clear and not thorough

The response choices are responsive to two different questions, which should be asked separately. As presented in the example, the response choices are unnecessarily complex and potentially confusing.

Another version of this problem is that a question should not be implied by embedding it among the response choices for another question. For example:

> Did you attend the presentation about binge drinking alcohol?
>> Yes, it was very helpful.
>> Yes, it was somewhat helpful.
>> Yes, but it was not helpful.
>> I did not attend.

This question asks for a simple "Yes/No" response regarding whether a respondent did or did not attend the presentation about binge drinking alcohol. However, the first three response choices are compound. They include an assessment of helpfulness in response to a question that was not asked. This format increases the respondent's burden. Also, it complicates processing and analysis because some response choices measure two variables. A better strategy is to first present a filter question asking if respondents attended the presentation. Then follow up with those who attended by asking them to assess the presentation's helpfulness.

Unidimensional

Response choices must refer to a single dimension. For example, consider the following question.

How would you describe your health care provider's explanation of your treatment?
   Clear
   Respectful
   Satisfactory

The response choices refer to three different dimensions of a health care provider's explanation. As presented, respondents may evaluate their health care provider on only one aspect. Moreover, there is no provision for respondents to reply that the explanation was not clear, not respectful, or not satisfactory. The solution is to ask three separate questions addressing the three dimensions of clarity, respect, and satisfaction.

Another version of this problem is that when a respondent is asked to provide a rating using an ordinal scale, the scale points should refer to a single dimension. For example, suppose respondents are asked to rate their health care provider's explanation of their treatment using an ordinal scale ranging from *Not clear* to *Very thorough*. One end of the scale refers to clarity while the other refers to thoroughness. Either the scale labels should be changed to refer to only clarity or thoroughness, or two questions should be asked, one about clarity and the other about thoroughness.

When appropriate, a unit of measure should be specified. For example, response choices for the frequency of performing a behavior should indicate whether the response is to be expressed in terms of number of times per day, per week, per month, and so on. Also, it is important not to confuse frequency and periodicity when asking about behaviors or events. For example, consider the following question.

How often does your health care provider ask you about your cigarette smoking?
   Never
   Sometimes
   Regularly
   Always

The response choices "Never," "Sometimes," and "Always" refer to ordinal levels of frequency. However, "Regularly" does not refer to a frequency. Instead, it refers to periodicity. Although sometimes a respondent or question writer may think "Regularly" means "Frequently," it does not. Indeed, "Regularly" could be infrequent.

Exclusive

Response choices must be exclusive, meaning they do not overlap with each other. Otherwise, respondents' answers might fall in more than one category. Consequently, respondents might select more than one choice, especially on a paper self-administered questionnaire. Alternatively, they might be confused and decide not to respond to the question. Typically, interval/ratio response choices are most susceptible to overlapping response choices. For example, age categories "18 to 30" and "30 to 45" both include age 30. Instead, they should be exclusive, such as "18 to 30" and "31 to 45." An ordinal example of overlapping response choices is that education categories might overlap. For instance, both "Some high school" and "1 to 3 years of high school" may apply to the same respondents. A nominal-level example is that employment status categories might overlap. For instance, respondents may be both "Retired" and "Employed full-time" or "Employed part-time." Thus, separate questions should be asked to determine if respondents are retired and if they are employed.

Exhaustive

Response choices must be exhaustive, such that there is an appropriate one for every respondent. Otherwise, respondents might select a response choice they consider is nearest to their answer but is not accurate. Alternatively, they might not respond to the question. Typically, the potential for nonexhaustive response choices occurs for interval/ratio response choices. For example, time categories "Less than 1 year ago" and "2 to 3 years ago" have a gap that excludes "1 year ago." Instead, they should be presented as "Less than 1 year ago" and "1 to 3 years ago" or "1 year ago or less" and "2 to 3 years ago." Ordinal response choices also might have gaps, such as "Not satisfied," "Mostly satisfied," and "Very satisfied," which do not provide an option for a respondent who feels "Slightly satisfied" or "Somewhat satisfied." The typical strategy for nominal response choices to be exhaustive is to include an "Other" category to capture responses that do not fit any of the specific response choices that are offered, as illustrated in the following example.

> If you were to choose <u>only one</u>, what would you say is your <u>favorite</u> fresh fruit?
> Apples
> Bananas
> Grapes
> Oranges
> Strawberries
> Another fruit (*please specify*)
> _____

Short and simple

Individual response choices should be as short and simple as possible. They should use as few words as necessary, and ones that are familiar and unambiguous. Similar to the guideline for wording questions, it is especially important for response choices to be short and simple for an interview. Also, response choices should not ask for more detail than is necessary to address the research question, or than is reasonable to expect respondents will be able and willing to provide.

Use "Don't know" cautiously

There is debate about whether and when to offer a "Don't know" or similar response choice, such as "Not sure" or "Don't remember" (Krosnick & Presser, 2010). Chapter 9 presented guidance on this matter regarding ordinal scales. It is advisable to offer a "Don't know" response choice for a question about knowledge or a fact for which it is plausible respondents might not know the answer, or they might not be able to answer with the degree of accuracy specified in response choices. Examples of such questions are

"How far is the nearest hospital from your home?" and

"When was the last time you visited a dentist to have a cavity filled?"

In general, it might be important to learn that respondents do not know such information. If a "Don't know" option is not offered, they might satisfice by selecting a response choice that does not represent their true answer, or they might not answer the question.

To prevent satisficing, it is advisable not to offer a "Don't know" response choice for a question about a topic that it is reasonable to expect respondents will be able to answer, such as "How many children under age 18 live in this household?" Also, it is appropriate not to offer "Don't know" for a question about a topic for which respondents are expected to have an attitude or opinion, such as what they think is the most serious problem the police should address in their community. For an interview questionnaire, an alternative strategy is to include a "Don't know" option on the questionnaire but flag it using a special type style, such as italics, that the interviewer is trained not to read aloud. However, the response is conveniently available for the interviewer to record it if a respondent answers "Don't know" voluntarily.

Nominal Level

Fill in the blank

Question 1 in Box 11.7 illustrates asking for a nominal-level response using the **fill-in-the-blank format**. This format is useful when it is not possible to identify the full range of possible responses in advance, such as when asking "What are the names of the streets at the major intersection nearest your home?" or when the range is known but is large, as it is for question 1. In a web questionnaire, the respondent may be presented with a drop-down list of states from which to choose instead of filling in a blank space.

BOX 11.7: NOMINAL QUESTION TYPES

1. What is the name of the state where you were born?............................. _____
   State

2. Are you <u>seriously</u> thinking about quitting smoking <u>within the next 30 days</u>?

   Yes 1
   No 2

3. What is your present martial status?

   Married 1
   Living with a partner 2
   Separated or divorced 3
   Widowed 4
   Never married 5

Dichotomous choice

The most common type of nominal-level dichotomous choice question asks for a "Yes/No" response, as in question 2 in Box 11.7. In an interview, "Yes/No" choices typically are not read aloud because they are implied by the question and reading them might appear condescending. However, they should be read aloud if a respondent is unsure how to respond. In other situations, dichotomous choices for an interview may be embedded in the question, such as "If you could receive only one employer-provided benefit, would you choose dental insurance or disability insurance?"

Multiple choice

Question 3 in Box 11.7 illustrates a multiple-choice nominal format. In an interview, it is essential for the interviewer to read aloud each response choice, and a transitional phrase should link the question and response choices. A script may be added to the end of the question, or the interviewer may be trained to make smooth transitions—for example, "What is your present marital status? Are you . . . ," followed by reading each response choice aloud.

Although there is no hierarchical order among nominal choices, several ordering strategies may facilitate the response process. When appropriate, the response choice(s) expected to be most common may be presented first, as in question 3 (for a general population study). However, care must be taken to ensure the respondent does not perceive the first choice as preferred or best. Otherwise, alphabetical order may be used. Alphabetical order also is effective when there are numerous response choices, such as a list of medical diagnoses. When appropriate, chronological order may be used, such as in a drop-down list in a web questionnaire asking for the respondent's birth month. Presenting the most socially desirable response choice(s) first should be avoided because it might introduce a social desirability response bias.

Sometimes it may be desirable to exclude a response choice if it is expected to be so dominant as to obscure other response choices from being selected. Two examples are presented below.

"Aside from cost, why don't you have health insurance?"

"Aside from dying, what is your main concern about how getting cancer would impact your life?"

When the number of response choices is large, presenting them all in a list imposes a heavy burden on a respondent and interviewer. A useful guideline is to offer explicitly only response choices that are expected to be selected by at least 10% of the respondents, based on field pretesting. Responses not included in the list still may be captured by including an "Other" response choice. This strategy also provides for capturing responses that are not anticipated. Whenever an "Other" response choice is presented, it is important to ask respondents to specify their response as illustrated below.

Other (*please specify*) _____

"Other" responses then may be coded into one of the offered categories or compiled to develop additional categories, as appropriate. Otherwise, they may be included in the analysis as "Other." It is important not to place overreliance on using an "Other" response choice. If a substantial portion of respondents fit in a category that is not offered, they might feel they are not valued. Moreover, respondents are less likely to provide a response that is not offered explicitly. Instead, they might satisfice by selecting the offered response choice they perceive as being closest to their true response.

Multiple response

Box 11.8 illustrates a multiple-response format (also called "check/mark all that apply"). A respondent may select as many choices that apply, instead of only one. Although this format is efficient and has been employed in many studies, it generally no longer is recommended (Bradburn, Sudman, & Wansink, 2004; Groves et al., 2009; Nicolaas, Campanelli, Hope, Jäckle, & Lynn, 2015; Rasinski, Mingay, & Bradburn, 1994; Sudman & Bradburn, 1982). Not being selected does not reliably indicate a response choice does not apply to a respondent. For example, one might have overlooked it, which is more likely as the number of choices increases. Moreover, it is difficult to administer a multiple-response question in a telephone interview because the respondent cannot see the list of choices. Consequently, there is a tendency for a respondent to select choices mentioned first and/or last, called **primacy and recency response effects**, respectively.

BOX 11.8: NOMINAL MULTIPLE-RESPONSE FORMAT

3. Thinking about the <u>past 2 weeks</u>, which of the following problems did you experience?
   Select all that apply

   a. Feeling unusually tired 1
   b. Stuffy nose/congestion 2
   c. Lack of energy 3
   d. Coughing 4
   e. Difficulty sleeping 5
   f. None 6

The recommended alternative to a multiple-response format is to present a series of individual dichotomous-choice questions ("Yes/No," "Applies to me/Does not apply to me," etc.), as illustrated in Box 11.9. This format prompts respondents to consider and reply to each item. For example, if an item does not apply, they will answer "No" instead of leaving it not selected. Also, item f ("None") no longer is needed in Box 11.9.

BOX 11.9: NOMINAL INDIVIDUAL-RESPONSE FORMAT

3. Thinking about the <u>past 2 weeks</u>, which of the following problems did you experience?

	Yes	No
a. Feeling unusually tired	1	2
b. Stuffy nose/congestion	1	2
c. Lack of energy	1	2
d. Coughing	1	2
e. Difficulty sleeping	1	2

Ordinal Level

Dichotomous choice

The simplest ordinal-level question presents two response choices that differ in terms of relative amount, as in Box 11.10, question 1. Typically, the best practice is to minimize the risk of social desirability bias by presenting ordinal categories from lowest to highest. However, question 1 presents the most positive category first because presenting the response choices as "do you oppose or favor" violates common conversational convention and likely would sound odd (Holbrook, Krosnick, Carson, & Mitchell, 2000). When presenting only two ordinal choices, both choices should be mentioned in the question. It may be difficult to interpret responses reliably if only one choice is mentioned explicitly and the other is implied. This concern is especially important for interviews because respondents typically do not see the response choices. For example, if a respondent is asked "Do you favor X?" a "No" response could mean the respondent is opposed, is undecided, or does not care about X.

Multiple choice

Question 2 in Box 11.10 illustrates a multiple-choice ordinal format. The response choices describe an ordinal hierarchy of household smoking restrictions. Unlike nominal-level multiple-choice questions, an "Other" category is not appropriate. All relevant ordinal response choices must be presented. In general, it is best to present ordinal response choices from lowest to highest. That order follows a natural progression. Also, higher response codes will correspond to higher-level response choices.

Rating scales

Chapter 9 discussed unipolar and bipolar rating scales in detail. Therefore, that information is not repeated here. For convenient reference, Box 11.11 presents examples of bipolar and unipolar ordinal rating scale formats.

Ranking

Another ordinal scaling technique is to ask a respondent to rank items in order, typically from highest to lowest. Ranking may be implemented in two ways. One is to ask a

---

BOX 11.10: ORDINAL DICHOTOMOUS- AND MULTIPLE-CHOICE QUESTIONS

1. For people who are convicted of murder, do you favor or oppose the death penalty?

    Favor 1

    Oppose 2

2. Which of the following best describes the rules about smoking in your household?

    There are no restrictions on smoking 1

    Smoking is allowed in some rooms/places only 2

    Smoking is not allowed at all 3

BOX 11.11: ORDINAL RATING SCALE FORMATS

Bipolar: Fully Labeled

Overall how do you rate the services you receive at your usual source of health care?

Very Dissatisfied	Somewhat Dissatisfied	Neither Satisfied nor Dissatisfied	Somewhat Satisfied	Very Satisfied
1	2	3	4	5

Bipolar: End Points Labeled

Overall how do you rate the services you receive at your usual source of health care?

Very Dissatisfied				Very Satisfied
1	2	3	4	5

Unipolar: Fully Labeled

Overall how do you rate the services you receive at your usual source of health care?

Not Satisfied	Slightly Satisfied	Somewhat Satisfied	Mostly Satisfied	Very Satisfied
1	2	3	4	5

Unipolar: End Points Labeled

Overall how do you rate the services you receive at your usual source of health care?

Not Satisfied				Very Satisfied
1	2	3	4	5

respondent to list a certain number of items in rank order using a fill-in-the-blank format as illustrated in Box 11.12, question 1. The goal is for respondents to rank items they identify as important rather than ones a researcher thinks are important. However, it involves a significant cognitive task, whereby the respondent must identify a pool of at least five items, select the five most important overall, and then place them in rank order. Some respondents might not be able to identify as many as five items, or whatever number is specified. They might satisfice by adding items to be compliant or not answer the question. Moreover, not every respondent will rank the same list of items, making comparisons in the analysis challenging. Question 2 illustrates a strategy that asks each respondent to rank-order the same list of items, which have been preselected with guidance from theory, practice, and/or prior research. That format significantly reduces the respondent's burden and facilitates comparisons.

> **BOX 11.12: RANK-ORDER QUESTION FORMATS**
>
> 1. Think about features that would be important if you were looking for a neighborhood to live in.
>
>   In the spaces below, please write in the <u>five</u> features you think are most important, starting with the one you think is most important of all (1), second most important (2), and so on.
>
>   1. _____
>   2. _____
>   3. _____
>   4. _____
>   5. _____
>
> 2. Five features of a neighborhood are listed below. Think about how important each one would be to you if you were looking for a neighborhood to live in.
>
>   In the space for each feature, please write a number from 1 to 5 to indicate the one you think is <u>most</u> important (1), second most important (2), and so on.
>
>   a. Crime rate .... _____
>   b. Grocery shopping .... _____
>   c. Health care access .... _____
>   d. Housing quality .... _____
>   e. Recreational facilities .... _____

Interval/Ratio Level

Fill in the blank

Box 11.13 illustrates questions that ask for exact quantities using the fill-in-the-blank format, which may be used when it is reasonable to expect respondents to know the exact information and are willing to provide it. A potential problem with question 1 in a self-administered paper questionnaire is a respondent might provide more than a single number, such as "14 or 15." An advantage of a web questionnaire is a drop-down list of ages may be presented from which the respondent may select only one. For an interview, interviewers should be trained to probe as to which of two such numbers is most accurate. When appropriate, it is important to indicate the desired units of measure for a fill-in-the-blank response, as illustrated in question 2.

> **BOX 11.13: FILL-IN-THE-BLANK INTERVAL/RATIO FORMAT**
>
> 1. How old were you when you started regularly smoking one or more cigarettes a day? _____
>   age
>
> 2. On average, about how much time does it take for you to travel from your home to your usual source of health care? _____ , _____
>   hours   minutes

Multiple choice

Most often, interval/ratio measures are presented using a multiple-choice format with grouped intervals as illustrated in Box 11.14. While this method does not obtain information that is as detailed as fill-in-the-blank questions, it reduces the respondent's burden and the item nonresponse rate. It also reduces the incidence of responses that are difficult to interpret and code for analysis, such as more than a single number or illegible writing on a paper self-administered questionnaire. Moreover, information collected using the fill-in-the-blank format often is recoded into grouped intervals for analysis and presenting results. It often is not possible to obtain an exact numerical response because such detailed knowledge or recall is not available to respondents. Furthermore, it is not necessary to collect exact numerical information if the analysis plan calls for processing it in grouped intervals. For example, that might be done to match policy eligibility requirements.

BOX 11.14: GROUPED-INTERVALS FORMAT

1. How old were you when you started regularly smoking one or more cigarettes a day?

    9 or younger 1

    10 to 13 2

    14 to 17 3

    18 to 25 4

    26 or older 5

2. On average, about how much time does it take for you to travel from your home to your usual source of health care?

    15 minutes or less 1

    16 to 30 minutes 2

    31 to 45 minutes 3

    46 to 60 minutes (one hour) 4

    More than one hour 5

Box 11.15 presents guidelines for constructing interval/ratio response choices. In general, it is desirable to construct intervals with equal breadth. However, that is not an essential requirement. It is more important to construct intervals that are responsive to the research question and analysis plan, and are familiar to and convenient for respondents. For example, instead of the response choices shown for question 2 in Box 11.14, most respondents are likely to find the following intervals as odd and cumbersome: 7 minutes or less, 8 to 24 minutes, 25 to 42 minutes, and so on. With the exception of discrete measures, such as the number of people living in a household, interval/ratio response choices typically are rounded to whole units. Although from a strict mathematical perspective there are fractional gaps between intervals in question 1, such as "10 to 13" and "14 to 17," generally that is not an issue.

> ### BOX 11.15: INTERVAL-/RATIO-LEVEL RESPONSE CHOICE GUIDELINES
>
> - Ensure response choices are responsive to the research question and analysis plan.
> - Present response choices that are familiar to and convenient for respondents.
> - Use numerals, not words.
> - Avoid using zero.
> - Do not use mathematical symbols.
> - Avoid percentages.
> - Present lowest to highest.

It is best to designate intervals using numerals, which are more efficient than words for respondents and interviewers to read. Also, the distance between interval boundaries should be indicated simply by the word *to* (e.g., 10 to 13) or a dash (e.g., 10–13). Wordy and awkward formulations such as "at least age 10 but younger than age 14" should not be used.

An exception to this guideline applies to the null category. In some situations, 0 may have a negative connotation. In others, it is better to use a word, such as *none* or *never*, instead of *zero*, which would sound odd in an interview. For example, in response to "During the past 7 days, how many drinks of alcohol did you have?" "None" is more conversational in tone than "Zero." Moreover, 0 is not appropriate for some variables. For example, "Zero" is an impossible response to "How long have you lived in this neighborhood?" Instead, the lowest value response choice must be something like "Less than 1 year" or "1 year or less."

It is best not to use mathematical symbols, such as <, >, ≤, or ≥, especially in a self-administered questionnaire, because some respondents might find them intimidating or not interpret them correctly. Also, in general, it is best not to ask for responses in terms of percentages because some respondents might not be comfortable with that abstract concept. It is better to ask for the number of times, and so forth, which may be converted into percentages during data processing and analysis. Moreover, responses reported in percentages when asked in a fill-in-the-blank format tend to be reported using only a few familiar points along the continuum from 0% to 100%, such as 10%, 25%, 50%, 75%, 90%, and 100%. Thus, respondents might treat what theoretically is a 101-point response range (0% to 100%) as comprising only a few discrete points. This response effect is called **response heaping**.

As illustrated in Box 11.14, the highest interval often must be "open" because it is not clear where it should be closed. So it does not appear too extreme, it should start at a level that might apply to at least some respondents but less than 10%. If the interval is expected to include substantially more than 10% of respondents, then it should be divided to avoid losing potentially important information. For example, if there is reason to expect a substantial portion of respondents to question 1 in Box 11.14 will have started smoking cigarettes at age 26 or older, then that response choice should be divided, such as "26 to 39" and "40 or older." Although the lowest interval may appear to be open in the examples, each is closed: "9 or younger" equals "0 to 9," and "15 minutes or less" equals "0 to 15." As described for ordinal-level response choices, in general, it is best to present interval/ratio response choices in a familiar progression from lowest to highest. Also, higher response codes then will correspond to higher-level response choices. It is more difficult for respondents to follow a countdown from high to low, especially in an interview.

CHECK YOUR UNDERSTANDING 11.4

- What are the general guidelines for developing closed question response choices?

Key Points

Closed Questions

Most questions in a structured questionnaire use a closed-response format that presents a predetermined set of response choices.

- **Advantages**
    - Standardization
    - Facilitation of data processing and analysis
    - Administration
    - Data quality

- **Disadvantages**
    - Construction
    - Vulnerability to satisficing
    - Restriction of spontaneity

Open Questions

Open questions ask respondents to answer in their own words.

- **Advantages**
    - Enabling spontaneity
    - Implying that a respondent's true feelings are valued
    - Capturing colorful aspects of a respondent's opinion or experience

- **Disadvantages**
    - Heavy administration burden
    - Challenging data processing
    - Challenging data analysis

Question Wording

Key aspects of wording questions to obtain reliable and valid responses are as follows:

- Vocabulary
- Tone
- Avoiding problem words

Question Structure

Key aspects of question structure are as follows:

- Keep it short and simple.
- Use complete sentences.
- Ask one question at a time.
- Do not use double negatives.
- Specify conditions at the beginning.
- Do not ask biased questions.
- Use appropriate strategies to ask about a sensitive topic.

Response Choices

General guidelines for response choices are as follows:

- Be responsive to the question.
- Present one response at a time.
- Ensure response choices are
  - unidimensional,
  - exclusive,
  - exhaustive, and
  - short and simple.
- Use "Don't know" cautiously.

Review and Apply

1. Prepare a draft of a structured questionnaire based on your outline from Chapter 10.
   a. Maintain a journal of key challenges your questionnaire presents and the reasons why you chose particular strategies to address them.
   b. Conduct five cognitive interviews to assess your questionnaire draft (Chapter 10). Respondents may be classmates, friends, or relatives.

c. Write a report about what the cognitive interviews revealed about any problems with your questionnaire draft and strategies for addressing them.

d. Prepare a revised draft of your questionnaire.

2. You have been engaged as a questionnaire design consultant to develop a self-administered paper questionnaire that will be administered with women age 18 and older who delivered a normal, live birth during the past six months. The sample will be women who already are known to be eligible for the survey. Therefore, there is no need to screen for eligibility. An initial rough draft of the questionnaire is presented below.

a. Prepare a constructive critique of the questionnaire draft in the form of a memo to your client.

b. Prepare a revised draft that addresses any problems you identify. Add questions only if they are essential to promote a smooth flow and coverage of topics (e.g., a filter question). Present a rationale for deleting any question(s). Do not delete a question because it is challenging to compose.

c. Prepare a report that describes how and why you revised the initial draft. This may be combined with part 2a in a single document.

Pregnancy Questionnaire

PART A

1. MARRIED? Yes _____ No _____   b. Living with father?

2. AGE:
    Teen
    Less than 30
    Over 30

3. How much education do you have?
    a. Less than H.S.
    b. H.S. Grad
    c. College Graduate

PART B

4. First pregnancy? _____ Yes _____ No?

5. How long were you pregnant when you found out you were pregnant this time? _____ weeks

6. Did you get any prenatal care from a doctor, nurse or anywhere else? _____ YES _____ NO

7a. What kind of place was this? _____ Private office _____ Health dept _____ Health ctr. _____ HMO _____ Other

7b. When was the . . . first time? _____ last time? _____

8a. How many drinks of alcohol did you have during the 3 months <u>before</u> you found out that you were pregnant?
    10 or more drinks a week _____   _____ 2 drinks a week
    6 to 10 drinks a week _____   _____ 1 drink a week
    3–5 drinks a week _____   _____ Less than 1 drink

(Continued)

(Continued)

8b. Did you change your drinking during this pregnancy?

_____ Yes, I was concerned about my baby. _____ Yes, my doctor or nurse told me to stop.

_____ No, no one told me. _____ Other _____

9. How many cigarettes did you have during the 3 months <u>before</u> you found out that you were pregnant? Average number per day

9b. Did you quit smoking when you were pregnant? _____ YES _____ NO _____ How long?

9c. How many cigarettes do you smoke now? _____ average number per day

10. How much did your baby weigh at birth? _____

11. Do you have a regular doctor or health care provider?
    - ☐ YES
    - ☐ NO
    - ☐ DON'T KNOW/NOT SURE
    - ☐ REFUSED

Hepatitis B

12. Have you ever heard of Hepatitis B?
    - ☐ YES
    - ☐ NO
    - ☐ DON'T KNOW/NOT SURE
    - ☐ REFUSED

13a. Hepatitis B is passed through genes (hereditary). ☐ True ☐ False

13b. Hepatitis B is passed from mother to child during birth ☐ True ☐ False

13c. HIV is passed through genes (hereditary). ☐ True ☐ False

13d. HIV is passed from mother to child during birth ☐ True ☐ False

14. How would you describe yourself?

    White-not Hispanic   Asian or Pacific Islander

    Black-not Hispanic   Native American or Alaskan

    Hispanic   Other

15. Overall, what would you say is the chance that you will get your baby all of its recommended shots?
    1. Almost 100% chance
    2. An 80% chance
    3. A 60% chance
    4. A 40% chance
    5. A 20% chance
    6. No chance
    7. DK

16. For each health factor, indicate whether it is or is not related, or unclear to a baby's health. Answer for each item.

	Is Related (1)	Not Related (2)	Unclear (3)
a. Smoking cigarettes	1	2	3
b. Emotional stress	1	2	3
c. Obesity	1	2	3
d. Exercise	1	2	3
e. First birth after age of 30	1	2	3
f. Not eating a good diet	1	2	3
g. High blood pressure	1	2	3

Study Further

Blair, J., Czaja, R. F., & Blair, E. A. (2014). *Designing surveys: A guide to decisions and procedures*. Los Angeles, CA: Sage.

Bradburn, N. M., Sudman, S., & Wansink, B. (2004). *Asking questions: The definitive guide to questionnaire design—for market research, political polls, and social and health questionnaires*. San Francisco, CA: Jossey-Bass.

Dillman, D. A., Smyth, J. D., & Christian, L. M. (2014). *Internet, phone, mail, and mixed-mode surveys: The tailored design method*. Hoboken, NJ: Wiley.

Krosnick, J. A., & Presser, S. (2010). Question and questionnaire design. In P. V. Marsden & J. D. Wright (Eds.), *Handbook of survey research* (2nd ed., pp. 263–313). Bingley, UK: Emerald Group.

Schaeffer, N. C., & Presser, S. (2003). The science of asking questions. *Annual Review of Sociology, 29*, 65–88.

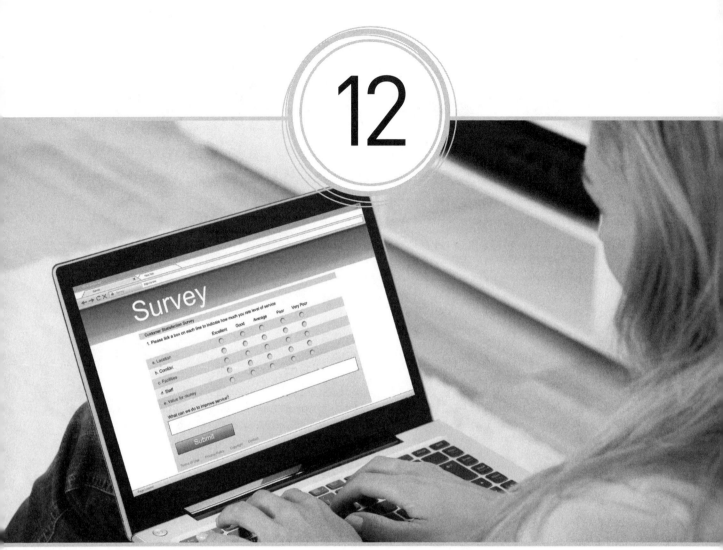

12

Survey Research Methods

Chapter Outline

Overview
Learning Objectives
Basic Concepts
    Survey Advantages
    Survey Disadvantages
    The Survey Process
Data Collection Modes
    Overview
    Comparison
    Additional Considerations
    Mixed Modes
    Computer-Assisted Modes
Conducting a Survey
    Mail
    Monitored
    Web
    Telephone Interviews
    In-Person Interviews
Interviewing
    General Guidelines
    Recording Responses
    Probing
    Interviewer Characteristics
    Interviewer Training
    Interviewer Supervision
Key Points

Learning Objectives

After studying Chapter 12, the reader should be able to:

- Decide when to employ survey research methods
- Select an appropriate survey data collection mode
- Develop an effective survey plan
- Conduct field pretesting to evaluate a survey plan
- Conduct a small-scale self-administered or interview survey
- Apply strategies to minimize bias

Overview

Surveys are one of the most commonly used methods for collecting information about health knowledge, attitudes, behaviors, and demographic characteristics. Health surveys may be used to assess needs, develop population profiles, monitor populations or cohorts longitudinally, or collect pretest and/or posttest measures in studies using experimental or quasi-experimental designs. Surveys may be conducted at the local, regional, national, or international level. Examples of well-known large-scale health surveys include the National Health Interview Survey (Centers for Disease Control and Prevention, 2018e), Behavioral Risk Factor Surveillance System (Centers for Disease Control and Prevention, 2018a), and National Health and Nutrition Examination Survey (Centers for Disease Control and Prevention, 2018g). Although there are several fundamental survey methods and many variations of them, a common characteristic of surveys is they collect information using a structured questionnaire (Chapter 10).

Basic Concepts

A **survey** is a method for systematically collecting self-reported information using a structured questionnaire. Research using a survey sometimes is described as using a "survey design," which most often refers to using a survey to collect information for a cross-sectional research design to describe a population at a single time point (Chapter 6). Indeed, survey methods probably are used most often with that design. However, there is no "survey design" in standard research design terminology. A survey is a *data collection method*, not a research design. As appropriate, a survey might be used to collect information at any observation point in any research design. Surveys often are used in trend and panel study designs. Moreover, they also may be employed in experimental and quasi-experimental research designs (Chapter 6). Instead of referring to a "survey design," clarity is gained by referring to a **survey plan** to distinguish how a survey is conducted from the research design in which it is applied.

Survey Advantages

Box 12.1 presents advantages and disadvantages of survey methods. Their primary advantage is standardization. In addition to the standardization in a structured questionnaire's wording, response choices, and ordering, a survey standardizes the data collection mode and the protocol for implementing it. Holding these factors constant allows them to be ruled out as alternative explanations for differences in responses across individuals and/or time. Surveys facilitate data processing and analysis because responses to most questions are numerically precoded (Chapter 10). Moreover, these aspects facilitate conducting replication and comparative studies.

Key Concept

The primary advantage of a survey is standardization.

Generalizing results to the target population is another advantage, provided a survey is conducted with a representative random sample of appropriate size (Chapter 7), which is the best practice. Also, by using self-reports, surveys provide a means for collecting information about variables that is not observable directly, such as attitudes, past behavior for which no records exist, and private, socially undesirable, or illegal activities. Because most surveys collect data rather quickly, they may provide timely information that enhances responsiveness to time-sensitive data applications, such as making decisions about initiating, revising, or terminating a health program, or advocating for health policies or legislation. Moreover, surveys are efficient for collecting information from a large number of participants, about a large number of variables, in relatively short time, and at low per-unit

BOX 12.1: SURVEY METHODS: ADVANTAGES AND DISADVANTAGES

Advantages	Disadvantages
• Standardization	• Ability to explore unanticipated aspects of a topic is limited.
• Replication and comparison	• Resource requirements may be significant.
• Generalizability/representativeness (with random sampling)	• Surveys may require substantial preparation time.
• Ability to collect information about variables not observable directly	• Large surveys require subcontracting with a professional survey organization.
• Speed/timeliness	
• Large data sets (participants and variables)	• Respondents might not be accessible.
• Low per-unit cost	• A low response rate may raise concerns about the validity of results.
• Broad geographic coverage	

cost. Finally, with the exception of in-person interviews, surveys enable collecting information across broad geographic areas efficiently.

Survey Disadvantages

A standardized approach limits a survey's ability to explore unanticipated aspects of a topic. Also, despite their per-unit-of-information efficiency, preparing for and conducting valid surveys may require a significant investment of resources in terms of time, financial support, staffing, and project management. The perception that conducting a survey generally is quick, easy, and inexpensive is not accurate. Exceptions are surveys that are very short, simple, about a salient topic, and conducted with an accessible, low-diversity population. An example is a web survey of college students in a single department, where there is free access to web survey software and email addresses, and the questionnaire is short, simple, and salient, such as to identify campus locations where students are concerned about their physical safety.

Conducting a large-scale telephone or in-person interview survey of the general population requires a large team of well-trained and supervised staff. Such studies typically are planned and conducted in collaboration with experienced professionals in academic or commercial survey research centers. Moreover, surveys are not necessarily appropriate for every population or topic. For example, it is difficult to identify and/or access some populations or subgroups using survey methods, such as injection drug users, homeless people, and institutionalized populations. Furthermore, a low response rate may raise concerns about the validity of results.

The Survey Process

Planning and conducting a survey is a process involving several integrated components. As depicted in Figure 12.1, once the research question and research design are specified and a survey is determined to be the most appropriate method, the first stage of the process is to develop a preliminary survey plan. A sampling frame must be identified, and a sample

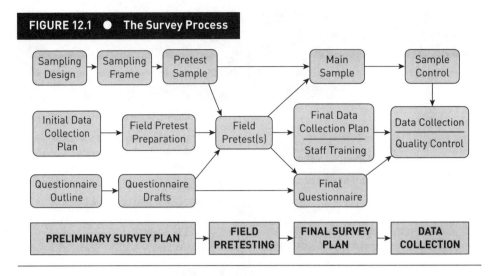

FIGURE 12.1 ● The Survey Process

selection design must be developed (Chapter 7); the most appropriate survey data collection mode must be selected; and a questionnaire outline and initial drafts must be prepared (Chapter 10). In addition, a time schedule and budget must be prepared, along with identifying necessary staff, equipment, supply, and requirements.

Box 12.2 lists key factors to consider when developing a survey plan. Typically, at this point, a proposal requesting funding support must be prepared and submitted to an appropriate agency. Going forward, the survey plan is assessed and refined by field pretesting (Chapter 10). When the survey plan is finalized, the main sample is selected, the final questionnaire is prepared for distribution, and the data collection staff are trained. Finally, data are collected while procedures are implemented to monitor and control allocating the sample, data collection integrity, and adherence to the budget and time schedule.

BOX 12.2: DEVELOPING A SURVEY PLAN

Target Population

- How can target population members be contacted?
- How likely is the target population to participate?
- How diverse is the target population?
- What is the geographic distribution of the target population?
- Does the target population present any special needs/problems?

Key Variables

- Will respondents be able to provide the information?
- Will respondents be willing to provide the information?
- Are there any sensitive topics?

- What data collection mode would be most effective?
- Can the information be collected more effectively by a method other than a survey?

Time Schedule

- By what time are the survey results needed?
- Are there any potential situational/historical threats to avoid?

Resources

- What funding support is required?
- What funding support is available?
- What staff and training are required?
- What equipment, supplies, and space are required?

CHECK YOUR UNDERSTANDING 12.1

- Consider the following research question:

  How do African American men identify and respond to heart disease symptoms?

  ○ What would be the main *advantages* of using a survey to address this question?

  ○ What would be the main *disadvantages* of using a survey to address this question?

Data Collection Modes

Overview

Surveys collect data using two basic modes: Respondents are asked to complete a **self-administered questionnaire (SAQ)** with no or minimal staff assistance, or an interviewer reads questions aloud and records a respondent's answers. The most common self-administered modes are mail, monitored, and web. A **mail survey** sends a paper questionnaire to respondents, typically at their residence by standard postal service, and they are asked to complete and return it using a postage-paid, preaddressed return envelope. For a **monitored self-administered questionnaire**, data collection staff distribute a paper questionnaire in-person to respondents individually or in a group, such as at a clinic, workplace, or school. Respondents are asked to complete the questionnaire while being monitored by data collection staff. Completed questionnaires are submitted to the staff or placed in a collection container.

A **web survey**, also called an **internet survey**, links respondents to a website where they may

> **Key Concept**
>
> *Surveys collect data using two basic modes: self-administered questionnaires and interviews.*

complete a questionnaire online. **Email surveys**, whereby a questionnaire is embedded in or attached to an email message, have been replaced almost entirely by web surveys.

Telephone interviews are the most widely used interview mode because of their versatility and time and cost efficiency. **In-person interviews**, also called "face-to-face" and "personal interviews," typically are conducted at a respondent's residence. They generally provide the best overall data quality of all survey modes. In-person interviews are the most expensive, challenging, and time-consuming to implement effectively.

Comparison

Table 12.1 presents a comparative summary of the main survey data collection modes in terms of administrative and resource considerations. Implications of data collection modes for questionnaire design were discussed in Chapter 10. A well-designed sample and questionnaire are assumed for this discussion that focuses on the data collection portion of the survey process.

TABLE 12.1 ● Data Collection Mode Administration and Resource Considerations				
Aspect	Mailed/Monitored SAQ	Web SAQ	Telephone Interview	In-Person Interview
Costs	**Low**	**Low**	Medium	High
Time	Long/medium	**Short**	**Short**	Medium/long
Geographic distribution	**Wide**/clustered	**Wide**	**Wide**	Clustered
Anonymity	**Very good**	Fair	Fair	Poor
Unit response rate	Low/medium	Low	Medium/**high**	**High**
Item nonresponse	Medium	Medium	Low	**Very low**

SAQ = self-administered questionnaire. Bolded items indicate methods with the greatest strength in general for each aspect.

Costs

There are no general formulas for estimating survey costs. Every survey, even controlling for mode, has unique features that must be taken into consideration, such as characteristics of the target population, sampling design, sample size, questionnaire length, questionnaire complexity, and use of incentives. Carefully estimating and monitoring data collection costs is vital because they involve the largest investment of resources for conducting a survey. Moreover, once data collection is well under way, typically it is a point of no return. If resources subsequently are found to be inadequate, a serious reduction in the sample size may be necessary. In the worst case, the study might have to be terminated.

Self-administered modes are the least expensive and interviews the most expensive in-person interviews. The main costs for a mailed survey include reproducing the questionnaire and cover letter, mailing supplies, and postage. For a large mail survey, staff must be hired, trained, and supervised. Costs for a monitored self-administered questionnaire include reproducing the questionnaire, staff, and travel to distribution sites.

The main costs for an interview survey are related to the interviewing staff. Both interview modes involve hiring, training, and supervising interviewers. For in-person interviews, costs also include interviewer travel time and expenses. Also, in-person surveys often offer a participation incentive. Singer and Ye (2013) found that survey participation incentives are most effective when they are prepaid instead of conditional on participation, monetary instead of a nonmonetary gift or service, and provided to all respondents instead of entering respondents in a lottery.

Time

The web is the fastest mode for a survey because it is administered electronically and requires minimal staff support. A web survey may be completed in as little as one or two weeks, although it is common to allocate an additional week or two in the time schedule to make follow-up contacts with sample members who have not responded. A telephone interview generally is the next fastest mode, typically requiring about three to six weeks, or longer. Although they involve interviewers and supervisory staff, most telephone interviews are conducted conveniently and efficiently from a calling center.

In-person interviews require more time because interviewers must travel from one respondent's location to another. In particular, they are much less efficient than telephone interviews for following up with respondents with whom an interviewer is not able to connect initially. Depending on how widely the sample is dispersed geographically and the size of the interviewing staff, in-person interviews generally require four to twelve weeks, or longer.

A monitored self-administered questionnaire survey generally may be completed in two to four weeks. However, collecting monitored questionnaires may take longer depending on the number of sites, their geographic dispersion, and the data collection staff size. Completing a mail survey generally requires about eight to twelve weeks. Questionnaires must be transmitted to and from respondents by postal service. Also, the typical mail survey plan involves sending multiple follow-up questionnaires to sample members who do not respond.

Geographic distribution

Mail, web, and telephone interview surveys may be distributed over wide geographic areas because they do not require staff presence and travel. Monitored questionnaires and in-person interviews are feasible only when the sample is clustered. However, that does not mean the target population must be geographically restricted. To obtain a representative sample of a widely distributed population for those modes, a cluster sampling design must be employed (Chapter 7).

Anonymity

A mailed questionnaire may provide the strongest protection of respondent anonymity if there are no identifiers in the questionnaire or on any of the return mailing materials. Anonymity for a monitored questionnaire may be facilitated by requiring respondents to seal their completed questionnaire in a plain envelope before submitting it to staff. Another strategy is to provide respondents a postage-paid, preaddressed return envelope in which they may independently send their completed questionnaire to the data processing staff. Although a web questionnaire may appear anonymous, respondents may be aware that the web is not an anonymous environment. When a telephone interview is conducted with a sample selected using random-digit dialing (see the "Telephone Interviews" section), the interviewer does not know respondents' identities, and respondents' telephone numbers should not be entered in the questionnaire because they are a potential identifier. Nevertheless, respondents may be wary that if it is possible to select their unlisted telephone number, it may be possible to identify them. Anonymity typically is not possible for an in-person interview because the sample usually is selected from a frame that includes the respondent's name and contact information. Moreover, the interview is conducted using a face-to-face protocol.

Unit response rate

The **unit response rate** is an indicator of survey data quality that generally is defined as the proportion of sample members who are known or assumed to meet a study's eligibility criteria from whom a completed questionnaire is collected (Kviz, 1977). The American Association for Public Opinion Research (AAPOR) (2016) has published standardized formulas for calculating response rates and other survey outcomes for a wide variety of survey situations. Some professional journals require employing them in reports of survey research results. A free Response Rate Calculator in a spreadsheet format is available from AAPOR at www.aapor.org/Standards-Ethics/Standard-Definitions-(1).aspx (accessed September 21, 2018).

In general, the higher the unit response rate, the more reliably the respondents will represent characteristics of the sample. **Nonresponse bias** may occur if nonrespondents differ from respondents systematically in a way that might influence a survey's results. For example, if nonrespondents tend to be less healthy than respondents, the less healthy segment of the population will be underrepresented. Moreover, unit non response reduces statistical power by resulting in an observed sample that is smaller than the desired sample size.

Interview surveys, especially in-person interviews, generally obtain the highest response rates owing to interviewer–respondent rapport. Interaction with a respondent generally is minimal or none for self-administered modes. In general, the unit response rate is lowest for web surveys.

Item nonresponse

Item nonresponse occurs when eligible sample members participate in a survey but do not provide a usable response to one or more questions that apply to them. That results in a condition called **missing data**, which may bias results if it is systematic. For example, if respondents who have several drinks of alcohol per day tend not to answer questions about their alcohol consumption, a survey's results may be biased in two ways. First, the proportion of "heavy" drinkers in the target population will be underestimated. Second, potential correlations between alcohol consumption and other variables, such as health status, may be distorted because they will be "censored" at the high end of the alcohol consumption range. In addition, statistical power is reduced for analyses that include variables for which there are missing data owing to item nonresponse.

Item nonresponse may occur for several reasons:

- Respondents refuse to answer a question.
- Respondents are unable to provide the requested information.
- Respondents or interviewers overlook a question.
- A question is not answered owing to unclear questionnaire navigation instructions.
- A response to a fill-in-the-blank or an open-response question is unusable owing to poor handwriting or being unintelligible.

Item nonresponse is lowest for interviews because the interviewers are trained and monitored to perform their tasks correctly. Also, interviewer–respondent rapport discourages respondent satisficing, such as by responding "Don't know" to avoid a challenging memory search. Item nonresponse for a self-administered mode may vary substantially depending on factors such as question and questionnaire complexity, questionnaire length, requests to refer to records, and asking questions about sensitive topics (Chapter 10).

Summary

Considering relative advantages overall, the lowest costs are associated with self-administered modes (mail, monitored, and web). Web and telephone interview surveys collect data most quickly. Mail, web, and telephone surveys enable collecting data from a population distributed over a broad geographic area. Mail and monitored questionnaires enable collecting data anonymously. Interviews obtain the highest response rates and lowest incidence of item nonresponse.

Regarding relative disadvantages, in-person interviews are most expensive, often prohibitively so. Mail and in-person interviews require the most data collection time. Monitored questionnaires and in-person interviews must be conducted with clustered samples. Self-administered modes generally yield lower response rates and more item nonresponse than interviews.

Additional Considerations

Compared to interviews, self-administered modes require fewer staff, are easier to administer, and are less intrusive. Mail and web surveys provide access to busy populations, and they enable respondents to complete the questionnaire at a time and place they choose. Mail surveys are familiar to most respondents, and web surveys are increasing in that regard. Once a web survey is set up, there are virtually no additional administrative costs regardless of the sample size or location. However, web surveys are limited to populations with web access and typically for whom email addresses are available. Monitored questionnaires may be implemented simultaneously with multiple respondents in multiple locations. However, self-administered modes are not appropriate for low literacy populations or subgroups. Also, web surveys are most vulnerable to "break-offs," where respondents stop completing the questionnaire for reasons such as it is long, uninteresting, or threatening.

Interviews generally provide the best data quality. In addition to the features listed in Table 12.1, Table 10.2 in Chapter 10 lists important advantages of interviews in terms of questionnaire design, especially for in-person interviews. However, interviews may be influenced by **interviewer variance** that may occur if there are substantial differences across interviewers in terms of reading questions, reading response choices, probing, or developing rapport with respondents. Typically, such issues may be addressed effectively through interviewer training and monitoring. However, sometimes an interviewer's personal characteristics (e.g., age, sex, or race/ethnicity) may influence whether or how respondents answer some questions. For example, respondents might answer questions about attitudes toward people of other racial/ethnic backgrounds differently depending on whether they perceive the interviewer to be of the same or a different background as them. Such a possibility should be assessed in a pilot study and/or field pretest. When appropriate, consideration should be given to matching interviewer and respondent characteristics.

Face-to-face interviewers may encounter difficulty gaining access to secure environments, such as apartment and office buildings. Also, precautions should be employed to protect interviewers' safety while they are in the field. In some situations, it may be advisable for interviewers to work in teams. If a community is deemed especially dangerous, either an alternative data collection mode, such as mailed questionnaires, should be considered for that community, or the community should be excluded from the target population.

> **CHECK YOUR UNDERSTANDING 12.2**
>
> - Focusing on administration and resource considerations, present an example for a situation in which it would be appropriate to employ each of the following survey data collection modes.
>
>   Briefly explain why the mode would be appropriate in that situation.
>   - Mailed self-administered questionnaire
>   - Monitored self-administered questionnaire
>   - Web self-administered questionnaire
>   - Telephone interview
>   - In-person interview

Mixed Modes

Two or more modes may be used in combination, called a **mixed-mode survey**, to take advantage of each mode's strength and offset its limitations. Modes may be implemented simultaneously or sequentially. One *simultaneous strategy* is to offer respondents a choice of modes. For example, for a questionnaire that is sent by mail, respondents may be offered the option to complete and return the paper version by mail, or to complete the questionnaire online at a link that is provided in the cover letter. Another simultaneous strategy is to employ different modes as appropriate for two or more population subgroups. For example, to increase population coverage for a survey where the primary mode is telephone interviews or a web survey, a questionnaire might be sent by standard mail to respondents for whom a telephone number or email address is not available, respectively.

A *sequential strategy* may be conducted in two ways. First, a *supplementary mode* may be employed to collect information that cannot be collected effectively, or at all, by the primary mode. For example, after completing a telephone interview, visual materials may be sent to the respondents by standard mail. Then, either a follow-up telephone interview may be conducted, or the respondents may be asked to complete a brief questionnaire about the visual material either by standard mail or online. A similar strategy may be employed with telephone interview respondents to collect information that requires them to consult household records and/or other household or extended family members. For an in-person interview, the interviewer may provide a paper self-administered questionnaire for the respondent to complete and return by mail.

During an in-person interview, the respondent may be asked to answer questions about a sensitive topic by completing a supplemental self-administered questionnaire. This may be done while the interviewer is present in two ways. One is that the respondent completes a paper questionnaire and submits it to the interviewer in a sealed envelope. Another strategy is for the interviewer to provide a portable device, such as a laptop computer or tablet, to answer questions about a sensitive topic.

Another type of sequential strategy is to employ a *follow-up mode* to increase the unit response rate. For example, a mailed questionnaire may be employed as the primary mode to take advantage of its low cost. Then, follow-up telephone interviews may be attempted with all or a random sample of individuals from whom a completed mailed questionnaire is not received. Box 12.3 presents an example of a study that implemented a sequential mixed-mode survey strategy.

> **BOX 12.3: EXAMPLE OF IMPLEMENTING A SEQUENTIAL MIXED-MODE SURVEY**
>
> **VALIDATION OF SELF-REPORTED COLORECTAL CANCER SCREENING BEHAVIOR FROM A MIXED-MODE SURVEY OF VETERANS**
>
> Partin et al. (2008) assessed the validity of self-reported colorectal cancer screening using the National Cancer Institute Colorectal Cancer Screening questionnaire. Participants were a stratified random sample of 890 patients, aged 50–75 years, selected from the Minneapolis Veterans Affairs (VA) Medical Center. A mailed questionnaire was the primary mode; a telephone interview was the secondary mode. The mail survey protocol included an initial mailing of a cover letter, the questionnaire, and a $2 cash incentive. A reminder postcard was mailed about one week later. Three to four weeks after the initial mailing, a second mailing, which did not include an incentive, was sent to sample members who did not return a questionnaire. Finally, a telephone interview was attempted with all sample members who did not return a questionnaire within three weeks of the second survey mailing. A total of 686 sample members participated in the study: A mailed questionnaire was completed by 627; a telephone interview was completed with 59.

Disadvantages of mixed-mode surveys include an increased administrative burden, increased preparation time, and potentially increased data collection time and costs. Moreover, the reliability and validity of results for mixed-mode surveys are threatened by potential **mode effects**, whereby respondents might answer the same question(s) differently depending on the mode. Methodological experiments do not provide consistent guidance about when or how it is effective to employ mixed-mode surveys (Blair, Czaja, & Blair, 2014; de Leeuw, 2005; Dillman, Smyth, & Christian, 2014; Groves et al., 2009). Therefore, mixed modes should be used prudently, and should be assessed by a pilot study and field pretesting prior to being implemented.

Computer-Assisted Modes

Technological advances have led to the introduction of computer-assisted methods for self-administered questionnaires and interviews. Web surveys are not included in this group because they are administered entirely via computer. Professional academic and commercial survey organizations conducting large-scale surveys typically employ proprietary software to administer computer-assisted modes. However, independently conducted small-scale surveys may emulate these methods by linking online to a web questionnaire.

The most frequent computer-assisted application is for conducting interviews. Indeed, most interviews conducted by professional survey organizations now are computer-assisted. The first applications were developed for telephone interviews. In a **computer-assisted telephone interview (CATI)**, instead of using a paper questionnaire, the interviewer reads questions and response choices displayed on a screen, usually a monitor connected to a computer in an interviewing center. The interviewer records responses as code numbers via a keyboard or mouse clicks. For a **computer-assisted in-person interview (CAPI)**, in which the *P* is derived from referring to in-person/face-to-face interviews as "personal" interviews), the interviewer reads questions and records responses in the same manner as CATI. However, for ease of portability, CAPI interviewers are equipped with a laptop/notebook or tablet device.

Computer-assisted self-interviews (CASI) are conducted by providing the respondents a device, typically a laptop/notebook or tablet, with which to self-complete a programmed questionnaire. Essentially, this is an electronic version of a monitored self-administered questionnaire, with staff present to explain and monitor respondents' use of the equipment and software. For an **audio computer-assisted self-interview (ACASI)**, the respondents also listen to a synchronized voice recording played over a speaker or headset of an interviewer reading aloud instructions, questions, and response choices. An option with ACASI is that an interviewer may be recorded in more than one language so respondents may choose the language they prefer. Other technological advances continue to be developed and tested, such as video interviewing, touchtone data entry, and voice-recognition data entry.

Advantages

Box 12.4 lists key advantages of computer-assisted modes. They automate questionnaire navigation, making following skip patterns invisible to both respondents and interviewers. This reduces their burden and eliminates skipping questions that should be answered or responding to questions that do not apply. Computer-assisted modes also enable inserting "fills" of a word, phrase, or value from responses to previous questions either in the same questionnaire or from another data source. For example, after respondents report the date of their most recent clinic visit, questions about that experience may refer to that date to aid recall.

> **BOX 12.4: COMPUTER-ASSISTED ADVANTAGES**
>
> - Automated questionnaire navigation
> - "Fills" from responses to previous questions
> - Customized wording
> - Accessing multiple language versions
> - Engaging interactive features
> - Presenting repeating question blocks
> - Automated real-time data entry and editing
> - Automated calculations
> - Automated real-time data quality checks

Question wording may be customized based on responses to previous questions. For example, after a roster of the first names of a respondent's children is entered, subsequent questions about each child's health may refer to the child by name. Another application is to insert the term respondents indicate they feel most comfortable using for a question about a sensitive topic. When a questionnaire is prepared in multiple languages, a computer-assisted mode may conveniently access the appropriate version selected by the respondent or interviewer, and there is no need to reproduce multiple copies of a printed questionnaire.

Computer-assisted methods enable using engaging interactive features that are not possible in a printed questionnaire, such as drop-down lists, radio buttons, pop-up instructions, and help screens, and presenting photographs, videos, and audio recordings. Sometimes the same block of questions may be asked about each of several related events. For example, the same block of questions might be asked about satisfaction with services received at each of several clinic visits. In a paper questionnaire, it is not possible to anticipate the number of such blocks that must be presented depending on the number of relevant clinic visits a respondent reports. However, the questionnaire for a computer-assisted mode may accommodate an unlimited number of such blocks.

Finally, responses are entered in real time into a data analysis file, reducing data entry time and costs. Calculations may be performed automatically and immediately, which avoids errors as well as saves time and costs. For example, respondents' age may be calculated immediately after they enter their birth date. Moreover, data quality checks may be performed in real time to flag problems such as responses that are out of the logical or acceptable range, responses that are not consistent with responses to earlier questions, and responses that are not entered in the correct format, such as a date.

Disadvantages

Employing a computer-assisted mode typically requires an investment in purchasing and maintaining equipment and software. Complex questionnaires require a substantial investment of programming expertise and time to ensure the accuracy of features such as navigation, "fills," automated calculations, and so forth. It is imperative to check that the programming handles appropriately all possible response conditions. For example, navigation errors may result in not collecting information about key variables for some respondents. A system for data file management and backup is essential. Also, consideration must be given to the risk of equipment theft and staff safety while transporting equipment in the field.

Conducting a Survey

Mail

General protocol

Table 12.2 presents a general protocol for conducting a mail survey. The timing includes sending materials to respondents, and allowing for them to complete and return the questionnaire. In most situations, the timing is not affected substantially by the sample's size or geographic distribution. It is best to avoid conducting a mail survey during major holiday and vacation periods. For all mailings, the best practice is to use first-class postage to speed delivery, take advantage of address correction and forwarding services, and avoid respondents associating the material with "junk mail" if bulk postage were used. To save costs, business reply mail, for which payment is made only for the return of completed questionnaires, may be used on return envelopes instead of using first-class postage on ones that are not returned. When preparing a budget, a mock-up sample of each mailing packet should be taken to a post office to verify postage costs. Also, mock-ups are essential for estimating costs of materials and staff time to prepare them.

In week 1, a cover letter, questionnaire, and preaddressed, postage-paid return envelope are mailed to the entire sample. The *cover letter* should be printed on the letterhead stationery of the agency under whose auspices the study is conducted. It should be prepared in a standard business letter format, not exceed one page in length, and be written with a cordial but professional tone. The salutation should include the respondent's full name

TABLE 12.2 ● Mail Survey Protocol

Week	Activity	Sample
1	Send an initial cover letter, questionnaire, and return envelope	All
2	Send a follow-up letter/postcard	All
3	Receive returns	
4	Send a second cover letter, questionnaire, and return envelope	Nonrespondents
5–6	Receive returns	
7	Send a third cover letter, questionnaire, and return envelope	Nonrespondents
8–9	Receive returns	
10	End data collection	

(e.g., "Dear Mary Smith"), if known, not his or her first name only, and a title should not be presumed if one is not known (e.g., Mr., Mrs., or Ms.). If the respondent's name is not known, the salutation should be generic, such as "Dear Illinois Resident," and it should not be inappropriately familiar, such as "Dear Friend."

The initial cover letter should present

- a brief description of the study's purpose and importance,
- a brief description of how the respondent was selected,
- a brief description of how the respondent's information will be used,
- an assurance of confidentiality,
- instructions for completing the questionnaire, and
- instructions for submitting a completed questionnaire.

It should be signed by the person with primary responsibility for conducting the study, and include that person's position and contact information (direct telephone number and email address). Also, contact information for the governing institutional review board (IRB) should be included, and the IRB protocol approval number and date should be included on all documents for each mailing (letters, questionnaires, and postcards). If one is available, a link should be provided to a study website for further information (e.g., FAQs). It is best not to include a deadline for returning a completed questionnaire unless there is a real deadline for closing data collection and delivering a report, such as for policy advocacy. Otherwise, a deadline undermines making follow-up contacts after it is elapsed.

In week 2 (or about five working days after the first mailing), a follow-up letter or postcard is mailed to the entire sample, thanking those who already have completed and returned a questionnaire, and reminding others of the importance of the study, encouraging them to complete and return the questionnaire as soon as possible, and thanking them in advance for their cooperation. Although a letter is more expensive than a postcard in terms of the cost of materials and postage, a letter conveys a sense of professionalism and importance a postcard does not.

During weeks 2 and 3, the first batch of completed questionnaires is received. The flow of returns should be monitored daily to identify when returns near zero, which usually occurs about the end of week 3. This procedure optimizes the timing of when to send out follow-up mailings. Also, it avoids incurring unnecessary costs from prematurely following up with respondents who will respond without a follow-up contact, or whose completed questionnaire already is in the mail. It is essential to assign each sample member a unique identification code that is recorded on his or her questionnaire and in a sample tracking log so follow-up contacts are attempted only with nonrespondents. That procedure saves costs, and avoids annoying or confusing sample members who already have returned a completed questionnaire.

In about week 4, a second mailing is sent to nonrespondents that includes a cover letter, questionnaire, and return envelope. The follow-up cover letter should be similar in format to the initial one, and emphasize the importance of the study and the value of obtaining information from everyone in the sample. Also, it should mention that another copy of the questionnaire is included for the respondents' convenience (also in case they discarded the initial one), and should encourage them to complete and return it as soon as possible. Subsequently, returns are received and their flow is monitored during weeks 5 and 6.

In about week 7, a third mailing is sent to nonrespondents that includes a similar but slightly different cover letter, questionnaire, and return envelope. Dillman et al. (2014) recommend as a means of motivation to indicate in the third mailing cover letter that this is the respondent's last chance to participate in the study. However, there is no consistent evidence in support of that procedure. Some respondents might feel relieved to know they will not be contacted again if they do not respond. Moreover, such a commitment invalidates any potential subsequent contact attempt with nonrespondents. The flow of additional returns is monitored. When it becomes apparent that very few if any further returns are likely to be received, usually about week 10, the data collection period is closed.

Preparing a budget for materials and postage requires estimating the cumulative number of sample members from whom a completed questionnaire is likely to be received at each point subsequent to the week 1 mailing. Such estimates may be obtained from conducting a pilot study, reviewing outcomes from other mail surveys using about a similar topic with a similar target population, and consulting with survey research professionals. A useful guide is to estimate the percent of the sample that will respond to the initial mailing, then multiply it by .5 to estimate the additional percent of the total sample that will respond to the second mailing, and then multiply that percentage by .5 to estimate the additional percent that will respond to the third mailing.

As illustrated in Table 12.3, suppose a completed questionnaire is expected to be received from 40% of the sample in response to the first mailing and follow-up letter (weeks 1 and 2). The second mailing will be sent to the remaining 60% of the sample that did not respond. By about the end of week 6, it is estimated that a completed questionnaire will be received from an additional 20% of the total sample (.5 × 40%), for a cumulative return from 60% (40% + 20%) of the total sample. The third mailing will be sent to the remaining 40% of the sample, from which it is estimated that by about week 10 a completed questionnaire will be received from an additional 10% of the total sample (.5 × 20%) for a cumulative return from 70% (40% + 20% + 10%) of the total sample. Attempting further follow-up contacts with the remaining 30% of the sample is likely to obtain a completed questionnaire from only about an additional 5% of the total sample (.5 × 10%). In most cases, the additional

TABLE 12.3 ● Mail Survey Estimated Recipients and Cumulative Returns

Week	Activity	Recipients	Cumulative Returns
1	Send an initial cover letter, questionnaire, and return envelope	100%	
2	Send a follow-up letter	100%	
3	Receive returns		40%
4	Send a second cover letter, questionnaire, and return envelope	60%	
5–6	Receive returns		60%
7	Send a third cover letter, questionnaire, and return envelope	40%	
8 & 9	Receive returns		
10	End data collection		70%

cost and time for doing that is likely to be deemed not worthwhile. Overall, the illustration in Table 12.3 calls for mailing a complete packet (cover letter, questionnaire, and return envelope) to 200% (100% + 60% + 40%) of the total sample. Moreover, the budget must include costs for postage, mailing labels, and assembling each packet. In addition, a week 2 follow-up letter (or postcard) will be sent to 100% of the total sample. Accordingly, if the total sample is 400, the budget must cover mailing 800 complete packets and 400 letters.

Options

About five working days prior to sending the first packet, a **prenotification** letter or postcard may be sent to all sample members to inform them about the study and that they should expect to receive a questionnaire within a few days. A benefit of prenotification is it helps identify bad addresses by receiving undeliverable returns from the post office. This saves costs for sending a complete packet to those addresses. Another useful aspect of prenotification, when appropriate, is to ask respondents in advance to locate any household records that may assist them in answering some questions. However, research results do not consistently support a general contribution of prenotification to increasing response rates or receiving returns more promptly (Groves et al., 2009; Nicolaas, Smith, & Pickering, 2015). Moreover, prenotification increases costs and data collection time. If it is employed, it is best not to ask sample members to provide consent (e.g., by marking and returning a postcard) to receive a questionnaire. That procedure generally leads to a lower unit response rate because potential respondents may refuse without the benefit of reviewing the questionnaire, and it eliminates making follow-up attempts with them.

If telephone numbers are available, nonrespondents may be called to encourage their participation and answer any questions they might have about a study. The optimal timing for such calls is one to two days after sending the third (and typically final) mailing packet (about week 7). The opportunity to send the third packet will be lost if calls are placed prior to that mailing and the sample member indicates he or she does not want to be contacted further about the study. Although such calls increase the budget, they have no effect on the time schedule. A decision must be made about whether staff making the calls should offer to conduct a telephone interview using the questionnaire, or be prepared to conduct an interview if the respondent requests one. If such interviews are to be conducted, they will add costs for interviewer training, supervision, and interview time. Also, they will require adding interviewer scripts to the questionnaire. Moreover, collecting information by mail from some respondents and by interview from others may introduce mode effects.

Sample

A current mailing address is necessary for each sample member. For some special populations, a sample might be selected from an existing list such as patient records or an employee directory. In the past, for the general population of the nation, states, counties, or cities, samples were selected from telephone directories or reverse street address directories. However, those methods are prone to bias because many households with telephone service are not included in such directories owing to unpublished or unlisted landline numbers, and the increasing prevalence of cell-phone-only households. As an alternative, **address-based sampling (ABS)** methods were developed, whereby a sample may be selected from the U.S. Postal Service (USPS) Delivery Sequence File (DSF). The DSF contains all delivery-point addresses serviced by the USPS, with the exception of general delivery. The USPS makes the DSF available in digital format through licensed sampling vendors (Iannacchione, 2011; Iannacchione, Staab, & Redden, 2003). In addition to residential addresses, the DSF includes addresses for businesses and institutions that must be purged for conducting a residential mail survey.

Monitored

When a monitored questionnaire is administered to individuals, staff approach potential respondents, such as community health fair visitors; introduce themselves; briefly describe the study; and ask if they are willing to participate. As appropriate, staff should ask questions to ensure each potential respondent meets the study eligibility criteria. In a clinic setting, the approach may be made by trained clinic or research staff. Each respondent should be given a single-page information sheet describing the study's purpose and importance, how he or she was selected, how his or her information will be used, assurance of confidentiality, and contact information for the person with primary responsibility for conducting the study and the governing IRB. The staff also explain how to complete and submit the questionnaire. They should supply each respondent with a pen or pencil, and either a clipboard or a table/desk on which to fill out the questionnaire. It is best to reproduce the questionnaire in a booklet format, which presents a professional appearance and facilitates proceeding from one page to another.

When a survey is administered to a group, an appropriate location and time should be arranged in advance. Potential respondents should be provided prenotification, and unless completing the questionnaire will take no more than a few minutes, an alternative activity should be arranged for any who choose not to participate. Whenever feasible, supervisory personnel (e.g., teachers, managers) should not be present to observe who does and does not participate. Moreover, their presence might influence some to participate who otherwise would choose not to participate, or influence how they answer questions that reflect on their relationship with them. For every question about a sensitive topic, there should be a response choice for every respondent, such as "Does not apply," to prevent others from observing who is and is not answering questions about the topic. Otherwise, observing who answers questions about a topic such as illegal drug use might imply who has or has not engaged in that behavior.

Similar to administering a questionnaire to individuals, staff should introduce themselves to the group, briefly describe the study, and ensure that all potential respondents are eligible to participate. To protect confidentiality, an alternative approach is to include eligibility questions in the questionnaire and discard questionnaires from any respondents who are not eligible. As for individual administration, each respondent should be given a single-page information sheet, regardless of prenotification. Staff should explain how to complete and submit the questionnaire, and supply each respondent with a pen or pencil and either a clipboard or a table/desk on which to fill out the questionnaire.

To the extent feasible, staff should control the environment to ensure respondents are not disturbed or distracted, and to discourage collaboration. To avoid some respondents completing questionnaire sections far in advance of others, the questionnaire should include an instruction to stop at the end of each section. Then staff may instruct the respondents to complete the next section. This procedure enables staff to address any issues about completing the questionnaire to the entire group as the respondents are completing the same section. For lower-literacy adult populations and schoolchildren, it is helpful for staff to read each question and its response choices aloud, allow time for everyone to record an answer, and then move on to the next question.

Web

The usual procedure for implementing a web survey is to send an email message, similar to a mail survey cover letter, inviting the sample members to participate by linking to a website where they may obtain further information and access the questionnaire. It is essential that a sampling frame with email addresses is available to select the sample. There is no general directory of email addresses. The frame must be provided by a third party, such as a school, clinic, workplace, or professional organization. Therefore, a web survey is not appropriate for obtaining data that are representative of the general population.

Similar to a mail survey, a reminder email message may be sent about three days after the first one. Receipt of completed questionnaires should be monitored daily to identify when they near zero. Then a follow-up email message should be sent to sample members who have not yet completed the questionnaire. Typically, that should be done during the second week of data collection. Additional follow-up messages may be sent at intervals of about five working days. Although sending follow-up messages is quick and inexpensive, follow-up contacts should be limited to three or four so sample members do not feel harassed. As for a mail survey, it is best not to include a deadline for completing a questionnaire unless there is a real deadline for closing data collection and delivering a report.

To prevent multiple entries by a single respondent, software should be used that assigns a password or personal identification number (PIN) to each respondent that must be entered to access the questionnaire online. The password or PIN may be provided in the email contacts, or it may be embedded in an extension to the web survey link, which reduces the respondent's burden and the potential for error. Also, the survey software should enable respondents to leave and return to the questionnaire if they do not have time to complete it entirely at one time. Respondents should be informed about this at the survey welcome and introduction page.

Telephone Interviews

General protocol

Table 12.4 presents a general protocol for conducting a telephone interview survey. Timing is not affected by the sample's geographic distribution. It is best to avoid major

TABLE 12.4 ● Telephone Interview Survey Protocol

Week	Activity
1	Send the prenotification letter, if addresses are available
1	Make initial contact attempts 3–5 days after sending the prenotification letter
2–3	Interview the most readily available sample members
2–6	Attempt contact with the remaining portion of the sample, as well as noncontacts, and keep appointments
3–6	Attempt to convert refusals, as appropriate
6	End data collection

holiday and vacation periods. When the sample is large or the interviewer staff is relatively small, the sample may be divided randomly into manageable-size batches that are processed in series. In that condition, the approximate timing shown in Table 12.4 will apply to each batch, and the overall data collection period must be extended by an appropriate number of weeks.

When addresses are available, a prenotification letter should be sent by first-class mail or email, with content similar to a mail survey cover letter and informing the sample member to expect an interviewer to call in the next few days. Prenotification helps legitimize the study and distinguishes it from telemarketing calls. Initial telephone contact attempts should be made three to five days later, allowing time for the prenotification to be received. Processing the sample in batches enables attempting contacts promptly after prenotification. If prenotification is sent to the entire sample at once, some might be contacted weeks later, diminishing its impact. Moreover, if prenotification includes visual aids or a request to retrieve information from records, respondents might discard the materials by the time they are contacted. Another benefit of processing the sample in batches is that when a new batch is allocated, a fresh group of relatively easy-to-complete cases becomes available, which motivates interviewers while they continue to work noncontacts from the previous batch.

Making contact

In general, most telephone interviews are conducted on weekday evenings and weekends. When an initial contact attempt is not successful, multiple follow-up attempts should be made, varying the day of the week and time of day. When several (e.g., at least five) contact attempts with a sample member are not successful on weekday evenings and weekends, attempts should be made during the daytime on weekdays. Although there is no standard minimum number of follow-up calls that should be made per sample member, professionally conducted telephone interview surveys usually attempt 10 to 15 calls before designating a sample member as a final noncontact.

A **contact log** should be maintained to record each attempt and its outcome. The log should be reviewed daily to identify patterns when contact attempts are most likely to be successful. If someone other than the sample member answers a call and the sample member is not available, the interviewer should inquire about when would be an appropriate time to call back. When a sample member who is willing to participate is contacted at an inconvenient time, the interviewer should attempt to schedule an appointment to call back. If a busy signal is received, several calls should be placed to that number shortly thereafter. Adequate time should be allowed for a telephone to be answered, such as 6 to 10 rings. If a call is not transferred to a messaging system, it generally is not productive to leave a voice message asking a sample member to call an interviewer.

When sample members are contacted and refuse an interview, the interviewer should attempt to identify the reason for the refusal and record it in the contact log. Unless sample members clearly indicate they wish not to be contacted about the study again, standard practice is to attempt to contact them once more several days later. Professional survey organizations typically assign "**refusal conversion**" cases to experienced and specially trained interviewers. In particular, interviewers for that assignment should be considered who have demonstrated in previous studies to effectively address concerns that might lead to a refusal. Moreover, it is essential to be sensitive so as not to make sample members feel they are being harassed.

Sample

Telephone interviews are appealing because in the United States they provide nearly universal coverage, with approximately 96% of households having telephone service (Blumberg & Luke, 2017). A current telephone number is required for each sample member. The most straightforward sampling strategy is to select a sample from an existing list such as patient records or an employee directory. However, there is no appropriate list for the general population. Even for smaller geographic units such as cities, many households with telephone service are not included in directories because their numbers are unpublished or unlisted. Moreover, landline service is declining, as the prevalence of cell-phone-only households (also called "wireless-only") continues to increase. As of January–June 2017, it was estimated that about 52% of households were wireless only and 38% were landline and wireless (Blumberg & Luke, 2017).

In response, **random-digit dialing (RDD)** sampling designs have been developed so a telephone interview sample may include both listed and unlisted numbers, as well as cell phone numbers (Blair et al., 2014; Dillman et al., 2014; Lavrakas, 2008; Levine & Harter, 2015). The most advanced RDD methods require subcontracting with a professional sampling vendor. That is done best by collaborating with a professional academic or commercial survey organization. Because interviewers do not know whom they are contacting with an RDD sample, they always must screen for eligibility, and it might be necessary to employ a procedure to randomly select one eligible household member to interview. Moreover, prenotification and sending visual aids in advance are not possible because addresses for members of an RDD sample are not available.

In-Person Interviews

General protocol

Table 12.5 presents a general protocol for conducting an in-person interview survey. As for the other data collection modes, it is best to avoid major holiday and vacation periods. If the survey is conducted in a geographic region where adverse weather conditions may be expected to hamper interviewer travel, those seasons should be avoided also. When the sample is distributed across a broad geographic area, interviewer travel time and costs may be reduced by establishing temporary local offices from which to operate. Similar to telephone interviews, when the sample is large or the interviewer staff is small, the sample may be divided into batches that are processed in series. However, instead of using random

TABLE 12.5 • In-Person Interview Survey Protocol

Week	Activity
1	Send the prenotification letter
1	Make initial contact attempts 3–5 days after sending the prenotification letter
2–4	Interview the most readily available sample members
3–10	Attempt contact with the remaining portion of the sample, as well as noncontacts, and keep appointments
3–10	Attempt to convert refusals, as appropriate
10	End data collection

selection, for in-person interviews batches should be designated as geographic clusters to reduce travel time and costs.

A prenotification letter should be sent by first-class mail or email, informing the sample member or household to expect an interviewer to call in the next few days. Prenotification is especially important for in-person interviews because most often they are conducted at the respondent's residence. However, they also may be done at schools, clinics, work sites, and other locations, as appropriate. Initial in-person contact attempts should be made three to five days later, allowing time for the prenotification to be received. The time schedule may be several weeks longer than depicted in Table 12.5, depending on factors such as the length of the interview, the sample size, the sample's geographic distribution and accessibility, travel conditions, and the size of the interviewer staff. For a special population, such as a survey of organizations or health professionals, an advance telephone call should be made to schedule an appointment. Otherwise, advance telephone calls are not advisable because it generally is easier to refuse an interview on a telephone than in person. Thus, advance telephone calls might undermine the advantage of in-person contact for gaining cooperation.

Making contact

In general, most in-person interviews are conducted on weekdays and weekends, from mid-morning through early evening. This pattern differs from telephone interviews to broaden the contact window and out of consideration for interviewer safety while traveling in the field. When an eligible respondent is contacted, the interviewer should attempt to conduct an interview or schedule an appointment. When an initial contact attempt is not successful, follow-up attempts should be made on different days of the week and times of day. Similar to telephone interviews, a contact log should be maintained and reviewed to identify patterns when contact attempts are most likely to be successful. When contact is made with someone other than the sample member, the interviewer should inquire about an appropriate time to call back.

After several unsuccessful contact attempts (e.g., three), the interviewer should attempt to verify that a dwelling unit is occupied and ascertain the best time to return by consulting a neighbor or building manager, as appropriate. Professionally conducted telephone interview surveys usually make at least five attempts before designating a sample member as a final noncontact. That number is much lower than for telephone interviews owing to the time and cost for interviewer travel. Additional contact attempts should be made as convenient when an interviewer is working other assignments nearby, which is another reason for selecting a clustered sample. If a telephone number is available, a final strategy is to place several calls (e.g., three) in an attempt to make contact and schedule an interview appointment.

As for telephone interviews, when a sample member refuses an interview, the interviewer should attempt to identify the reason for the refusal and record it in the contact log. In addition, an in-person interviewer may record on-site observations about characteristics of the sample member, dwelling unit, and community that may be used in assessing potential nonresponse bias. Unless sample members clearly indicate they wish not to be contacted about the study again, standard practice is to assign a "refusal conversion" interviewer to attempt contacting them once more several days later.

Sample

In-person interviews require a current address for each sample member. It is most convenient when a sample may be selected from an existing list, such as patient records or an employee directory. If a list sampling frame is broadly distributed geographically, it should be stratified geographically to select a sample. Sometimes a population is clustered naturally, such as parents of children in a particular school district. Alternatively, in consideration of available data collection resources, the target population might be respecified to include only one or more geographic areas.

In the past, samples of the general population of the nation, states, counties, or cities were selected using area-probability methods. For example, a multiple-stage cluster sample design using probabilities proportionate to size (Chapter 7) would select a series of geographic segments, such as states, counties, cities/towns, census tracts, and blocks. Then staff in the field would list every dwelling unit on those blocks, from which a sample of dwelling units would be selected. Instead, virtually all professionally conducted in-person interview surveys currently use ABS from the USPS DSF, as introduced in the mail sample section.

CHECK YOUR UNDERSTANDING 12.3

- Select one of your survey mode examples from Check Your Understanding 12.2 and draft a protocol for administering that survey (try to do this without looking at the general protocol examples in the preceding sections).
- Write a brief description of and explanation for your protocol draft.

Interviewing

General Guidelines

Box 12.5 presents general guidelines for conducting a survey interview using a structured questionnaire. Deviations from these guidelines contravene the standardized approach to developing a structured questionnaire and threaten the validity of comparisons across individuals and/or time. An interviewer must read aloud, clearly and slowly, every question and response choice exactly as it appears in the questionnaire. Interviewers must not substitute for or omit any word. They may not define a term, or explain the meaning of a question or response choice, unless they are given explicit permission and instruction for doing so during interviewer training. In addition, an interviewer must present every question and response choice exactly in the order as it appears in the questionnaire, and present every question and response choice that applies to each respondent. Thus, interviewers must be precise, and may not tailor any part of an interview according to their perception of aspects that might be irrelevant, discomforting, or too difficult for a respondent.

> **Key Concept**
>
> *A survey interviewer must read aloud every question and response choice exactly as it appears in the questionnaire.*

BOX 12.5: GENERAL INTERVIEWING GUIDELINES

- Read aloud, clearly and slowly, every question and response choice exactly as it appears in the questionnaire.
- Present every question and response choice exactly in the order as it appears in the questionnaire.
- Present every question and response choice that applies to each respondent.
- Assume and maintain control of the interview and conditions as much as possible.
- Be professional, but not impersonal.

An interviewer must assume and maintain control of the interview as much as possible. More control is possible for in-person than telephone interviews. Interviewers should seek a private setting in which they and the respondents will be comfortable. They should suggest eliminating distractions (e.g., turning off a television) or moving away from them. An interviewer's conduct must be professional, patient, respectful, and nonjudgmental. All questions and response choices must be read in a neutral tone, except when the questionnaire indicates emphasizing certain words or phrases.

However, interviewers must not be impersonal. They should engage in casual conversation to establish rapport to encourage the respondents to answer each question accurately and completely. Interviewers must teach the respondents their role by establishing the question/response pattern and controlling the interview's pace. If respondents offer a response prematurely, interviewers should politely ask them to please wait until they read the entire question and/or all response choices. When a question involves a visual aid, interviewers should retrieve it as soon as respondents answer the question to prevent them from being distracted by it. Interviewers must not react to any response by expressing approval, disapproval, surprise, amusement, and so forth, by means of spoken words, tone of voice, facial expression, or body language. They should provide neutral reinforcement of appropriate respondent behavior, such as "Thank you for that response," not "That's a good answer."

Recording Responses

An interviewer must record a "response" for every question that applies to a respondent. If a respondent is unable to answer a question, the interviewer should record a "Don't know" response if it is included in the questionnaire. Otherwise, standard practice is to enter the abbreviation DK or a predesignated code. To minimize missing data, best practice

> **Key Concept**
>
> *A survey interviewer must record a "response" for every question that applies to a respondent.*

is not to include "Refused" as a response outcome. If a respondent refuses to answer a question, the interviewer may record the abbreviation "Ref" or a corresponding predesignated code. A common practice for a single-digit coding scheme is to designate 8 for "Don't know" and 9 for "Refused," leaving available values for up to seven response choices (ignoring zero). A double-digit coding scheme should be used for more than seven choices, designating 98 for "Don't know" and 99 for "Refused," leaving available codes for up to 97 response choices.

Every response should be recorded immediately to record it accurately and prevent leaving a question blank. Interviewers never should record a response from memory. If they neglect to record a response, they should ask the respondent to repeat his or her response. If a blank is discovered after an interview is completed, the interviewer should attempt to contact the respondent to obtain his or her response. Responses to open questions and "Other—please specify" response choices should be recorded verbatim while respondents are speaking. Interviewers should not paraphrase or summarize a response. They may use abbreviations to facilitate verbatim recording. When appropriate, they should ask respondents to speak more slowly, pause, or repeat part of a response so they may record it accurately. Moreover, such procedures indicate the respondents are providing valuable information, which generally enhances their cooperation.

Probing

Probing is employed most often when asking an open question or when a response to a closed question falls in an "Other—please specify" category. Nevertheless, probing also may be employed with closed questions for which there is no such response choice. As appropriate, after asking a question, an interviewer should probe to

- encourage a response,
- clarify a response, and
- obtain a complete response.

All probes should be presented in a neutral manner so as not to influence a response. Probes should be encouraging and reaffirming, and express neither approval nor disapproval. Probing never should make a respondent feel pressured or coerced to answer a question. Frequently used, effective probing techniques are

- silent probe,
- encouragement,
- reassurance,
- rereading the question,
- rereading the response choices,
- playing back the respondent's words,
- requesting clarification, and
- asking "What else?"

To facilitate coding responses and assessing an interviewer's performance, all probes should be recorded on the questionnaire, either in parentheses or in another special way, to distinguish probes from responses. This is especially important when an interviewer probes an open question or an "Other—please specify" response. Probes may be recorded using abbreviations, such as RQ for *repeating the question*, RC for *repeating response choices*, and *Time* for "Take some time to think about it."

Encouragement

The first strategy an interviewer should use to encourage respondents to answer a question is the **silent probe**, whereby the interviewer allows time for respondents to process their response. There is no standard length of time for a silent probe, but generally it is several seconds. A long pause is likely to create an uncomfortable atmosphere. The interviewer may determine an appropriate time based on factors such as the interview pace, the extent to which respondents appear engaged in the topic, facial expressions, and body language.

All "Don't know" responses should be probed, first using a silent probe. Instead of indicating the respondent is unable to answer the question, an initial response such as "Oh, I don't know" might mean "Give me a moment to think about that." Other techniques are encouraging respondents to take some time to think about their answer, rereading the question, asking for their best estimate, reassuring them they are not being judged ("There are no right or wrong answers"), and reminding them that all responses are confidential. Also, virtually all initial refusals to both closed and open questions should be probed. A brief explanation about why the information is being requested often is effective. In addition, the interviewer might reassure the respondents that they will not be judged and all responses will be confidential.

Clarification

When a respondent answers a question, the interviewer's first responsibility is to ensure the response is clear. For a closed question, the interviewer must assess whether it fits one of the response choices. For example, suppose an interviewer asks,

> When was the last time you tried to stop smoking and you did not smoke even one puff for at least 24 hours? Was it within the last 30 days, 1 to 6 months ago, 7 to 12 months ago, or more than 1 year ago?

If the respondent says, "It was several months ago," the interviewer should probe for clarification. In this instance, the interviewer should read all the response choices again. Subsequently, suppose the respondent says, "I think it was about six or seven months ago." Then, the interviewer should probe by saying, "Would you say it was more likely to be six or seven months ago?" In another situation, a respondent might say, "I've tried to stop smoking so many times I can't remember them." That indicates the respondent might not have heard or interpreted the question correctly. It did not ask how many times the respondent tried to quit ever. The most appropriate probe would be to reread the question, emphasizing that it is asking about "the last time" the respondent tried to stop smoking.

For an open question, interviewers should assess whether the response is sufficiently clear that they would be confident placing it in an analysis category. For example, suppose they ask, "What would you say is the most important problem in this community?" and the respondent says, "It's not safe." There are many ways in which a community may be perceived as "not safe." An appropriate probe would be to play back the respondent's words, such as "How is it 'not safe'?" The interviewer never should suggest a reason why it might not be safe, such as "Are there any problems with gangs?" Respondents might be concerned about other issues, such as traffic, rodents, abandoned buildings, air pollution, or a contaminated water supply. A probe about gangs or any other example might distract them from what *they* think is "the most important problem." Similarly, responses in an "Other—please specify" category for a closed question should be probed for clarity. Examples are as follows:

- How was it "difficult"?
- What do you mean when you say "it makes you worry"?
- Why do you say it is "not convenient"?

Completeness

For an open question, after probing for clarification of an initial response, as appropriate, the interviewer should explore whether there are additional comments respondents might share about the topic. The best practice is to use a probe that is a form of "What else?" to express an expectation the respondents might have more to say. Examples are "What else can you tell me about that?" "What else happened that time?" and "What else would you like to say about that?" Asking if there is "anything else" may express the response is sufficient and the interviewer is ready to move on to the next question. Consequently, the respondents are not likely to provide additional information, which might be more valuable than what they shared thus far. When respondents provide additional information, the interviewer should probe for clarification as appropriate, then probe again for completeness.

Interviewer Characteristics

Box 12.6 lists essential characteristics for an interviewer using a structured questionnaire. Although interviewers must read every question and response choice exactly as it appears in a questionnaire, they must be able to apply general interviewing principles in a variety of situations to gain cooperation, establish rapport, control the interview situation, and probe responses. That requires a substantial degree of self-confidence and interpersonal skill. At the same time, interviewers must be able and willing to follow instructions and accept supervision. Also, a background check should be conducted to ensure each interviewer is trustworthy and honest.

Interviewers must be adept in reading out loud. They must be accurate, clear, and well paced, and provide emphasis as appropriate. In particular, a telephone interviewer must have a strong, clear voice and good enunciation. All interviewers must be good listeners, and have good clerical skills to record responses accurately and probe effectively. When a computer-assisted mode (CATI or CAPI) is employed, interviewers must be appropriately computer literate.

In addition, interviewers must be reliable, and available on days and at times of day when interviewing is most likely to be successful. Moreover, they must be available and committed for the duration of the data collection period. In general, it is best to hire and pay an interviewing staff instead of using volunteers (e.g., students or senior center clients) in the interest of reducing costs and/or providing experience. Volunteers tend to be less reliable than paid staff. For example, they might assign a higher priority to other matters (e.g., preparing for a school examination), they might not be available during inclement weather, or they might resign if they become bored or frustrated with attempting to contact hard-to-reach sample members.

> **BOX 12.6: INTERVIEWER CHARACTERISTICS**
>
> **Personal**
> - Able to apply general principles in diverse situations
> - Self-confident
> - Able to follow instructions and accept supervision
> - Trustworthy and honest
>
> **Skills**
> - Reading out loud
> - Listening
> - Clerical ability
> - Computer literacy, as appropriate
>
> **Availability**
> - Reliable
> - Available on days and at times of day when interviewing is most likely to be successful
> - Available and committed for the duration of the data collection period

Interviewer Training

Interviewer training typically requires at least one full day and may require several days, depending on the length and complexity of the questionnaire, the nature of the target population, and other study design features. There are two types of interviewer training. First, interviewers must be trained in basic interviewing principles. This should include classroom instruction, self-study, and modeling appropriate interview techniques. Experienced interviewers should be required to review the basic principles.

Second, all interviewers must be trained for the specific study. This includes introducing themselves, explaining the study's purpose and how respondents were selected, and assurance of confidentiality. It is helpful to prepare an anticipatory list of frequently asked questions (FAQs) respondents are likely to ask, and guidelines or scripts for responding to them. Next, the questionnaire should be reviewed thoroughly, including every script, question, response choice, and skip pattern, as well as how to record responses. Then interviewers should practice by conducting **mock interviews**, in which a trainer plays the respondent role and the interviewer receives immediate feedback about his or her performance. Mock interviews may be done individually or in a group. Finally, each interviewer should conduct at least two successful practice interviews in the field, monitored by a trainer/supervisor.

Interviewer Supervision

All interviewers should be monitored to ensure they are performing appropriately, and to maximize productivity, minimize errors, and prevent falsification. This is done most effectively at a telephone interviewing center using CATI, where a supervisor may remotely listen to interviewer–respondent interactions and observe data entry on a remote monitor. Otherwise, telephone interviews may be monitored through a conference call. Monitoring in-person interviews requires a supervisor to accompany interviewers in the field. In all situations, the respondent must be informed the interview may be monitored for quality control.

A general guideline is to randomly select throughout the course of data collection 10%–15% of each interviewer's assignments for monitoring. The supervisor should provide the interviewer prompt feedback about his or her performance. In addition, validation contacts should be made with 5%–10% of each interviewer's completed interview respondents to confirm the interview was completed and conducted properly. For convenience, in-person interview respondents may be contacted by telephone. However, if data collection includes on-site observations, a portion of in-person interview validations should be done in the field.

CHECK YOUR UNDERSTANDING 12.4

- What are the five general guidelines for conducting a survey interview?
- What are the four essential personal characteristics for an interviewer using a structured questionnaire?
- What are the four skills a survey interviewer must have?

Key Points

Basic Concepts

A survey systematically collects self-reported data using a structured questionnaire.

- **Key Advantages**
  - Standardization
  - Ability to collect information about variables not observable directly
  - Speed/timeliness
  - Large data sets (participants and variables)
  - Low per-unit cost
  - Broad geographic coverage
- **Key Disadvantages**
  - Ability to explore unanticipated aspects of a topic is limited.
  - Resource requirements may be significant.
  - Respondents might not be accessible.

Survey Modes Comparison

- Costs typically are lowest for self-administered questionnaires (mail, monitored, and web).
- Web and telephone interview surveys collect data most quickly.

- Mail, web, and telephone interviews enable collecting data over a broad geographic area.
- Mail and monitored questionnaires enable anonymity.
- Interviews obtain the highest response rates and lowest item nonresponse.
- In-person interviews are most expensive.
- Mail and in-person interviews require the most data collection time.
- Cluster samples are best for monitored questionnaires and in-person interviews.

Conducting a Survey

- **Mail:** Several mailings are sent out over about a 10-week period.
- **Monitored:** Staff distribute questionnaires and receive completed ones.
- **Web:** Sample members complete a questionnaire online.
- **Telephone interviews:** Interviews are conducted over a telephone.
- **In-person interviews:** Interviews are conducted in-person.

General Interviewing Guidelines

- Read aloud, clearly and slowly, every question and response choice exactly as it appears in the questionnaire.
- Present every question and response choice exactly in the order in which it appears in the questionnaire.
- Present every question and response choice that applies to each respondent.
- Assume and maintain control of the interview and conditions as much as possible.
- Be professional, but not impersonal.

Interviewing Training

- First, interviewers must be trained in basic interviewing principles.
- Second, interviewers must be trained for the specific study.

Interviewing Supervision

- About 10%–15% of each interviewer's assignments should be selected randomly for monitoring.
- About 5%–10% of respondents to each interviewer's completed interviews should be selected randomly for validation.

Review and Apply

1. Prepare a protocol for administering the structured questionnaire you developed in the "Review and Apply" section of Chapter 11.
   a. Describe the rationale for your data collection plan, including how you would take into account any special factors of your target population, setting, and so forth.
   b. Draft a prenotification letter (even if your protocol does not include one).

2. Suppose you are an interviewer and you just asked the following question:

   "In general, how would you describe the condition of buildings in this neighborhood?

   Would you say they are in very good, good, poor, or very poor condition?"

   How would you handle each of the following responses? (Recommended techniques are listed after "Review and Apply" item 5.)

   a. "They're all right."
   b. "There are some that really need work."
   c. "The one on the corner is in bad shape, but in general they're in good condition."
   d. "When I first moved here, they were in good condition."
   e. "What do you mean by 'very good condition'?"
   f. "I really haven't thought about it much."
   g. "I'm not sure; what do you think?"

3. If you developed your questionnaire to be self-administered (mail, monitored, or web), revise it by adding scripts so it could be used to conduct a telephone or in-person interview. If your questionnaire already is designed for an interview, go to "Review and Apply" item 4.

4. Prepare an interviewer training manual specific to your questionnaire and mode (telephone or in-person). Use the example at the end of this section for a follow-up telephone interview with HMO smoking cessation participants as a model. Note: The example assumes a paper questionnaire.

5. Review your training manual with at least one other person, such as a classmate, and conduct mock interviews using your questionnaire. Alternate playing the roles of interviewer and respondent. Discuss positive and problematic aspects of each interviewer's performance.

Recommended Techniques for Exercise 2

a. Reread the response choices.
b. Say, "In general, would you say they are [read response choices]?"
c. Record "good."
d. How would you describe them now? Would you say they are [read response choices].
e. "'Very good' is whatever it means to you."
f. Silent probe. "Take some time to think about it."
g. "My opinion isn't important. We would like to know your opinion."

Interviewer Manual

HMO Smoking Cessation Follow-up

Purpose

- This study seeks to conduct telephone interviews to ask questions about attitudes about smoking and stopping smoking, recent smoking behavior, and how the HMO can best help people who would like to stop smoking.

Sponsors

- The XXX University and XXX HMO.
- Funding source(s) also may be provided.

Supervision

- Interviewing will be supervised by [supervisor name].
  - Office phone: (xxx) xxx-xxx Room xxx
  - Cell phone: (xxx) xxx-xxx
  - Email: XXXX@XXX.XXX
- The Project Director is [name and title].
  - Office phone: (xxx) xxx-xxx Room xxx
  - Cell phone: (xxx) xxx-xxx
  - Email: XXXX@XXX.XXX
- All interviewing assignments will be distributed and monitored by [supervisor name].
  - Any and all questions about interviewing procedures should be directed to [supervisor name]. Do not ask other interviewers about questions or problems with interviewing.
  - [Project director name] should be contacted only in cases of emergency when [supervisor name] is not available.

Time Schedule

- Interviewing will start [day of the week], [month and day, year].
- The goal is to complete all interviews by [month and day, year].

Sample

- Respondents will be adult HMO members (N = nnn) who smoke cigarettes and during the period [month and day, year] through [month and day, year]:
  1. Completed a baseline self-administered questionnaire, and
  2. Participated in a smoking cessation program (self-help manuals, nurse consultations, and optional classes) offered by the HMO.

According to the study and HMO records, all sample members are expected to be eligible to participate in the study. Nevertheless, each respondent's eligibility should be verified using the script in your portfolio before starting an interview.

Prenotification

- All sample members will be sent a prenotification letter informing them about the study and telling them that they will be called by an interviewer (see the example included in your portfolio).
- For each sample member, the letter will be mailed three days prior to the sample member being assigned to an interviewer.
- Start attempting to contact each sample member assigned to you promptly, while the impact of the letter is current.

Voluntary Participation

- Participating in the interview is entirely voluntary.
- If any sample member decides not to participate in the interview, this will not affect the quantity or quality of services the individual will receive in the future at the HMO. Explain this if a sample member expresses concern about it.

Respondent Dignity and Sensitivity

- Always deal with respondents in a professional and courteous manner.
- Some respondents may be upset that someone is calling to check on their smoking behavior.
  - Emphasize that the study is not judging anyone—there are no right or wrong answers to any of the questions.
  - For continuing smokers, emphasize that we understand it is very difficult for most people to stop smoking, and the purpose of this study is to learn about ways to help them and other people like them.

Confidentiality

- ALL information every respondent provides will be treated as strictly confidential.
  - No information provided during any interview will become part of any respondent's HMO record.
  - No information provided during any interview will be reported to any respondent's health care provider.
  - The results will be analyzed and reported in the form of group statistics, after information from all the participants are combined.
  - Results will be used for research purpose only.
  - No report of the results will include the name of any respondent.
- Although you may discuss your work and experiences as an interviewer in general with other persons, you may not show or discuss any interviewer report form (IRF) or completed (or partially completed) questionnaire to/with anyone who is not a member of the study staff.
- You may not identify any respondent by name or by any other identifying characteristic to anyone who is not a member of the study staff

Institutional Review Board (IRB)

- The project was reviewed and approved by the institutional review boards of the XXX University (protocol #XXXX-XXXX) and the XXX HMO (protocol #XXXX-XXXX).
- Sample members who have questions or concerns about their rights as participants in this study may contact:
  - The Project Director, [name and title], at (xxx) xxx-xxxx.
  - The XXX University Office for Protection of Research Subjects at (xxx) xxx-xxx.

Making Contact

- A minimum of 10 attempts will be made to contact each sample member.
- All callback attempts should be on a different day of the week/different time of the day.
- Be considerate of respondents' time and privacy. Do not call at times that typically would be inappropriate unless you are explicitly invited to do so by the respondent or another member of the respondent's household.
- It is essential to keep appointments for conducting interviews—call the respondent promptly at the appointed time.
- Do not leave messages on answering machines or voice mail systems. If you repeatedly contact only an answering machine/voice mail system for a respondent, bring this to the attention of [supervisor name].
- Resist accepting refusals from any person other than the designated sample member.

Interview Length/Duration

- On average, interviews are expected to last about 15 minutes.
- Because each interview will vary according to respondent characteristics, do not promise an exact time for an interview. Instead, if asked, provide a range, such as the following:

"It varies from person to person. In most cases it will take about 10 to 20 minutes."

Editing and Returning Completed Interviews

- Review thoroughly and edit carefully each interview as soon as possible after you complete it.
- Be sure that all questions that appear relevant to the respondent are answered, and are recorded appropriately and legibly on the questionnaire.
- If necessary, recontact the respondent as soon as possible to obtain any missing information or to clarify any problems.
- Return completed and edited questionnaires as soon as possible to [supervisor].

Study Further

Aday, L. A., & Cornelius, L. J. (2006). *Designing and conducting health surveys* (3rd ed.). San Francisco, CA: Jossey-Bass.

Blair, J., Czaja, R. F., & Blair, E. A. (2014) *Designing surveys: A guide to decisions and procedures*. Los Angeles, CA: Sage.

Dillman, D. A., Smyth, J. D., & Christian, L. M. (2014). *Internet, phone, mail, and mixed-mode surveys: The tailored design method*. Hoboken, NJ: Wiley.

Groves, R. M., Fowler, F. J., Jr., Couper, M. P., Lepkowski, J. M., Singer, E., & Tourangeau, R. (2009). *Survey methodology* (2nd ed.). Hoboken, NJ: Wiley.

Johnson, T. P. (Ed.). (2015). *Handbook of health survey methods*. Hoboken, NJ: Wiley.

13

Qualitative Research Methods

Chapter Outline

Overview
Learning Objectives
Basic Concepts
    Key Characteristics
    Limitations
Qualitative Interview Methods
    Unstructured Interviews
    Semistructured Interviews
    Structured Open-Ended Interviews
    Focus Groups
    Qualitative Interviewing Techniques
Observation Methods
    Participant Observation
    Nonparticipant Observation
    Reactivity
    Recording Observation Data
Sampling
    Purposive Sample
    Key Informants Sample
    Referral Sample
    Convenience Sample
    Sample Size
Mixed Methods
    Concurrent Designs
    Exploratory Sequential Designs
    Explanatory Sequential Designs
    Confirmatory/Generalizability Sequential Designs
    Monomethod Designs
Key Points

Learning Objectives

After studying Chapter 13, the reader should be able to:

- Decide when to employ a qualitative research method
- Identify the advantages and limitations of qualitative methods
- Select an appropriate qualitative data collection mode
- Develop a qualitative data collection plan
- Conduct a small-scale study using at least one qualitative interview method
- Conduct a small-scale study using at least one qualitative observation method
- Decide when and why to employ a mixed methods design

Overview

Qualitative research methods use varying degrees of unstructured data collection techniques to develop an in-depth understanding of a problem's nature and scope. They employ a holistic and context-specific approach to collect and interpret data primarily from participants' perspectives in natural settings. They are used to gain insight into how people experience, interpret, and respond to relationships, conditions, and events in their real-life context. Qualitative methods focus on describing and understanding how factors such as knowledge, beliefs, behaviors, social support, and access to services are correlated with particular needs or outcomes. Examples of research questions for which qualitative methods might be applied are as follows:

- *What* motivates Asian American women to get a mammogram?
- *Why* do some low-income parents not complete their child's immunization schedule?
- *How* do African American men identify and respond to heart disease symptoms?

Basic Concepts

Key Characteristics

As the name implies, qualitative research methods primarily collect qualitative data. Nevertheless, they also may collect quantitative measures, such as people's ages or the time since their most recent clinic visit. Moreover, they go beyond categorical nominal-level measurement (Chapter 8), using formats such as interview narratives, field observation notes, and audio and visual recordings. **Qualitative methods** use an inductive approach (Chapter 1) that affords substantial flexibility for following wherever the pursuit of relevant information leads.

> **Key Concept**
>
> Qualitative methods use an inductive approach to follow wherever the pursuit of relevant information leads.

Typically, collecting qualitative data is an iterative and responsive process, whereby as data are accumulated, they continually are reviewed. Among the purposes for employing qualitative methods are to

- identify emergent topics,
- explore a topic in greater depth,
- identify protocol modifications to enhance subsequent data collection, and
- identify participants or settings to include in subsequent research.

Qualitative methods commonly are employed with small nonprobability samples to enable focusing in depth on specific types of people, events, and conditions. They are not well suited for estimating population parameters or testing hypotheses about program or treatment outcomes. However, they excel in generating theory and hypotheses. Software, such as ATLAS.ti and NVivo, developed specifically for qualitative data greatly facilitates their analysis (Chapter 15). Qualitative research methods predominantly employ an observational design (Chapter 6), which may be cross-sectional or longitudinal.

Box 13.1 presents a summary of key qualitative research methods characteristics and limitations.

BOX 13.1: QUALITATIVE METHODS CHARACTERISTICS AND LIMITATIONS

Characteristics	Limitations
• Primarily unstructured, qualitative data	• It is challenging to combine or compare data across participants, situations, or time.
• Holistic and context-specific approach	
• Natural settings	• Data do not indicate size of differences.
• Inductive approach	• Data collection in natural settings tends to compromise internal validity.
• Iterative and responsive process	
• Typically small nonprobability samples	• It is not efficient for large samples or the general population.
• Predominantly observational designs	• Small nonprobability samples may not be generalizable.

Limitations

It is challenging to combine data collected by qualitative methods from multiple participants or in different situations. They do not necessarily collect the same information from every participant or about every situation (Patton, 2015). Indeed, they may deliberately elicit different information in diverse contexts to develop a holistic understanding of a problem. Moreover, qualitative data may not be comparable even when information is collected about the same aspects. For instance, unlike a structured questionnaire (Chapters 10 and 11), differences in qualitative interview responses may be confounded with differences in question wording and order. Additionally, participants may give unique expression to similar concepts when using an open-response format as opposed to selecting from closed response choices. Such differences may render it difficult to compare data even from the same participant across time.

> **Key Concept**
>
> *Qualitative methods do not necessarily collect the same information from every participant or about every situation.*

Similar challenges may result from differences in how data are recorded in the field. For instance, observers may differ in what they observe or how they record observations. As described in Chapter 8, qualitative (nominal-level) data do not indicate the size of differences. While collecting data in natural settings enhances external validity, it tends to compromise internal validity because extraneous variables typically are not controlled (Chapter 5). The in-depth approach characteristic of qualitative methods makes them inefficient for collecting data from large samples, and the nonprobability samples they typically study do not provide a reliable foundation for generalizing results.

> **CHECK YOUR UNDERSTANDING 13.1**
>
> - Consider the following research question:
>
>   *How do African American men identify and respond to heart disease symptoms?*
>   - What would be the main *advantages/benefits* of using qualitative methods to address this research question?
>   - What would be the main *limitations* of using qualitative methods to address this research question?

Qualitative Interview Methods

Table 13.1 summarizes key characteristics, strengths, and limitations of four basic types of qualitative interviews. A common characteristic is they ask questions in an **open-response format** (also called "open-ended"), whereby participants are encouraged to respond in their own words, typically at length, and freely speak about whatever comes to mind regarding a topic. For example, women might be asked to describe any problems (barriers) they may have encountered in getting a mammogram. In contrast, using a yes/no format in a structured questionnaire (Chapters 10 and 11), women might be asked if they have encountered each of several specific potential problems when getting a mammogram.

Key Concept

Qualitative interviews primarily ask questions in an open-response format.

A qualitative interviewer (or focus group moderator) employs probes similar to those for asking open questions in a structured questionnaire (Chapter 12). Also, the interviewer asks follow-up questions to explore a topic in greater depth or explore a new topic raised by a participant. Qualitative interviews typically are conducted in person. They also may be conducted by telephone or online video chat to eliminate travel time and costs, and include participants distributed across a wide geographic area. However, in-person generally is preferred because it enhances interaction and enables interviewers to observe nonverbal cues, such as facial expressions and body language, and surroundings. Most qualitative interviews are conducted one-on-one, with the exception of focus groups, which typically are conducted with about six to ten participants at a time.

Unstructured Interviews

An **unstructured interview**, also called an **in-depth interview**, is a guided conversation that proceeds naturally and interactively to explore relevant topics from the participant's perspective (Patton, 2015). This technique is especially appropriate when initially exploring the nature and scope of a problem about which there is little prior knowledge (Saldaña & Omasta, 2018). An unstructured interview offers great flexibility to pursue a research question in whatever relevant direction the interviewer–participant interaction leads. Nevertheless, being unstructured does not mean an interview is not focused. The interviewer should have a general plan of inquiry and may refer to a list of intended topics (Patton, 2015).

Unlike a structured questionnaire (Chapters 10 and 11), neither question wording nor question order is predetermined. Essentially, the interviewer is the data collection

TABLE 13.1 ● Qualitative Interview Methods

Method	Characteristics	Strengths	Limitations
Unstructured[a]	The interviewer has a general plan of inquiry, and may use a list of topics. Neither question wording nor question order is predetermined.	The interviewer takes a familiar conversational approach. Question wording and order is tailored to the participant and context.	There is heavy interviewer burden. Data collection is time-consuming. Data may not be comparable across individuals or time.
Semistructured[a]	The interviewer uses an interview guide that lists topics in prospective order. The interviewer may change topic order and question wording.	Using the interview guide • ensures all topics are addressed, • reduces interviewer burden, and • enhances comparability across individuals or time.	Flexibility in question wording and topic order may reduce comparability across individuals and time.
Structured Open-Ended[a]	Question wording, order, and topic predominantly are predetermined.	Using a structured interview guide enhances comparability across individuals or time. It is efficient for a large sample.	It is assumed that standard question wording and order is equally appropriate for all participants. Interaction is reduced.
Focus Groups	The moderator typically has flexibility to determine topic order and explore other relevant topics.	A group discussion is familiar and efficient. Using a semistructured guide ensures all topics are addressed.	Data may not be comparable across groups. Individual-level analysis is not appropriate.

[a]Typically conducted one-on-one.

"instrument," tailoring questions and topic order to the participant and context. However, an unstructured interview places a heavy burden on the interviewer, who must be an engaged listener while skillfully guiding the conversation to address topics related to the research question. Also, an unstructured interview is time-consuming, typically lasting one hour or longer. In addition, processing and analyzing unstructured data is challenging and time-consuming. Moreover, the free-flowing format may cover different topics across individuals or time, which makes it challenging to aggregate or compare data reliably owing to variation in topic/question order (Patton, 2015).

Semistructured Interviews

In a **semistructured interview,** also called an "interview guide approach," the interviewer uses an **interview guide** that lists topics in prospective order (Bernard, 2000). Some prior knowledge about the research problem is necessary to provide a foundation for preparing an interview guide. For example, such knowledge might be derived from unstructured interviews in a pilot study. The interview guide serves as a checklist to ensure all intended topics are addressed and to promote a smooth, logical flow across topics.

Typically, the interviewer has flexibility to change the topic order according to the natural flow of an interview and explore other relevant topics raised by the participants (Barbour, 2014; Patton, 2015).

An outline serves as a convenient interview guide format, as illustrated in Box 13.2. The interviewer typically is free to word questions in a conversational style and tailor them for the participant and context. However, the wording of some questions may be specified in advance, as illustrated by items IIA and IIB in Box 13.2, which are highlighted in italics. An interview guide reduces the interviewer's burden. Also, by ensuring that the same basic topics are addressed with each participant, it enhances data comparability across individuals or time, and facilitates data processing and analysis. However, comparability depends on the extent of variation in question wording and topic order. Compared to an unstructured interview, a semistructured interview tends to be somewhat less conversational in tone and is less likely to identify unanticipated issues.

> **BOX 13.2: SEMISTRUCTURED INTERVIEW GUIDE: NEIGHBORHOOD SAFETY AND STREET VIOLENCE**
>
> I. General attitudes about living in the neighborhood
>   A. What the participant likes most
>   B. What the participant likes least
>
> II. Concerns about safety on neighborhood streets
>   A. *How would you describe how safe you feel on the streets in your neighborhood?*
>   B. *Would you tell me why you feel that way?*
>
> III. Physical attacks on others in the past 12 months
>   A. Know/heard about
>   B. Witnessed firsthand
>
> IV. Physical attacks on oneself in the past 12 months
>
> V. How to improve neighborhood safety

Structured Open-Ended Interviews

A **structured open-ended interview** uses an interview guide with open-ended questions similar to those that might be included in a structured questionnaire (Chapters 10 and 11). For every participant, each question is worded the same and is presented in the same order (Patton, 2015). This approach rules out attributing response variation to differences in question wording and/or order. Also, it ensures all intended topics are addressed and promotes a smooth, logical flow across topics. As with a semistructured interview, some prior knowledge about the research problem is necessary to prepare an interview guide.

A structured open-ended interview is efficient for collecting qualitative data from a relatively large sample and at multiple sites. It reduces interviewer burden and potential interviewer effects, and it facilitates data processing and analysis. However, compared to unstructured and semistructured interviews, structured open-ended interviews are less conversational in tone. Although interviewers may have flexibility to change the topic order according to the interview flow and/or explore a relevant topic raised by participants, they are less likely to identify unanticipated issues. Box 13.3 presents an example of a structured open-ended interview guide based on the semistructured interview guide in Box 13.2.

BOX 13.3: STRUCTURED OPEN-ENDED INTERVIEW GUIDE: NEIGHBORHOOD SAFETY AND STREET VIOLENCE

1. When you think about your neighborhood overall, what things do you like <u>most</u> about living in your neighborhood?

2. When you think about your neighborhood overall, what things do you like <u>least</u> about living in your neighborhood?

3. How would you describe how safe you feel on the streets in your neighborhood?

    Would you tell me why you feel that way?

4. Thinking about the past 12 months, has someone <u>you know</u> been physically attacked in your neighborhood?

    Would you tell me what happened?

5. During the past 12 months, have you <u>heard</u> about <u>someone else</u> who was physically attacked in your neighborhood?

    Would you tell me what you heard?

6. During the past 12 months, have <u>you seen</u> someone being physically attacked in your neighborhood?

    Would you tell me what you saw?

7. During the past 12 months, have <u>you</u> been physically attacked in your neighborhood?

    Would you tell me what happened?

8. What do you think could be done to make your neighborhood safer?

Focus Groups

A **focus group** is conducted by a *moderator* who uses a semistructured guide and encourages a small group of participants to interactively respond to questions about a narrowly defined topic. The goal is to explore the range and depth of participants' perspectives about the topic in the context of others' perspectives. It is not to build consensus, solve a problem, make a decision, or conduct a debate (Patton, 2015). The format is not a "group interview," in which the moderator might ask a question to which participants respond individually and sequentially. Instead, participants are encouraged to freely share their perspectives, build on each other's responses, and comment respectfully on those expressed by others. The dynamics of group interaction may reveal aspects of the topic that might not emerge from a series of one-on-one interviews, or even from a group interview.

A focus group is not an open discussion about a broad topic. For example, instead of asking a group of cigarette smokers to discuss their experience as smokers in general, Kviz et al. (2003) asked smokers to discuss their perceptions of symptoms that might be correlated with cigarette smoking. Box 13.4 presents excerpts from the transcript for one such focus group with male Korean American cigarette smokers aged 45–74. In addition to asking questions, the moderator may ask participants to comment on photographs, video clips (e.g., to refine a video-based intervention), audio recordings, or vignettes, which are brief descriptions of a relevant event. For instance, following an open discussion, Kviz et al. (2003) asked participants to comment on a list of symptoms that might be associated with cigarette smoking based on a review of the literature and clinical guidelines.

> **BOX 13.4: FOCUS GROUP EXCERPTS: PERCEPTIONS ABOUT SMOKING-RELATED SYMPTOMS AMONG MALE KOREAN AMERICAN CIGARETTE SMOKERS**
>
> **M:** Some people say that some symptoms might be caused by smoking. What do you think about that?
>
> **A2:** Generally, many say smoking is bad. I have such a healthy constitution that I don't have to worry about it. It depends on an individual's physical condition.
>
> **A7:** As A2 said, it depends not only on an individual's physical constitution, but also on one's environment. If you sleep in a room with dry or dusty air, even a healthy person will cough as you get up in the morning. In my opinion, this is not related with smoking problem.
>
> **A5:** People close to me say smoking is bad for my health.
>
> **A7:** Generally smoking is known to be bad for health, so they say, "quit, quit."
>
> **A3:** I don't have anybody telling me, "You seem to have this or that symptom because of smoking." One of my close friends died of lung cancer five years ago. He never smoked in his entire life, but he suddenly died of lung cancer.
>
> **A5:** TV and newspapers constantly say smoking is bad, but I've never heard of anybody who died of smoking. I heard a lot of death from drinking. I discuss with other people about this a lot. I don't know if it is because I am very healthy even if I am smoking.
>
> **A2:** Two of my friends who hadn't smoked are already dead. Rather than having problems, those friends who smoke are alive and well. Certainly, as I told you before, you cannot relate health with smoking.
>
> **M:** Are you saying that, compared to nonsmokers, smoker friends seem to be healthier?
>
> **A7:** Friends who like to drink and smoke are all healthy. They look healthy. People who don't smoke or drink make me think that they don't do so because they have some health problems. Indeed there are my friends who cannot smoke because of health problems. Many people have problems like feeling chest pain among those who do not smoke.
>
> **M:** So, you are saying people experience symptoms that are not necessarily related with smoking?
>
> **A3:** People with high blood pressure would have these problems such as short breath, chest pain. So smoking has nothing to do with these symptoms.
>
> **A2:** I am saying that there are only a few people who would experience bad health effects of smoking. If you feel these symptoms, you should quit. Most smokers wouldn't feel any need to quit because smokers themselves cannot feel that smoking is affecting their health.
>
> **A4:** That sounds right.
>
> M = moderator; A = participants

The moderator's role is to facilitate an environment that encourages participants to share their perspectives and comment respectfully on others' responses to the questions. In addition to asking questions to initiate discussion, the moderator may ask follow-up questions and probe, as appropriate. The moderator should be a skilled manager of group dynamics who is able to assume and maintain control to keep the discussion on track.

A group's time is used most productively by restricting questions to those that are most relevant to the study topic. In addition to asking questions, the moderator must be a gracious host who sets a welcoming, respectful tone. The moderator must be able to deal tactfully with participants who are overly talkative or reserved, and ensure every participant is respected and has an opportunity to contribute to the discussion.

When feasible, professional moderators may be hired to take advantage of their expertise and maximize neutrality. It is essential for moderators to focus on facilitating group discussion. Therefore, one or two assistants should be available to attend to matters such as supplying refreshments; adjusting room conditions; distributing materials; operating audio/video equipment; writing key points on a flip chart, whiteboard, or smart board; dealing with distractions; and so forth.

Typically, a focus group is conducted with six to twelve participants. Including fewer than six participants tends to capture less diverse perspectives. Including more than twelve is difficult to manage and reduces contributions from reserved participants. It is advisable to recruit three or four potential participants more than the goal to allow for some loss owing to nonattendance. Participants should be relatively homogeneous in terms of their background characteristics because they tend to be more likely to share information when interacting with people who are similar to them (Bernard, 2000; Patton, 2015). Aspects defining similarity may vary depending on a study's focus (Bernard, 2000). For example, Kviz et al. (2003) conducted focus groups with participants who were all males (gender) and Korean Americans (ethnicity). However, they conducted separate groups with those who were current smokers and former smokers. Moreover, whenever feasible, participants should be strangers to one another, which encourages frank sharing of information and helps to protect participants' confidentiality.

Focus groups typically run about one to two hours. As illustrated by the agenda in Box 13.5, in addition to the topical discussion, planning a focus group must allow time for welcoming and registering, administering informed consent (Chapter 2), presenting an overview of the group's purpose, specifying procedures and ground rules (Box 13.6), doing introductions and icebreaker warm-ups, and wrapping up. In consideration for participants' time, effort, and travel costs, they typically are paid a cash honorarium when the group discussion is finished. Assuming eight to ten participants, the agenda in Box 13.5 estimates a total of about 20 minutes will be used for matters other than discussing the study's topic. That leaves about 40 minutes for discussion in a one-hour session and about 70 minutes for discussion in a one-and-a-half–hour session.

BOX 13.5: FOCUS GROUP AGENDA

I. Welcome and registration (5 minutes)

II. Administration of consent form (3 minutes)

II. Study overview (1 minute)

III. Procedures and ground rules (3 minutes)

IV. Self-introductions and icebreaker (3 minutes)

V. Group discussion

VI. Wrap-up (5 minutes)

Source: Based on Kviz et al. (2003).

> **BOX 13.6: FOCUS GROUP PROCEDURES AND GROUND RULES**
>
> Now I would like to go over some rules for the group discussion.
>
> 1. All your opinions are important to us. You might not agree with one another about some things. That's okay. We want to hear about your different experiences and ideas. If you disagree with others, please be respectful of them.
> 2. It's important to speak one at a time. Please do not interrupt each other. Let others finish what they're saying. Then you will have your chance to speak.
> 3. We have a limited amount of time, so please understand that sometimes I might have to cut short what someone is saying so we can stay focused on the topic or give others a chance to speak.
> 4. It's important that we all respect each other's privacy. What you say during the group discussion is for the purposes of the research study only. Please do not tell other people what you hear someone say during the group discussion.
> 5. Another person is with us [introduce the observer]. [Observer] will be helping me in several ways, such as distributing materials and taking notes to be sure that we don't miss anything you say. The notes will not include any identifying information about you.
> 6. Some of the researchers for this project will be in a room next door to observe the group discussion through a one-way mirror and by listening to a speaker. This is so they can get a firsthand idea about the important things you say.
> 7. We will audio record the discussion to keep track of everything you say. [Point out the microphone's location.] Please speak strongly and clearly so it picks up your voice.
> 8. When you refer to someone who is a group member or someone who is not a group member, please use his or her first name only to help protect confidentiality.
> 9. You will receive an honorarium of [insert] for your participation today. We will pay you in cash when the group discussion is finished.
> 10. Does anyone have any questions before we begin the group discussion?
>
> *Source:* Based on Kviz et al. (2003).

Focus groups must be conducted at a site where appropriate facilities are available. Minimum requirements are a private, quiet, comfortable space of adequate size where participants may communicate face-to-face with the moderator and each other. A conference room at a clinic, school, workplace, community center, or university generally is appropriate. In addition, the site should be reasonably accessible by all participants. Priority should be given to maximizing convenience for participants, not the research staff. Although it is not essential, whenever feasible it is best to conduct focus groups in a facility specifically designed for them, with features such as audio and/or video equipment and an observation room with a one-way mirror and speaker. Such facilities may be available in a university social science research center or at a commercial research firm.

CHECK YOUR UNDERSTANDING 13.2

- What would be the relative *strengths* and *limitations* for using each of the qualitative interview methods listed below to address the following research question?

  How do African American men identify and respond to heart disease symptoms?
  - Unstructured interview
  - Semistructured interview
  - Structured open-ended interview
  - Focus group

Qualitative Interviewing Techniques

The main qualitative interviewer role is to engage participants in a topic and guide a discussion about it. The typical qualitative interview pattern is iterative, as follows.

- Ask a question.
- Probe, as appropriate, for clarity and completeness of response.
- Ask follow-up questions, as appropriate.
- Ask a new question.

This process requires the interviewer to be an attentive listener and permit participants to speak as long as they address a relevant topic. Interviewers must be patient and allow participants time to process a question and formulate their response. Also, interviewers must tactfully keep the discussion on track by redirecting participants who drift off topic.

Key Concept

The main qualitative interviewer role is to engage and guide participants in discussion about a topic.

As discussed in Chapter 11, wording questions may be challenging even when preparing them in advance. A qualitative interviewer must be skilled at spontaneously composing questions and appropriate follow-ups while interacting with participants. That requires them to be well familiar with the study's goal, relevant theoretical constructs, and prior research results. For that reason, unstructured interviews typically are conducted by members of the research team instead of hired staff. Moreover, all interviews might be conducted by a single interviewer to maintain continuity and maximize sensitivity to emerging topics. However, when using an interview guide for semistructured and structured open-ended interviews, it is feasible to use multiple interviewers, including hired staff (Bernard, 2000).

Although qualitative interviews have a conversational tone, interviewers must be as neutral as possible to avoid influencing the nature of the information participants provide. They must refrain from expressing their opinions and solicit the participants' opinions instead. As appropriate, they must emphasize that it is the participants' experiences and opinions that are important for the study, not those of the interviewer. Moreover, they must not express in words, facial expressions, or body language that they are being judgmental regarding anything a participant says. However, they should affirm appropriate participation, such as by saying "Thank you" or "That's helpful." Interviewers must show respect for the participants and appreciation for their participation. They should be courteous, and make generous use of terms such as *please* and *thank you*. They never should be demanding, even unintentionally. For example, instead of saying "Tell me what you think about . . . ," it is better to ask "Would you please tell me what you think about . . . ?"

Whenever feasible, interviews should be conducted in a private, comfortable place, removed from distractions and the potential for being overheard by others. Location priority should be to maximize convenience for participants. Qualitative interviews typically run about one to two hours. At the outset, interviewers introduce themselves, describe the nature and purpose of the study, explain how and why the participants were selected, explain when and how the participants might be paid for participating, and obtain informed consent to proceed. Also, they must obtain participants' permission if the interview will be audio and/or video recorded. Next, interviewers should ask a few initial questions that are engaging and easy to answer. That helps to establish the question–response pattern, set participants at ease, and build rapport.

In general, questions should be relatively broad to elicit an in-depth response. For example, if cigarette smokers are asked "When did you start smoking?" a likely response is the age when they smoked their first cigarette. More information about getting started as a cigarette smoker is likely to be elicited by asking "Could you please tell me about how you became a cigarette smoker?" Questions should be avoided that participants may answer in only one or a few words, such as "Yes" or "No." It is especially important not to ask such questions when starting an interview or opening discussion about a topic. For example, if the focus group moderator opened the discussion in Box 13.6 by asking "Do you think smoking cigarettes causes health problems?" it is likely the general response simply would have been "No." That would have made it difficult to encourage further discussion about the topic because it would appear the moderator was not accepting the participants' response.

As appropriate, interviewers should probe responses for clarity and completeness, using strategies similar to those described in Chapter 12. Probing also helps participants to understand the scope and depth of information that is being sought. Often, an effective follow-up question is to ask for a specific example that illustrates a participant's viewpoint or experience. A useful technique for assessing the reliability of understanding a response is to paraphrase it and ask the participant to confirm its accuracy.

Typically, qualitative interviews are audio recorded and subsequently transcribed verbatim to facilitate the analysis. In addition, audio recording frees interviewers to focus on conducting the interview and maintain eye contact with participants, instead of trying to write down most or all of what they say verbatim. Despite making an audio recording, the interviewer and/or an assistant should take notes for several reasons. One is to serve as a backup in the event the audio recording is corrupted or lost. Another reason is that participants observing that a note is being made of what they are saying affirms that they are making a valuable contribution to the study. In addition, notes may include follow-up questions to ask when participants are done speaking, they may flag an emergent topic to explore in greater depth, or they may be a reminder to return to a topic that temporarily is passed over in the flow of an interview. Notes also may record participants' nonverbal gestures, interruptions, and other factors that might help interpret their responses. For example, a note might state that a participant was upset or thought something was funny.

CHECK YOUR UNDERSTANDING 13.3

- Describe the typical qualitative interview iterative pattern.

Observation Methods

Information from interviews may be incomplete, inaccurate, or biased owing to factors such as recall error, lack of awareness, selective reporting, or participants reporting their perceptions of what happened. Observations collect information about behaviors and events firsthand, in their physical and social contexts. In particular, observation methods are effective for studying how interactions among people vary depending on the setting, participants, activities, and communication modes. Table 13.2 presents examples of the types of features that might be observed, depending on a study's purpose.

> **Key Concept**
>
> *Observations collect information about behaviors and events firsthand, in context.*

There are two fundamental types of qualitative observation methods, participant observation and nonparticipant observation. In **participant observation**, the observer becomes, or already is, a member of a group being studied to gain experiential knowledge (Bernard, 2000, p. 365) as an *insider*. In **nonparticipant observation**, the observer is an *outsider* and does not participate in the group's activities. Table 13.3 presents a comparative summary of key characteristics, advantages, and limitations for these two observation methods.

Participant Observation

The primary application of participant observation is to observe social processes as people interact in their natural context. Participating in the activities of a group under study in its natural setting enables an observer to experience directly how the group functions. In addition, a participant observer may have opportunities to observe activities that otherwise might not be accessible. Collecting information as a participant observer provides an insider's view, which anthropologists call the emic perspective. As described by Patton (2015, p. 338), "the participant-observer not only sees what is happening but also feels what it is like to be a part of the setting or program." In addition to what they see and hear, observers' feelings as participants are part of the data.

TABLE 13.2 • Types of Features to Observe

Setting	Participants	Activities/Events	Communication
Geographic features	Demographic characteristics (e.g., age, gender, race/ethnicity)	Type	Mode (verbal or nonverbal)
Structural features		Planned or spontaneous	Format (formal or informal)
Layout	Manner of dress	Duration	Content (e.g., informational, questioning, affirming, criticizing)
Sociopolitical environment	Number	Outcome(s)	
	Location in the setting		

TABLE 13.3 ● Observation Methods

Method	Characteristics	Strengths	Limitations
Participant	The observer becomes, or already is, a member of a group being observed. Observations are made in a natural setting.	An insider's perspective to understanding group activities and interactions is provided.	The observer may influence what is observed. There is heavy observer burden. Data collection is time-consuming. Data are difficult to analyze.
Nonparticipant	The observer is an outsider, and does not interact with people being observed. Observations may be made in a natural or controlled setting.	Observation may • be semistructured, and • include multiple groups and/or settings.	There is less comprehensive coverage of activities, times, or conditions. It is difficult to infer motivations and emotional reactions.

Participant observation data are collected in an unstructured format, primarily recorded as **field notes**. Similar to unstructured interviewing, a participant observer must be well familiar with the study's goal and sensitive to relevant topics. For that reason, a participant observer typically is a member of the research team instead of hired staff. The goal of participant observation is not to record every detail of all activities. A participant observer should have a plan of inquiry that is focused on the research question, such as observing certain types of activities, situations, and participants. Typically, the scope of observation initially is broad and increasingly becomes focused on certain aspects to understand them as fully as possible.

Various degrees of participation are possible. As **complete participants** (Patton, 2015), observers become fully engaged in a group's activities. For example, complete participants might join and fully participate in a community organization focused on reducing gang-related activities. Box 13.7 presents an example of a complete participant study. **Limited participants** (Hoyle, Harris, & Judd, 2002) are fully engaged in a group's activities except in certain situations, such as negotiating an understanding that they will not participate in activities that are dangerous or illegal, or that they regard as immoral. For example, observers might adapt a limited role to study injecting drug users or sex workers.

Participating observers (Bernard, 2000, p. 321) gain access to a setting but collect data primarily as outsiders, perhaps because they are not qualified to participate fully or to record observations objectively. For example, a nonclinician might be embedded in a clinic to observe clinical staff implementing safety precautions. Box 13.8 presents an example of a participating observer study.

The degree of participation may change over the course of a study. For instance, an observer initially might assume a participating observer role to develop a basic understanding about the types of activities that occur in a particular context, and then become increasingly engaged in those activities as a complete observer. Alternatively, an observer might begin as a complete participant to experience group membership fully, and then gradually withdraw participation to assume a participating observer role to record observations from a more distant perspective.

To the extent that observers maintain an outsider's perspective, they may not truly experience events from the participants' perspectives. However, if observers become totally

> ## BOX 13.7: COMPLETE PARTICIPANT
>
> Greifinger, St. Louis, Lunstead, Malik, and Vibbert (2013) collected information about youth living with HIV/AIDS to make recommendations for program design. Two observers who were experienced working with young people living with HIV/AIDS attended a five-day residential conference that brought together 32 youths aged 16–25 and living with HIV/AIDS from throughout the United States. The conference consisted of peer-led activities focused on psychosocial issues, leadership, and life-skills education. It also provided opportunities to engage in dialogue with one another.
>
> The observers attended full-group sessions and small-group workshops, and engaged with conference participants outside those settings. They used a list of topics and issues meriting special attention. During sessions, they typed brief notes on laptop computers and then expanded on their notes in private at the end of each day. Note-taking during sessions was deemed not to be disruptive of activities because it was common for participants to take notes.
>
> The analysis identified four broad themes: "1) the power of peer support in helping young people living with HIV/AIDS develop confidence, self-esteem and a notion of community; 2) disclosure of HIV status, with particular attention to sexual partners; 3) building positive and healthy relationships; and 4) finding new ways to discuss adherence to medication" (Greifinger et al., 2013, p. 243). In conclusion, the authors called for more youth-led, peer-based programs focused on support for disclosure of HIV status, self-esteem in relationships, and medication adherence.

immersed as participants, sometimes called "going native," they might lose objectivity. For example, they might not report activities that may embarrass a group. Moreover, the more observers are immersed as participants, the more likely their participation may influence activities in ways that might differ from what otherwise would happen.

Various factors may limit the extent to which an observer may become a participant, or even whether a participant role is possible. For example, if group members already know each other intimately, or they engage in behaviors they do not wish to be revealed, they might be unwilling to accept a new member, especially one who appears to be a social or cultural outsider (Patton, 2015). Administrators or program staff might object to an observer's presence if it is perceived as burdensome, an intrusion, or threatening. Demographic factors such as age, gender, and race may create barriers to participant observation. For instance, an adult cannot assume a child's role. Health status or health behaviors may be restrictive characteristics. For example, an observer cannot fully participate in a breast cancer survivor group if she has not been diagnosed with breast cancer.

Another limitation of participant observation is that typically there is only a single observer because embedding multiple observers often is not feasible. Thus, most often there is no means for checking the reliability of observations within a single study. Data might not be comparable across settings or time owing to the primarily unstructured observation format. In addition, generalizing results typically is limited by studying small, nonrandom samples that most often are single groups selected because they are convenient and accessible. Participant observation places a heavy burden on the observer, who must discern what activities and features are relevant to record. Moreover, depending on a study's purpose and the nature of the setting, collecting data by participant observation typically requires a substantial time investment, which may extend across several days, weeks, months, or even years. In addition, typically it is difficult and time-consuming to analyze participant observation data.

> **BOX 13.8: PARTICIPATING OBSERVER**
>
> To contribute to developing patient teaching programs, Barber-Parker (2002) studied the process of integrating patient teaching into daily care among the nursing staff of a 42-bed acute care oncology unit at a U.S. community hospital. Patient teaching was defined broadly as "any communication from the nurse providing health information to the patient and/or family including, but not limited to, information about diagnosis and treatment, self-care activities related to diagnosis and treatment, medications and side effects and other health-related issues, such as smoking cessation and community resources" (Barber-Parker, 2002, p. 108).
>
> A single observer participated in the role of a "known observer" and accompanied three experienced registered nurses as they provided care over twelve months. Although the observer already was employed at the hospital, she was not a member of the oncology unit staff and had no supervisory relationship with the unit staff. The nurse manager encouraged and supported staff nurse participation. Written informed consent was obtained from the three nurses.
>
> The analysis found that communication across disciplines was ineffective at times. Family members often were not present "when nurses intermittently provided teaching during other direct care activities" (Barber-Parker, 2002, p. 111). Much of the patient teaching was based on preconceptions of patient education needs instead of individual learning needs assessments. Evaluation of patient learning was limited. In conclusion, the author identified three areas for developing strategies to improve acute care patient education: "staff nurse knowledge, structure for teaching and reinforcement of teaching behaviors" (Barber-Parker, 2002, p. 112).

Nonparticipant Observation

Nonparticipant observers are outsiders, or spectators, who do not interact with the people they observe. Nonparticipant observation is used to collect information in a systematic manner that is more objective compared with participant observation. A nonparticipant observer may use an observation guide, similar to a semistructured interview guide, to ensure that relevant topics are addressed; enhance comparability across individuals, settings, or time; and facilitate data processing and analysis. Also, in addition to making field notes, the observer may use a structured instrument such as a checklist or tally sheet to record observations.

Compared with participant observation, nonparticipant observation is less likely to discover unanticipated issues and relationships. Also, nonparticipant observation generally is less comprehensive because it may not be feasible to observe all relevant activities as a nonparticipant, such as ones that are private or illegal, and observation opportunities may be limited to certain time periods or conditions. Moreover, it is difficult to know a person's motivations and emotional reactions without interacting within them.

The systematic approach reduces the observer's burden and data collection time, and enables employing more than one observer to check reliability. Also, observations may be collected in multiple settings, which may be selected randomly in some situations, to enhance the generalizability of results. Although nonparticipant observation typically is conducted in a natural setting, it also may be employed in a controlled setting. Table 13.4 presents examples of types of settings in which nonparticipant observation may be employed.

Collecting data in a natural setting enhances external validity (Chapter 5) because people are more likely to display their typical behavior as compared with a controlled setting. However, it is difficult to identify potential causal relationships because typically

TABLE 13.4 ● Nonparticipant Observation Settings

Setting	Example
Unscheduled natural	Parental supervision of children at a public beach
Scheduled natural	Visitors at a community health fair
Arranged natural	Presentation of a violence prevention curriculum in a school classroom
Controlled	Children playing in an observation laboratory with a one-way mirror and audio/visual recording equipment

extraneous variables (Chapter 5) are not controllable in a natural setting. In a controlled setting, such as a university psychology laboratory, a researcher may employ random assignment and manipulate factors such as environmental conditions, activities, and participant characteristics (Chapters 6 and 7). Depending on the situation, similar controls may be implemented in settings such as school classes, clinics, or workplaces. However, while such controls enhance internal validity (Chapter 5), they compromise external validity. Thus, whenever feasible, a more comprehensive understanding about a topic may be obtained by collecting observations in both natural and controlled settings. For example, the internal validity of relationships inferred from observations in a natural setting might be assessed by subsequent observations in a controlled setting. Box 13.9 presents an example of nonparticipant observation conducted in an unscheduled natural setting; Box 13.10 presents an example in an arranged natural setting.

BOX 13.9: NONPARTICIPANT OBSERVATION IN AN UNSCHEDULED NATURAL SETTING

Greenberg-Seth, Hemenway, Gallagher, Ross, and Lissy (2004) used nonparticipant observation to evaluate the short-term effect of a community-based intervention (Kids in the Back/Niños Atrás) to increase the proportion of children aged younger than 12 years seated in the rear of motor vehicles in a low-income Hispanic community. They observed child rear seating patterns at pre- and postintervention (2 years later) at six intersections each in one intervention city and two control cities. They defined a child passenger as aged younger than 12 years, which observers determined by appearance and height. A motor vehicle was defined as a noncommercial vehicle.

Observers were trained in the use of standardized observation forms. Two observers were stationed at opposite corners of each intersection to observe motor vehicles traveling in all directions. The observers did not stop any motor vehicles. Preintervention observations were recorded for 1,393 vehicles in the intervention city and 3,428 in the control cities. Postintervention observations were recorded for 1,960 vehicles in the intervention city and 4,290 in the control cities.

They found that child rear seating increased in all three cities. However, the increase was greater in the intervention city (33% to 49%) than in the control cities (28% to 41%). They concluded that such community-based interventions "can have a significant effect in improving child passenger safety behavior independent of legislation" (Greenberg-Seth et al., 2004, p. 1013).

> **BOX 13.10: NONPARTICIPANT OBSERVATION IN AN ARRANGED NATURAL SETTING**
>
> Booth, Davidson, Winstanley, and Waters (2001) used nonparticipant observation to compare the interventions of nurses and occupational therapists during morning care of stroke patients at a rehabilitation unit. A single impartial observer, who was neither a nurse nor an occupational therapist, observed two morning care sessions for each of 10 patients, one when care was provided by an occupational therapist and one when care was provided by a nurse. The study was approved by the ethics committee, and informed consent was obtained from each patient. The observer was allowed to engage in normal social conventions but explained the need to focus on recording observations during patient care. The observer recorded observations at the end of 20-second intervals using a coding scheme of predetermined categories for physical interaction and activities (the categories and their definitions are available in two appendices in Booth et al., 2001).
>
> The analysis found many similarities between nurses and occupational therapists. However, occupational therapists used prompting, instructing, and facilitation techniques more than nurses. Nurses preferred supervision techniques, as compared with occupational therapists. The authors recommended that health care professional education should aim to achieve consistency of effort in providing care to improve therapeutic outcomes.

Reactivity

Reactivity is a limitation of observation that may occur when people are aware or suspect that they are being observed, and consequently act differently than they would otherwise. For instance, they might be less animated or less aggressive, or they might be more generous or more polite. The potential for such artificial and temporary changes threatens the validity of observations. In general, reactivity is most likely to occur when people wish to make a positive impression with an observer or to conceal attributes that might jeopardize their social, economic, or legal status. For example, clinical staff members might perceive being observed while performing their duties as a potential threat to their employment status. However, when the same people are observed repeatedly over the course of a study, they tend to become accustomed to an observer's presence and are increasingly likely to return to their usual behavior patterns the longer they are observed (Bernard, 2000, pp. 325, 382; Patton, 2015, p. 411). Thus, reactivity effects are likely to be greatest during the early stages of such studies, and observations collected later are likely to be more reliable.

In most situations, when it is feasible and deemed ethical, reactivity may be avoided by conducting **covert observation**, that is, so people are not aware they are being observed. That strategy is most feasible when observing nonsensitive behavior in public places (Chapter 2). It is important for covert observers to be inconspicuous in terms of their location in a setting, their physical appearance, and their behavior. For example, it would not be effective for an observer of parental supervision of children at a public beach to sit close to a family, wear street clothes, and write notes on a clipboard while obviously watching them. However, ethical concerns arise when covertly observing nonpublic and sensitive behavior, such as by eavesdropping or using a hidden recording device. In some situations, people may have a reasonable expectation of privacy, such as observing hand washing in a public restroom. Ethical concerns arise also when observers are complete participants if they do not disclose that they are collecting information for research purposes to gain access and/or avoid reactivity effects. Such concerns should be assessed by an institutional review board (Chapter 2) in terms of the following considerations (U.S. Department of Health and Human Services, 1993):

- Whether an invasion of privacy is acceptable in consideration of any reasonable expectations of privacy in the situation under study
- Whether the potential importance of the research justifies an invasion of privacy
- Potential harms associated with an invasion of privacy
- Procedures for protecting participants' confidentiality
- Whether the research could be conducted using methods that do not involve an invasion of privacy

CHECK YOUR UNDERSTANDING 13.4

- What would be the relative strengths and limitations for using participant observation compared with nonparticipant observation to address the following research question?

    What are the key factors that contribute to effective collaboration between community health clinic staff and a grassroots community organization to develop and implement strategies for reducing substance abuse among teens?

Recording Observation Data

Field notes are the main body of observation data. There are two fundamental types of field notes:

- **Descriptive notes** are an account of what is observed.
- **Reflective notes** are an account of the observation process, and insights about the potential meaning and significance of what is observed.

Box 13.11 lists aspects typically recorded in **descriptive** and **reflective** field notes.

BOX 13.11: ASPECTS TO RECORD IN FIELD NOTES

Descriptive	Reflective
• Date and time	• Emerging topics
• Location and its physical characteristics	• Topics not worth pursuing further
• Social, political, and other characteristics of the setting	• Modifications to the observation protocol
• Participants (number, characteristics, placement in the setting, roles)	• Potential meaning and significance of what is observed
• Events, activities, and behaviors	• Potential reactivity
• Statements and conversations	• Potential observer bias
	• Ethical issues

When recording notes, it is essential to differentiate between the two types for analysis purposes. When feasible, it is best to record them in separate documents. If notes are recorded in a single document, then a strategy should be employed to indicate which type of note is being entered. Examples are to use different-color ink for handwritten notes, or to insert representative symbols, such as *D* (descriptive) and *R* (reflective). As soon as possible after an observation session, the two types of field notes should be extracted and saved in separate documents. Most often, especially when conducting participant observation, field notes are recorded initially in a handwritten format and typed later. When conducting nonparticipant observation, sometimes it may be feasible to type field notes. Usually, typing is faster, and word processing macros may be created to enter key words or phrases quickly and accurately. Moreover, typed notes are easier to read, and their content may be searched electronically.

Field notes should be recorded as unobtrusively as possible to avoid reactivity effects. When feasible, field notes should be recorded as observations are being made. Otherwise, they should be recorded as soon as possible thereafter to ensure accuracy and avoid losing information that might not be recalled. Recording notes in real time is most likely to be feasible when conducting nonparticipant observation because the observer is not involved with participating in the observation setting.

When appropriate, a checklist or grid format, combined with alphabetic or numeric codes, may facilitate recording accurately and avoid missing relevant information. Another strategy is to use a shorthand system to indicate certain activities, behaviors, conditions, communication patterns, nonverbal communication, and so forth. The confidentiality of speakers or actors should be protected by using symbols, such as *F1* = female #1 and *M3* = male #3. When recording statements, notes should indicate who is the speaker and to whom he or she is speaking. When feasible, important statements should be recorded as exact quotes indicated by quotation marks. Otherwise, a symbol should indicate if a note is a paraphrase (e.g., *P*) or summary (e.g., *S*) of a statement. If the exact content of what participants say is not important, codes might be used to indicate the nature of what is said, such as *Q* = asked a question, *R* = responded to a question, *S* = offered a suggestion, *A* = affirmed, *C* = criticized, and so forth.

Descriptive notes should be factual and comprehensive, while being focused on information that is relevant for analysis. For example, if one is observing how parents attend to their children when crossing a street together, the presence of a passing vehicle is relevant, but the vehicle's brand is not relevant. Moreover, attending to irrelevant details may distract from observing truly important aspects of a situation. It is helpful to anticipate what might be observed in a setting and what is likely to be relevant to the analysis. However, observers should be open to recording any relevant aspects they observe and not be restricted by a preconceived checklist. The best practice is initially to record everything that might be relevant. As a study progresses, observers should review their descriptive and reflective field notes to identify aspects that do not merit attention during subsequent observation sessions.

Depending on the nature of a study, other methods of recording observations may be employed in addition to handwritten or typed field notes. These may include audio recordings, video recordings, photographs, drawings, maps, and so forth. While these may be very helpful, in most situations they should be treated as supplemental to field notes. A serious concern is the potential for losing information owing to equipment failure. It is essential to be competent in using and attentive in maintaining recording equipment (e.g., charged batteries, clean lenses, ensuring adequate memory capacity is available), and backup equipment and/or accessories should be available when feasible. Moreover, field notes may include information that might not or cannot be captured by a recording device. For instance, an audio recording cannot include nonverbal clues. A video or photograph cannot capture information outside a camera's field of view. Before analyzing data from audio recordings, they must be transcribed verbatim.

Owing to factors such as the observation method, topic, participants, and setting, the use of some recording devices may not be feasible or ethical. For example, participant observers generally do not use audio or video recording devices because they are likely to introduce reactivity effects and raise ethical concerns. Sometimes participant observers record brief notes, called *jottings*, on cards or in a small notebook, and write expanded field notes based on them in private as soon as possible following an observation session. Whatever method(s) are used for recording observations, at least one backup copy should be stored separately from the original, in a different location and/or on a different device. For instance, it is not adequate to store original and backup word processing files in separate folders on the same computer. In addition, all observation data must be stored in a secure manner approved by an institutional review board (Chapter 2).

Sampling

Most qualitative research methods use nonprobability (nonrandom) sampling strategies, which are based on judgment, to focus in depth on certain settings, individuals, and events. Probability (random) sampling (Chapter 7) often is not appropriate or feasible for qualitative research because it is not efficient for selecting special groups, events, or conditions that typically are the focus of qualitative research. Examples are parenting a child born with Down syndrome, dealing with a household member who is an injecting drug user, or caring for a spouse diagnosed with Alzheimer's disease. There is no reliable sampling frame for such populations, and qualitative interviewing and observation methods typically require negotiating access to collect data about such issues. Moreover, as a qualitative study progresses, sample selection criteria and strategies may change to pursue certain topics in depth and explore emergent topics. However, sometimes random sampling may be combined with nonprobability sampling, such as randomly selecting students at a school, or time periods to observe activities at a clinic.

The primary goal of qualitative research is to represent content and context relevant to the research question, rather than represent a target population, as typically is the goal for quantitative research using probability sampling. Nevertheless, the validity of results from nonprobability samples may be challenged based on alternative subjective perspectives about what constitutes an appropriate sample. Moreover, qualitative research samples may be biased toward selecting settings that are most accessible and participants who are expected to be willing to cooperate, are well familiar with the topic, and are able to articulate their insights effectively. There are no systematic strategies for effectively assessing the nature and degree of such potential bias.

> **Key Concept**
>
> *The primary goal of qualitative research is to represent content and context relevant to the research question.*

Purposive Sample

Purposive sampling, also called **purposeful sampling** or **judgmental sampling**, selects units (e.g., individuals, groups, organizations, settings, or events) based on factors such as their characteristics, activities, experience, relationships, location, and so forth that lead to an expectation that they will provide the type of information that will serve a study's purpose. A key aspect of purposive sampling is that it requires knowledge of which units of study are most appropriate. At the start of a qualitative study, such knowledge must be available for at least some units of the target population, such as from conducting a pilot study, reviewing records, or referrals. Other units of study often may be identified as a study progresses. Most qualitative research uses a form of purposive sampling, either in its entirety or in combination with another nonprobability sampling strategy. Some of the most frequently used purposive sampling strategies, which often are employed in combination, are described below.

Typical case sample

Units (cases) are selected to focus on ones that represent the average or normative condition. For example, for program planning or policy purposes, it generally may be more relevant to understand typical, majority situations instead of the minority that are exceptionally good or poor.

Atypical case sample

Units (cases) are selected to focus on ones that deviate from the average or normative condition to understand why they differ from the typical situation. An **atypical case sample** also is called a "deviant case sample," "special case sample," "extreme case sample," or "outlier sample." This strategy is most effective when it is employed in combination with a **typical case sample** to conduct a comparative analysis and develop strategies for addressing disparities.

Homogeneous sample

A **homogeneous sample** selects units to focus on ones that are similar regarding characteristics that are relevant to a study's purpose. This strategy enables studying one or more groups of units in depth. Focus groups typically use homogeneous samples to stimulate discussion among participants who share a similar background and experience. For example, in the previously described focus groups conducted by Kviz et al. (2003) with Korean American men aged 45–74, the participants were similar in race/ethnicity, gender, and age. Also, separate focus groups were conducted with current and former cigarette smokers. That strategy enabled studying each group in depth and conducting a comparative analysis, and it avoided potential discord owing to differences in participants' smoking status. Focus group participants most often are volunteers who are recruited through advertising. Another strategy is to recruit focus group participants through referral by key informants or chain referral, both of which are described in following sections.

Heterogeneous sample

A **heterogeneous sample** selects units to capture the diversity of characteristics that are relevant to a study's purpose. This strategy is particularly useful in the initial stage of studying a problem to understand the nature and range of differences in the target population. Other sampling methods may be employed subsequently to select subsets of the target population that warrant investigating in depth. A **quota sample** is a strategy for ensuring a sample reflects similar proportions as the target population regarding key variables. Typically, an interviewer or observer selects a quota sample in the field by convenience, which is described in a following section. Therefore, the selection criteria must be easily identifiable, such as gender or location. Otherwise, an interviewer must screen potential participants for eligibility. Similar to stratified random sampling with proportionate allocation (Chapter 7), the distributions of the selection criteria in the target population are analyzed first. Then the same proportions of individuals are selected in the sample. For example, if 30% of the target population is female and aged 50–64, then 30% of the sample is selected to include females aged 50–64, and so forth.

Key Informants Sample

Key informants are individuals who are selected because they have special insight about a research problem. This strategy often is used in the initial stage of a study to understand the nature and scope of a problem. Also, key informants may help interpret results and confirm/disconfirm conclusions and recommendations. It generally is best to select as diverse a sample of key informants as possible to obtain multiple perspectives. Examples of key informants are community leaders/activists, long-term community residents, gang leaders, organization administrators, union leaders, local police community liaison officers, business leaders, health care professionals, teachers, religious leaders, and social workers.

Referral Sample

A referral sample selects units by referral from others. This strategy is especially useful when target population members are difficult to identify and contact, such as homeless people, injecting drug users, sex workers, and men who have sex with men. One approach to obtaining referrals is to interview key informants, who may identify appropriate individuals or settings.

Chain referral/snowball sample

Another approach, called a **chain referral sample** or snowball sample, is to interview an initial sample of *seed cases* that might be identified by key informants or from records. Then, those participants are asked for referrals to other target population members, who are interviewed and asked for referrals, and so on.

Respondent-driven sample

Respondent-driven sampling (RDS) is a relatively recent variation of chain referral sampling (Heckathorn, 1997, 2002; Magnani, Sabin, Saidel, & Heckathorn, 2005). After a sample of seed cases is interviewed, the participants are asked to *recruit*, rather than make referrals to, other target population members, who are interviewed and asked to recruit others, and so on. Typically, participants are paid an incentive for recruiting participants. However, informed consent and data collection are done by the interviewer.

Convenience Sample

A **convenience sample** selects units because they are conveniently accessible. For example, a convenience sample might select a clinic based on having an existing relationship with administrators and/or staff, which may enhance accessibility and collaboration, and/or because it does not require extensive travel. Individuals might be selected because they happen to be present at a particular place and time, such as shoppers in the fresh produce section of a grocery store. This latter type of convenience sample sometimes is called an "accidental," "haphazard," "incidental," or "intercept" sample. Selecting a group of individuals, such as students in a fifth-grade classroom, sometimes is called a "captive" or "captive-audience" sample.

A convenience sample is most appropriate when the target population is homogeneous regarding a study's key variables, which minimizes differences across units that might be selected. Thus, a study's findings are not expected to differ substantially depending on which units are selected. The representativeness of a convenience sample may be enhanced by combining convenience with purposive selection of settings in which individuals will be studied. For example, to study fresh produce shoppers, if access to the grocery stores in a particular community is similarly convenient, then one might be selected because it is considered to be a typical case setting. Moreover, a multistage strategy might be used, where a grocery store is selected by convenience in the first stage. Then days of the week and times of day might be selected by convenience or randomly. Finally, individual shoppers might be selected sequentially using a systematic interval (Chapter 7), such as selecting every 10th one. Such a design is likely to obtain a more representative sample of shoppers and make collecting data more manageable than attempting to interview or observe all shoppers.

Sample Size

For qualitative research, the sample size typically is not predetermined, such as by mathematical calculations for quantitative research using random sampling (Chapter 7). Instead, it is based on judgment. Data collection generally continues as long as new information that is relevant to the research question is obtained. Data collection is stopped when it appears that it is not likely to yield substantial new information, which is called the **saturation point**. Samples for qualitative research often are small, such as in the range of 20 to 50 cases. Typically, a larger sample is required the more complex the research topic and the more heterogeneous the target population. Focus group studies generally require conducting three or four groups (Krueger & Casey, 2015; Stewart & Shamdasani, 2015).

> **CHECK YOUR UNDERSTANDING 13.5**
>
> - Give an example for a situation in which it would be appropriate to employ each of the following qualitative sampling methods, and briefly explain why the method would be appropriate in that situation:
>   - Purposive typical case sample
>   - Purposive atypical case sample
>   - Purposive homogeneous sample
>   - Purposive heterogeneous sample
>   - Key informants sample
>   - Referral sample
>   - Convenience sample

Mixed Methods

Mixed methods research designs use at least one qualitative and one quantitative method to investigate a research problem from an integrated perspective. The methods may be implemented concurrently or sequentially. Mixed methods designs take advantage of each method's unique contributions to understanding a research problem. The most commonly employed designs are addressed below. Useful reviews of the history and continuing development of mixed methods research are available from several sources, notably Creswell and Plano Clark (2011); Johnson, Onwuegbuzie, and Turner (2007); and Small (2011). Many definitions of mixed methods have been suggested in the research methodological literature. Johnson et al. (2007) collected current definitions of mixed methods from 19 leading mixed methods research methodologists. Based on their analysis of those definitions, Johnson et al. (2007, p. 118) offered the following general definition for mixed methods research:

> Mixed methods research is the type of research in which a researcher or team of researchers combines elements of qualitative and quantitative research approaches (e.g., use of qualitative and quantitative viewpoints, data collection, analysis, inference techniques) for the broad purposes of breadth and depth of understanding and corroboration.

In addition, they proffered that "a *mixed methods study* would involve mixing within a single study; a *mixed method program* would involve mixing within a program of research and the mixing might occur across a closely related set of studies [italics added for emphasis]" (Johnson et al., 2007, p. 123).

Typical purposes for employing a mixed methods design are to

- obtain a more comprehensive understanding of a research problem,
- enhance validity of findings,
- use one method to develop the plan for another method,
- use one method to interpret the findings from another method, and
- use one method to assess the generalizability of findings from another method.

Not all combinations of qualitative and quantitative methods constitute a mixed methods design. It has long been common practice for qualitative research to collect some data in a quantitative format and for quantitative research to collect some data in a qualitative format. Box 13.12 presents some such routine strategies that are not mixed methods research designs.

BOX 13.12: STRATEGIES THAT ARE NOT MIXED METHODS DESIGNS

- Asking qualitative interview or observation participants to complete a brief structured questionnaire to collect quantitative background characteristics, such as age
- Qualitative observation that records quantities, such as the number of times a particular activity occurs during a specific time interval
- Including a few open-ended questions in a structured questionnaire, or an open-ended question at the end of a structured questionnaire requesting additional comments
- Conducting cognitive interviews or behavior coding to assess a structured questionnaire draft (Chapter 10)

Several typologies have been proposed for classifying mixed methods designs, notably by Creswell and Plano Clark (2011), Johnson and Onwuegbuzie (2004), Morgan (1998), Morse (1991), and Teddlie and Tashakkori (2006). In general, such approaches organize mixed methods in terms of two dimensions: timing and priority. Drawing upon these sources, Box 13.13 presents one of the most commonly used mixed methods research designs.

> **BOX 13.13: MIXED METHODS DESIGNS**
>
> **Concurrent Designs**
>
> Equivalent design: QUAL + QUAN or QUAN + QUAL
>
> Complementary design: QUAL + quan or QUAN + qual
>
> **Sequential Designs**
>
> Exploratory design: qual → QUAN or quan → QUAL
>
> Explanatory design: QUAN → qual
>
> Confirmatory/generalizability design: QUAL → quan
>
> Notation:
>
> *QUAL* or *qual* indicates a qualitative method.
>
> *QUAN* or *quan* indicates a quantitative method.
>
> When both methods are uppercase, they are given equal priority.
>
> When one method is uppercase and the other is lowercase, the uppercase method is the main priority.
>
> A plus sign (+) indicates the methods are employed concurrently.
>
> An arrow (→) indicates the methods are employed sequentially.

Concurrent Designs

Concurrent mixed methods designs, also called "convergent designs" (Creswell, 2015), employ qualitative and quantitative methods simultaneously, or with a minor time lapse to avoid a potential historical threat to validity (Chapter 5). In an equivalent concurrent design, the methods are given equal priority: QUAL + QUAN or QUAN + QUAL. They are conducted and analyzed separately. Similarity or convergence of results from different methods that concurrently investigate the same research question, sometimes called *triangulation*, enhances confidence in both sets of results. However, dissimilarity does not necessarily indicate that either or both results are invalid. Different methods and different types of data may be sensitive to different aspects of a research problem. Thus, it is possible for both results to be valid, and differences may indicate paths for further investigation. Results also may be integrated, drawing on each method's unique insights, to derive a more comprehensive understanding of the research problem than may be drawn from either method alone. A limitation of mixed methods designs is that it is challenging to implement and analyze two full-scale methods simultaneously. Box 13.14 presents an example of an equivalent concurrent mixed methods design.

An alternative to implementing two full-scale methods is to use a *complementary concurrent design* (QUAL + quan or QUAN + qual), which gives priority to one method. Accordingly, a full-scale version of the priority method is implemented, and a small-scale version, typically with a smaller sample size, of the other method provides insight from another perspective. For example, as a complement to conducting nonparticipant observation at a community health fair, participants might be asked to complete a brief self-administered questionnaire.

> **BOX 13.14: EQUIVALENT CONCURRENT MIXED METHODS EXAMPLE**
>
> Guthrie, Auerback, and Bindman (2010) used a concurrent mixed methods design to assess the impact of the California Medicaid pay-for-performance incentive program on the quality of health care. They conducted semistructured qualitative interviews to understand the *perceived* impact from the perspective of health plan senior staff. In addition, they examined the program's *quantitative* impact for certain health conditions according to five HEDIS (Healthcare Effectiveness Data and Information Set) quality measures for care delivered before and after program implementation.

Exploratory Sequential Designs

In an exploratory sequential design, results from the first method are used to plan and implement the second method. This design often is implemented by using results from an initial qualitative investigation to plan a subsequent quantitative investigation: qual → QUAN. Common purposes for employing this design are to

- explore the nature and scope of the research problem,
- identify key constructs and generate hypotheses,
- specify variables,
- identify appropriate sites and populations,
- guide selecting an appropriate quantitative method, and
- guide selecting/developing a quantitative instrument.

For example, survey research professionals commonly use results from focus groups and cognitive interviews (Chapter 10) to guide developing a structured questionnaire to ensure it addresses key topics and uses appropriate language for wording questions and response choices.

Another application of the exploratory sequential design is to use results from a quantitative investigation to plan a qualitative one: quan → QUAL. Common purposes for employing this design are to

- identify topics that should be explored in depth,
- identify types of or specific population members to study,
- obtain contact information for specific participants, and
- identify appropriate sites.

Initial quantitative results typically are obtained by conducting a survey or analyzing existing survey data or institutional records (Chapter 14). The quantitative results may be used to identify topics that should be investigated in depth based on factors such as incidence and/or prevalence rates, health disparities, and demographic characteristics. In other situations, the quantitative results may identify appropriate sites, such as clinics with different incidence rates for childhood diseases, or street intersections with high rates of vehicle-related injuries.

Explanatory Sequential Designs

In an explanatory sequential design, after analyzing results from the first method, a second method is employed as a follow-up. This design may be implemented in two ways. One is to employ a qualitative method following a quantitative investigation: QUAN → qual. The qualitative follow-up may be conducted to help explain or elaborate the quantitative results in general, or it may target certain results or target population members. The follow-up may be especially useful to help explain unexpected results and for planning further research. The qualitative data may be collected either from a sample of participants in the quantitative investigation or from a separate sample of the target population. A common application of this design is to conduct follow-up qualitative interviews either with a sample of survey respondents or with a separate, parallel sample selected from a survey's target population, as presented in the example in Box 13.15.

> **BOX 13.15: EXPLANATORY SEQUENTIAL MIXED METHODS EXAMPLE (QUAN → qual)**
>
> Mayoh, Bond, and Todres (2012) conducted a self-administered survey of 100 adults with chronic health conditions about their experiences seeking health information online. Then, to avoid potential reactivity effects, they conducted qualitative interviews with a parallel sample of 60 participants to obtain in-depth descriptions of their experiences seeking online health information regarding six aspects that were identified in the survey results.

Confirmatory/Generalizability Sequential Designs

In a confirmatory/generalizability sequential design (QUAL → quan), after analyzing results from an initial qualitative method, a quantitative method is employed to assess the generalizability of the qualitative results in a representative sample of the target population. For example, a survey with a random sample of the target population might be conducted subsequent to completing qualitative interviews. The quantitative method might estimate the prevalence and describe the distribution of issues identified by qualitative results. Also, inferential statistics may be applied when analyzing the quantitative data to test hypotheses generated by the preceding qualitative investigation.

Monomethod Designs

Often, two or more qualitative or quantitative strategies are combined. Such combinations are *monomethod designs*, not mixed methods designs. The following are some common examples:

- A participant observer conducts qualitative interviews with participants in addition to observing their activities (QUAL + QUAL).

- A nonparticipant observer conducts qualitative interviews with participants after observing an event (QUAL + qual).

- A researcher conducts a mixed-mode survey (QUAN + QUAN, or QUAN + quan) (Chapter 12).
- A researcher conducts in-person survey interviews with a subsample of respondents who report certain characteristics in response to a self-administered questionnaire (QUAN + quan).

Key Points

Basic Concepts

Qualitative research methods

- primarily collect qualitative data;
- use a holistic and context-specific approach;
- collect data primarily in natural settings;
- use an inductive, iterative approach; and
- do not necessarily collect the same information from every participant or about every situation.

Qualitative Interview Methods

Qualitative interview methods primarily are conducted one-on-one, in person, using an open-response format.

- **Unstructured interview:** A guided conversation proceeds naturally and interactively to explore relevant topics from the participant's perspective.
- **Semistructured interview:** The interviewer uses an interview guide that lists topics in prospective order.
- **Structured open-ended interview:** The interviewer uses an interview guide with open-ended questions.
- **Focus group:** A moderator uses a semistructured guide and encourages a small group to respond interactively to questions about a narrowly defined topic.

Qualitative Observation Methods

- **Participant observation:** The observer becomes, or already is, a member of a group being studied to gain an insider's perspective.
- **Nonparticipant observation:** The observer is an outsider and does not participate in a group's activities.
- **Descriptive notes:** The observer records a factual and comprehensive account of what is observed.
- **Reflective notes:** The observer records an account of the observation process, and insights about the potential meaning and significance of what is observed.

Qualitative Sampling Methods

Most qualitative samples use nonprobability strategies based on judgment.

- **Purposive sample:** Units are selected based on factors that lead to an expectation they will provide the type of information that will serve a study's purpose.
  - **Typical case sample:** Units represent the normative condition.
  - **Atypical case sample:** Units deviate from the normative condition.
  - **Homogeneous sample:** Units are similar.
  - **Heterogeneous sample:** Units are diverse.
- **Key informants sample:** Individuals have special insight about a problem.
- **Referral sample:** Units are referred by others.
- **Convenience sample:** Units are conveniently accessible.
- **Sample size:** Samples are typically small; data collection continues until it appears it is not likely to yield substantial new information, called the saturation point.

Mixed Methods

Mixed methods designs use at least one qualitative and one quantitative method that may be implemented concurrently or sequentially.

Minor or routine inclusions of another method are not mixed methods designs.
Combinations of two or more qualitative or quantitative strategies are monomethod designs.

Review and Apply

1. Review the research plan you developed in the "Review and Apply" sections of the previous chapters. Prepare a protocol for addressing your topic by conducting qualitative interviews using one of the four methods described in this chapter, or conducting participant or nonparticipant observation.

   OPTION: Instead, do this activity for another health-related problem that interests you.

   a. Describe how the method you select might enhance your understanding about your topic.
   b. Describe your rationale for choosing the qualitative method you would use.
   c. Draft an outline of topics and an interview guide, a moderator's guide, or an observation guide as appropriate for your data collection plan.
   d. Develop a sampling plan and describe your rationale for choosing it.

2. Experience is the best way to develop interviewer skills. Take turns with your classmates, conducting unstructured interviews with each other. This might be done in class or outside class. When it is not your turn to play the interviewer or interviewee role, observe the interviewer's performance and provide feedback to reinforce positive performance and suggest ways to improve. Write a summary of what you learned from being an interviewer and your observation of other interviewers.

Each interviewer should choose a topic about a familiar activity that is not sensitive. Nevertheless, all responses should be treated as confidential. The following are some suggested topics:

Educational history	Favorite vacation place(s)
Employment experience	Favorite type(s) of music and performer(s)
Volunteer experience	Favorite movies or television shows
Postgraduation goals and plans	A family holiday or birthday tradition
Social media use	Favorite fruit(s) and vegetable(s)
Recreational activities/hobbies	Favorite dessert(s)

3. Experience is the best way to develop observer skills. Conduct a total of at least one hour of nonparticipant observation. Record descriptive and reflective field notes. Write a summary of what your observations reveal and your experience as a nonparticipant observer.

Choose a topic to conduct nonparticipant observation of behavior at a public or semipublic place. The topic should not involve sensitive behavior, and your observations should not invade participants' privacy. The following are some suggested topics:

Behavior of adult observers at a children's sports event (e.g., soccer or baseball)	Behavior of individuals waiting for and boarding public transportation (e.g., bus, train, or subway)
Behavior of individuals or adults with children at a public park, forest preserve, or beach	Behavior of individuals or adults with children placing orders inside a fast-food restaurant
Behavior of individuals or adults with children at a zoo, museum, arboretum, or botanic garden	Safety and law-abiding behavior of bicyclists riding on a busy city street

Before entering the field:

  a. Develop a list of the types of activities, people, and other things you will observe. Keep in mind that it is not feasible to observe everyone and every activity. Also be prepared to record information you did not anticipate observing.
  b. Develop a plan for the time(s) and location(s) where you will make observations.
  c. Develop a strategy for recording descriptive field notes, such as a grid system, categories, and/or coding scheme (e.g., letters, numbers, or tallies).

4. Review the qualitative research study summaries in Box 13.9 and Box 13.10. Assess the potential for reactivity as a validity threat to each study's result. Suggest at least one strategy that might reduce each reactivity threat you identify.

5. Describe how you might use a mixed methods design to address the topic you specified in the first "Review and Apply" activity in this chapter. Explain how your mixed methods design might enhance understanding your research problem.

Study Further

Barbour, R. (2014). *Introducing qualitative research: A student's guide* (2nd ed.). Thousand Oaks, CA: Sage.

Creswell, J. W., & Plano Clark, V. L. (2011). *Designing and conducting mixed methods research* (2nd ed.). Thousand Oaks, CA: Sage.

Hesse-Biber, S. N. (2017). *The practice of qualitative research* (3rd ed.). Thousand Oaks, CA: Sage.

Miles, M. B., Huberman, A. M., & Saldaña, J. (2014). *Qualitative data analysis: A methods sourcebook*. Thousand Oaks, CA: Sage.

Patton, M. Q. (2015). *Qualitative research and evaluation methods: Integrating theory and practice* (4th ed.). Thousand Oaks, CA: Sage.

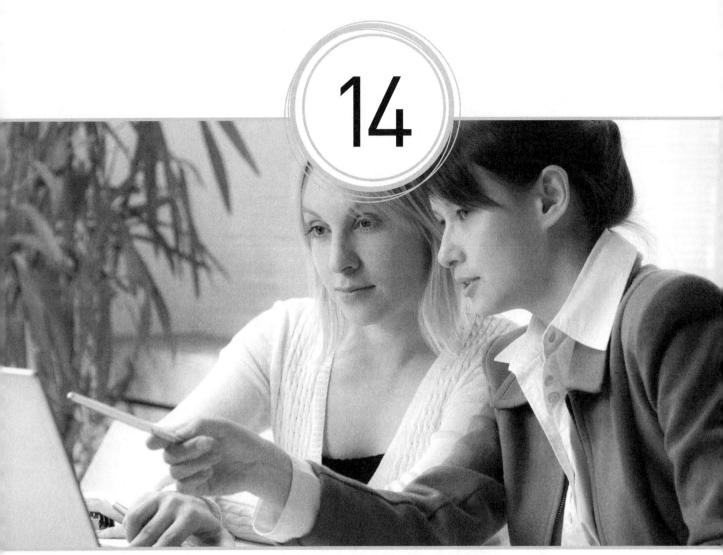

14

Secondary Analysis and Existing Data

Chapter Outline

Overview
Learning Objectives
Basic Concepts
The Secondary Data Analysis Process
Advantages, Limitations, and Ethics
    Advantages
    Limitations
    Ethics
Secondary Data Sources
    Major Sources
    Qualitative Data
    Documents and Records
    Big Data
Synthesizing Results From Multiple Studies
    Narrative Review
    Systematic Review
    Meta-analysis
Key Points

Learning Objectives

After studying Chapter 14, the reader should be able to:

- Decide when it is appropriate to conduct a secondary data analysis
- Implement the secondary data analysis process
- Explore and evaluate sources for conducting a secondary data analysis
- Understand and assess strategies for synthesizing results from multiple studies

Overview

Conducting research does not necessarily require collecting data. Valuable research may be done using existing data that are available from an increasing number and range of sources. The main use of existing data for research is **secondary data analysis**, which involves analyzing research data previously collected and analyzed by others for another purpose. Other types of existing data, such as administrative records and government statistics, which were not necessarily collected for research purposes, also may be analyzed. In addition, a variety of documents, such as community organization meeting minutes and clinic policies, may be reviewed to systematically extract data from them. Recently, internet use and real-time electronic recording systems have contributed to amassing extremely large data sets, referred to as **big data**, about behaviors such as where and how people seek health information online, where and what groceries people buy, and attitudes about current events posted at social media sites. Such existing data sources may be useful for conducting a study in its own right or for a pilot study (Chapter 1), or they may be combined with or supplement new data. This chapter presents guidelines and strategies for selecting and using existing data sources. Also, it describes **systematic reviews** and **meta-analysis**, which comprise strategies for synthesizing results across multiple studies about the same research question.

Basic Concepts

When researchers design a study and collect and analyze the data, the data analysis addresses the *primary* research question. *Secondary data analysis* is the analysis of data previously collected and analyzed by others. An important distinction is that a secondary data analysis is not a replication of the original analysis to assess its reliability (see Chapter 1). However, a secondary data analysis may assess the generalizability of findings from one data set by using data from another data set. In some situations, the secondary analysis research question may be related to the primary one. For example, it might compare results across demographic subgroups that were not a focus of the primary research question. In other situations, a secondary data analysis might employ a different statistical technique and/or add data about variables from another source.

> **Key Concept**
>
> Secondary data analysis is the analysis of data previously collected and analyzed by others.

Other times, the secondary analysis question may be unrelated to the primary one, such as to examine the association between different independent and dependent variables that were measured by the study. For example, while the primary analysis might have assessed the association between social support (independent variable) and outcomes for a smoking cessation intervention (dependent variable), a secondary analysis might examine the association between household composition (independent variable) and social support (dependent variable). Moreover, the term *secondary* should not be interpreted as implying the result from a secondary data analysis is less valuable than a primary analysis result. Box 14.1 presents an example of a secondary analysis of national survey data.

BOX 14.1: SECONDARY ANALYSIS OF NATIONAL SURVEY DATA

Leung et al. (2018, p. 11) conducted a secondary analysis of data from the 2012 National Health Interview Survey (NHIS) "to determine prevalence of the use of special diets, the individual characteristics associated with their use and reasons for use." The NHIS (www.cdc.gov/nchs/nhis/index.htm, accessed November 12, 2018) is a cross-sectional household interview survey of a nationally representative sample of nonhospitalized U.S. adult populations. It is conducted periodically by the National Center for Health Statistics (NCHS) at the U.S. Centers for Disease Control and Prevention (CDC). The 2012 survey data set includes 34,525 cases. The dependent variables Leung et al. analyzed were the use of any of five special diets for health reasons for a period of two weeks or more, *ever*, and use of any of the special diets *during the past 12 months*. Independent variables were participant demographics, common conditions associated with diet, mental health conditions, body mass index (BMI), and lifestyle behavior.

The analysis found lifetime and 12-month prevalence of using a special diet were 7.5% and 2.9%, respectively. Characteristics of individuals who were most likely to have used a special diet in the past 12 months were female, not married, college educated, and depressed. Special diet users were more likely to also use herbal products, as well as nonvitamin and vitamin supplements. Different individuals reported using different special diets for different reasons. The most commonly used special diets were vegetarian and the Atkins diet. The main uses of a special diet were "to improve overall health (76.7%) or for general wellness/prevention (70.4%)" (Leung et al., 2018, p. 11). About one-third of special diet users reported they did not disclose their use to their health care provider.

The Secondary Data Analysis Process

Conducting a secondary data analysis does not involve a complete shortcut through the research process (Chapter 1), such that one simply acquires an existing data set and analyzes it. Figure 14.1 presents an overview of the secondary data analysis process. As for any research investigation, secondary data analysis requires a plan that starts with specifying the research question and conceptual approach. Also, prior to searching for a suitable data set, it is necessary to specify a research design, a target population, key variables, and measurement and data collection strategies that will adequately address the secondary analysis research question.

FIGURE 14.1 ● The Secondary Data Analysis Process

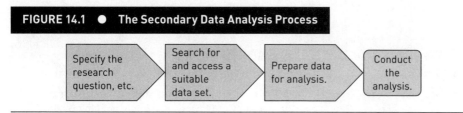

Next, a search must be conducted to identify and access a suitable data set. Most data sets available for secondary analysis may be found by an internet search or through an online portal, as discussed in a following section. Others may be identified by referral or contacting authors of reports based on data that might be suitable for a secondary analysis. It is essential to obtain and carefully review as much documentation as is available about a prospective data set to assess aspects such as when, where, how, by whom, and from whom the data were collected, and how the data set is structured. As appropriate and available, such documentation may include

- unpublished reports;
- papers presented at professional conferences;
- published reports;
- data collection instrument(s), such as questionnaire(s);
- data collection protocol;
- data collector's training manual and handbook; and
- data codebook (a description of how each variable was measured and its format).

In addition, it is very useful to interview key members of the primary research team, especially the lead researcher(s) and data collection and data processing supervisors, to gain further insight about a data set, especially regarding its limitations. For example, data from a large study, such as a national survey, that used a complex sampling design (Chapter 7) typically requires applying weights to adjust for differences in probabilities of selection and reflect the target population's distribution on key demographic characteristics (Bell et al., 2012). A secondary data analyst must be able to either obtain the sampling weights that were applied, or obtain the information necessary to compute them. Consulting or collaborating with a statistician who is experienced working with such data and appropriate analysis software is recommended.

Other issues relate to accessing a data set and reporting secondary analysis results. Many data sets may be downloaded from the internet and even analyzed over the internet. However, some might be available on computer tapes, disks, or paper format. Typically, one must register to access a data set and agree to certain conditions for its use, such as maintaining confidentiality, appropriately citing its source, original funding support, technical assistance, or restrictions on how the data may be used. Also, it should be determined whether a fee must be paid to access the data. It is essential to establish at the outset a clear, written understanding regarding conditions for accessing a data set and disseminating the results of a secondary analysis of it.

Finally, prior to analyzing a data set that has been accessed, it must be prepared for the secondary analysis. This step may include addressing issues such as deleting ineligible cases (e.g., not in the specified age range), imputing missing values, recoding variables (e.g., combining nominal-level categories), and computing multiple-item scale scores. Data analysis file preparation is discussed in further detail in Chapter 15.

CHECK YOUR UNDERSTANDING 14.1

- Describe how the secondary data analysis process is similar to and different from the general research process where a study is designed and implemented to collect primary data (Chapter 1).

Advantages, Limitations, and Ethics

Advantages

Box 14.2 presents the main advantages and limitations of secondary data analysis. The most obvious advantage is that the data already are available, which eliminates time for developing a study design, preparing and submitting a proposal to obtain funding, developing measurement instruments, and collecting data. In addition, in most situations, a data analysis file already is available. Moreover, most data sets that are available for secondary analysis are free or may be accessed for a modest fee. Thus, secondary analysis saves the substantial financial costs for sampling, data collection, and initial data analysis file preparation.

Typically, data sets that are archived to be available for secondary analysis are from studies with large, representative samples, and that measured large numbers of variables. Also, such studies typically are well designed and conducted, often by full-time methodological

BOX 14.2: ADVANTAGES AND LIMITATIONS OF SECONDARY DATA ANALYSIS

Advantages	Limitations
• Data already are available.	• It might not cover the desired population.
• A large, representative sample is available.	• Key variables might not be included.
• There is a large number of variables.	• Key variables might not be measured in an acceptable format.
• Data quality is high.	• Data might not be current.
• Longitudinal data may be available.	

experts using state-of-the-art methods at academic or commercial research centers, or at nonprofit or government agencies. Thus, the data quality generally is high. Finally, secondary data analysis may facilitate longitudinal analysis. Collecting longitudinal data is challenging, expensive, and time-consuming (Chapter 6). Trend analysis may be conducted with cross-sectional data collected periodically, such as by the National Health Interview Survey (NHIS) series (Centers for Disease Control and Prevention, 2018e). Repeated-measures analysis may be conducted using data from a panel study, conducted with the same individuals at multiple **observation points**, such as by the Longitudinal Studies of Aging (LSOAs) (Centers for Disease Control and Prevention, 2018d).

Limitations

Overall, secondary data analysis is limited by the likelihood that a study conducted by someone else, for another purpose, rarely will have been conducted in all ways the secondary data analyst would prefer. Secondary data analysis typically involves a trade-off between reaping the advantages of using an existing data set, and accepting and taking into account its limitations in the same way as if the analyst him- or herself collected the data. Thus, although analyzing an existing data set substantially saves time and money, preparing to conduct a secondary data analysis requires an investment to identify, access, and thoroughly understand all its aspects.

As shown in Box 14.2, a key issue is whether the desired population is covered adequately. In addition to the sampling frame and sample selection procedure, this concern includes the target population definition. For example, suppose the initial secondary data analysis research question focuses on women aged 40–65, but a primary data set included only women aged 45–60. A compromise might be to redefine the target population as women aged 45–60 and acknowledge not being able to include those aged 40–44 and 61–65 as *a limitation of the secondary data analysis*; it would not be a limitation of the primary data set. Alternatively, if a data set includes women aged 18–80, the secondary analysis might focus only on those aged 40–65, provided the data set includes a sufficient number of women in that age category to address the secondary analysis research question.

Additional concerns are whether all key variables (independent, dependent, mediators, and moderators) for a secondary data analysis were measured, and whether they were measured in an acceptable format. For example, the wording of survey questions and response choices should be assessed carefully (Chapter 11). Also, secondary data analysis inherently involves using data that might not be as current as would be ideal.

The elapsed time between when the data were collected and when they are made available for secondary analysis, especially for large, complex studies, may be two years or longer. For example, as of November 2018, the most recent release of data from the NHIS was for the year 2017. Moreover, definitions or terminology for key variables may change over time, as exemplified by measures of race/ethnicity, sexual orientation, and gender identification.

Ethics

Although the data were collected by someone else, a secondary data analyst still is responsible for protecting the privacy of the individuals who provided the data (Chapter 2). Whenever possible, the best practice is to request a copy of the data set that is de-identified, meaning individual identifiers (e.g., name, address, telephone number, or patient/employee/student identification number) have been removed. Otherwise, the secondary data analyst must treat the data with the same concern for protecting confidentiality as when analyzing primary data. It is not sufficient that the primary researcher's institutional review board (IRB) approved the study. Secondary analysts must comply with any requirements of their own IRB regarding their data access and analysis plans. Generally, secondary analysis of de-identified data qualifies for IRB exempt status. An additional ethical aspect for secondary data analysis is that the source of the data must be acknowledged in any report of results.

> **CHECK YOUR UNDERSTANDING 14.2**
>
> - Consider the following research question:
>
>   *How do African American men identify and respond to heart disease symptoms?*
>
>   ○ What might be the main *advantages/benefits* of conducting a secondary analysis of *quantitative* data to address this research question?
>
>   ○ What might be the main **limitations** of conducting a secondary analysis of *quantitative* data to address this research question?

Secondary Data Sources

Major Sources

The most frequently used sources for secondary data analysis are large-scale surveys conducted by academic, commercial, and government organizations. Moreover, many such data sets may be searched and accessed over the internet at data repositories, data archives, and portals. Table 14.1 presents a list of major sources of secondary analysis data. Other data sets are available from individual study or organizational websites. Still others must be accessed by contacting the original researcher(s) directly.

When searching for a secondary data source, it is important to ascertain whether data are available at the aggregate or individual level. Government statistics, from the U.S. Census for instance, typically are available at the aggregate level, such as for a state, county, city, or census tract. For example, aggregate data might be available for the percent of women in a city who visited a health care provider during the past year. Survey data, including from surveys conducted by government agencies, typically are available at the individual level. For example, data might be available to estimate the percent of women in the United States who visited a health care provider during the past year and who have a particular health history.

TABLE 14.1 ● Major Sources of Secondary Analysis Data

Source	Description/Examples
Area Health Resources Files (AHRF), Health Resources & Services Administration (HRSA), Data Warehouse: https://data.hrsa.gov/	County-, state-, and national-level files in eight areas: health care professions, health facilities, population characteristics, economics, health professions training, hospital utilization, hospital expenditures, and environment.
Behavioral Risk Factor Surveillance System (BRFSS), Centers for Disease Control and Prevention (CDC): www.cdc.gov/brfss/	Completes more than 400,000 adult survey interviews each year about health-related risk behaviors, chronic health conditions, and use of preventive services. Collects data in all 50 states as well as the District of Columbia and three U.S. territories.
CDC Wonder: https://wonder.cdc.gov/	A portal to wide-ranging, integrated online data for public health research.
Data.gov: www.data.gov/health/	The U.S. government's open data source.
Inter-university Consortium for Political and Social Research (ICPSR), University of Michigan: www.icpsr.umich.edu/icpsrweb/	An international consortium of more than 750 academic institutions and research organizations. Maintains a data archive of more than 250,000 files of research in the social and behavioral sciences.
National Center for Health Statistics (NCHS), Centers for Disease Control and Prevention (CDC): www.cdc.gov/nchs/nchs_for_you/researchers.htm	Downloadable public-use data files for several large-scale national health surveys and vital statistics, such as • Longitudinal Studies of Aging (LSOAs) • National Ambulatory Medical Care Survey (NAMCS) • National Health Interview Survey (NHIS) • National Health and Nutrition Examination Survey (NHANES) • National Hospital Discharge Survey (NHDS) • National Survey of Children's Health • National Vital Statistics System (NVSS)
National Opinion Research Center (NORC), General Social Survey (GSS): http://gss.norc.org/	Started in 1972, collects data on contemporary American society to monitor trends in attitudes, behaviors, and attributes.
Society of General Internal Medicine (SGIM), Dataset Compendium: www.sgim.org/communities/research/dataset-compendium	Assists investigators conducting research on existing data sets, with an emphasis on health services research, clinical epidemiology, and medical education.
U.S. Census Bureau: www.census.gov/data.html	Extensive data for the United States at the individual and household levels.
USA.gov: www.usa.gov/statistics	Data and statistics about the United States.
World Health Organization (WHO), Global Health Observatory data repository: http://apps.who.int/gho/data/node.home	WHO's gateway to health-related statistics for more than 1,000 indicators for its 194 member states.

Qualitative Data

Most data available for secondary data analysis are quantitative. It is much easier to archive and reproduce copies of quantitative data as compared to qualitative data that includes field notes, unstructured interviews, narratives, and so forth. Moreover, conducting a secondary analysis of qualitative data is substantially limited in that the analyst is not able to engage in the iterative process that is a hallmark of qualitative research methods (Chapter 13). Nevertheless, the number of archived qualitative data sets is increasing. In particular, the Inter-university Consortium for Political and Social Research (ICPSR) at the University of Michigan data archive includes a growing population of studies that collected at least some qualitative data. A search for "qualitative data" at www.icpsr.umich.edu/icpsr-web/ICPSR/index.jsp in November 2018 returned 907 results. Tate and Happ (2018) present an excellent overview and example of conducting secondary analysis of qualitative data. The UK Data Service QualiBank (https://discover.ukdataservice.ac.uk/QualiBank) provides access to over 350 collections (as of May 2018) that contain qualitative or mixed methods research data.

Documents and Records

Documents (e.g., institutional policies) and records (e.g., hospital admission and discharge records) may be available at either the aggregate or individual level. They typically are neither designed nor maintained for analysis by external investigators. It may be necessary to extract, code, and enter such data in a database to analyze them, which would increase the analysis time and costs. Also, gaining access to such data typically is more challenging than accessing data from a data archive (e.g., ICPSR) or a data portal (e.g., CDC Wonder). Moreover, records may have empty data fields for some individuals. As Patton (2015, p. 390) has cautioned, "Client files maintained by programs are notoriously variable in quality and completeness, with great detail in some cases and virtually nothing in others." Box 14.3 presents an example of a secondary analysis of electronic records data.

BOX 14.3: SECONDARY ANALYSIS OF ELECTRONIC RECORDS DATA

Simons, Unger, Lopez, and Kohn (2015) conducted a secondary analysis of electronic health records to estimate human papillomavirus (HPV) vaccine series completion rates and examine predictors of completion among adolescents and young adults. They used electronic health records from 119 health centers in 11 U.S. states for 9,648 patients who initiated HPV vaccination between January 2011 and January 2013. Their analysis focused on two dependent variables: vaccine completion within 12 months and time to completion. They found that almost one-third of vaccine initiators completed the three-dose vaccine series. Patients who were male, younger, or non-Hispanic Black, or who had public insurance, were less likely to complete the series within 12 months, and those who completed it took longer than patients who were female, older, or non-Hispanic White, or who had private insurance. The authors recommended health care providers should work with patients to identify potential barriers to vaccination completion and develop an action plan to mitigate them. They also suggested that vaccination inequities might be addressed through tailored interventions among the subgroups at greatest risk for noncompletion.

Big Data

Electronic formats for communication, data capture, and data storage have given rise to massive data sets about human behavior that generally are referred to as big data. Such data are not collected deliberately for research. Instead, they are "organic" (Groves, 2011) in nature and *captured* from a wide variety of sources (Couper, 2013), such as purchasing groceries and other consumer items, filling a medical prescription, traveling while using a global positioning system (GPS), accessing electronic health records, browsing the internet, and posting and accessing content at online social media/networking sites. For example, as of May 2018, on average Google was processing over 40,000 search queries every second and over 3.5 billion searches per day (Google Search Statistics, 2018); on average, 1.49 billion people who are considered "active users" log on to Facebook each day, and 510,000 comments are posted every 60 seconds (Zephoria Digital Marketing, 2018). Such data sources increasingly are being explored to identify trends and patterns in human behavior nearly in real time.

Although some have suggested that big data eventually might replace much of traditional data collection methods, such as surveys and qualitative interviews (e.g., Savage & Burrows, 2007), others (e.g., AAPOR Big Data Task Force, 2015; Couper, 2013; Daas & Puts, 2014) have raised cautions about several aspects of big data that must be taken into consideration:

- **Coverage bias.** Big data are not derived from representative random samples. If the target population is users of a particular system or device, such as people who purchase dietary supplements online at Amazon.com, then big data might be well representative of that population. However, if the target population is all people who purchase dietary supplements, big data will not include people who pay cash to purchase items at a brick-and-mortar retail store.

- **Selection bias.** Big data are more likely to include information about people of higher socioeconomic status as compared with the general population. For example, not everyone has a Facebook account. Participating in Facebook requires access to an appropriate electronic device and a certain degree of competence navigating online.

- **Measurement bias.** Big data may not include the same variables for all people, variables may be measured or expressed differently for/by different people, and some variables may be missing for some people. Moreover, demographic/background variables may not be included in some big data sets.

- **Measurement limitations.** Big data primarily capture information about behavior; little information is collected about variables such as attitudes, feelings, beliefs, motivations, expectations, and intentions.

- **Accessibility.** It is difficult to access much of big data for research purposes because it is proprietary and is used for commercial or institutional purposes.

- **Artefactual effects.** Changes in the methods for collecting big data, such as web page design and search algorithms, may artificially induce differences in data patterns that are not attributable to human behavior.

Box 14.4 presents a summary of a notorious cautionary tale about using big data.

> **BOX 14.4: THE SUCCESS AND FAILURE OF GOOGLE FLU TRENDS**
>
> Google Flu Trends (GFT) estimated influenza incidence from internet searches using Google's search engine for flu symptoms, flu remedies, and other flu-related key words. GFT estimates correlated remarkably well with flu incidence in the United States reported by the U.S. Centers for Disease Control and Prevention (CDC) for the years 2009–2011. Indeed, the GFT estimates matched almost exactly the CDC's surveillance data, and the GFT estimates were available sooner than those from the CDC. This gave rise to the concept of "nowcasting," which is near real-time forecasting of flu vaccine needs, and also might be extended to other public health issues. However, for the 2012–2013 flu season, GFT predicted more than double the proportion of physician visits for flu-like symptoms than were reported by the CDC for that period (Butler, 2013). One reason proposed to explain the disparity between GFT estimates and CDC surveillance data is there was widespread media coverage of the 2012–2013 flu season, including a declaration by New York State of a public health emergency. These conditions may have triggered an inordinate number of searches for flu-related content by people who were not experiencing any flu-related symptoms (Butler, 2013). Another reason is the GFT search algorithm was modified such that when a search included flu-related terms such as *fever* or *cough*, the user was referred to sites with information about flu symptoms and remedies. Thus, the number of flu-related searches was artificially inflated (Lazer, Kennedy, King, & Vespignani, 2014). The AAPOR Big Data Task Force (2015) observed: "In survey research, this is similar to the bias induced by interviewers who suggest to respondents who are coughing that they might have flu; then asking the same respondents if they think they might have flu."
>
> As of November 2018, an online search for "Google Flu Trends" yields the following message at www.google.org/flutrends/about/:
>
> > Google Flu Trends and Google Dengue Trends are no longer publishing current estimates of Flu and Dengue fever based on search patterns. The historic estimates produced by Google Flu Trends and Google Dengue Trends are available below. It is still early days for nowcasting and similar tools for understanding the spread of diseases like flu and dengue—we're excited to see what comes next.

CHECK YOUR UNDERSTANDING 14.3

- Consider the following research question:

  How do African American men identify and respond to heart disease symptoms?

  - Which types of sources for secondary data analysis might be appropriate to address this research question?
  - Briefly describe why you might use the source(s) you suggest to address this research question.

Synthesizing Results From Multiple Studies

As stated in Chapter 1, scientific evidence derives validity from the preponderance of results from multiple independent studies addressing the same problem. Synthesizing results from multiple studies is essential for developing evidence-based best-practice guidelines. Three methods may be used to synthesize research results:

- Narrative review
- Systematic review
- Meta-analysis

> **Key Concept**
>
> *Synthesizing results from multiple studies is essential for developing evidence-based best-practice guidelines.*

These methods are similar in the sense that the existing "data" they assess are the results of completed studies that addressed the same, or very similar, research problems and outcome measure(s). They differ in how they select studies, and how they assess and report their results. If individual-level data are available from studies meeting the literature search inclusion criteria, then it is more effective to conduct an individual-level secondary data analysis of a combined data set instead of a narrative review, systematic review, or meta-analysis.

Narrative Review

A **narrative review** is a scholarly summary of completed studies that includes comparisons and interpretations of results, critiques of strengths and limitations, and recommendations for further investigation. It is the most familiar format for summarizing results across completed studies. In virtually every research proposal or report, one of the first sections is a narrative review of results from previously conducted relevant studies. Although more extensive narrative reviews presented as reports themselves previously were quite common, preference generally has shifted toward systematic reviews and meta-analyses.

Typically, a narrative review describes each study individually in terms of its design, key findings, strengths, and limitations. A summary highlights the main points of agreement, disagreement, strengths, limitations, and gaps in the studies to establish the context for and potential significance of the current study. Ideally, a literature review would be comprehensive and balanced, covering all relevant studies and presenting results from ones with both positive and negative results. However, the scope of a narrative review embedded in a research proposal or report is limited owing to space limitations and the need also to present the main study design, measurement and analysis strategies, results, discussion, and conclusion. Even when presented as an independent report, a narrative review typically does not provide comprehensive coverage of all relevant studies. Instead, the focus of a narrative review tends to be biased toward the most notable studies (e.g., in terms of factors such as size and outcomes). Moreover, study selection criteria tend to be subjective, and inclusion criteria rarely are specified, making it difficult to assess the representativeness of the studies reviewed. Of greatest concern is the potential for *reviewer selection bias*, whereby studies may be included because they are in accord with the reviewer's theoretical and/or policy perspective.

Systematic Review

A systematic review assesses and summarizes results from all completed studies that meet explicit, prespecified inclusion criteria. The studies are identified through an extensive search to ensure to the extent it is feasible that all relevant studies are included and minimize selection bias. In addition, prespecified evaluation criteria are employed, typically by two or more independent reviewers for reliability, to assess and synthesize results from the selected studies. Examples of potential study eligibility criteria are

- research design,
- target population,
- key variables,
- time frame, and
- publication type.

Examples of potential study evaluation criteria are

- sample size,
- participation/response rate,
- measurement reliability and validity,
- analytical methods,
- size of outcome differences/associations, and
- limitations.

These aspects generally render the results from a systematic review as more valid and reliable than a narrative review. Although a scoring system may be employed to assess various aspects of each study, a systematic review primarily is qualitative because the studies' results are not combined and analyzed using statistical methods, as is the case for a meta-analysis (discussed in the next section). The Preferred Reporting Items for Systematic Reviews and Meta-Analyses (PRISMA) statement (Moher et al., 2015) provides useful guidelines for conducting and reporting a systematic review. Box 14.5 presents excerpts from a systematic review that followed the PRISMA guidelines.

BOX 14.5: EXAMPLE OF SYSTEMATIC REVIEW PROCEDURES

Search strategies. The search for relevant studies was performed using the following databases: CINAHL, MEDLINE, PUBMED, EMBASE, the Cochrane Methodological Register, Cochrane Database of Systematic Reviews, PsycInfo, Social Sciences Abstracts, ERIC, and HEALTH STAR. The keywords used in the search included recovery phase, post-operative, coronary artery bypass graft (CABG), valve/valvular replacement (VR), heart surgery, post-surgical, post-operative behaviors, web-based interventions, self-care, self-care behavior. Following initial searches, the results were combined with the operands AND and OR. Reference lists of studies retrieved were examined for additional studies that address the post-operative recovery period of patients who have had heart surgery. A total of 352 articles were found to have addressed web-based patient education. Seventy-two were duplications, which were removed. An additional 261 articles were excluded because the reported study assessed the effectiveness of a combined pre- and post-web-based educational intervention and non-surgical web-based patient education intervention. A total of 19 studies met the selection criteria and were included in the systematic review (articles included in systematic review are indicated in Reference list with an asterisk).

Study selection: Inclusion criteria. Studies were included in the systematic review if they met the following selection criteria: (a) the sample represented adult ($\geq$ 18 years) patients who underwent heart surgery, (b) the outcomes assessed relate to the number and type of self-care behaviors performed during the post-hospital discharge recovery period, and (c) the study report was published in English between 2000 and 2012 and used non-experimental, experimental, or randomized clinical trial (RCT), quasi-experimental, mixed methods, and qualitative designs.

Data Abstraction

The research team extracted data from all articles screened (Table 1). Interrater reliability was assessed to demonstrate consistency in data extraction. This was accomplished by two members of the research team who were familiar with the data abstraction process. They independently abstracted data from 10% of the articles retrieved and then compared results to determine the degree to which they are equivalent. A value of .80 or greater was considered an acceptable value of inter-rater reliability, as this is a commonly accepted value in nursing research (Fredericks & DaSilva, 2010). The interrater reliability score of .93 was obtained.

Measurement of Outcome

The following information was gathered about each study: year of publication, country in which the study was conducted, study design (non-experimental, quasi-experimental, experimental, qualitative, mixed method), sample size (total, and for each study group, if relevant), sample demographics (age, sex, marital status, co-morbid condition, type of surgery), drop-out rate, and number and type of study groups (control or comparison and treatment, or two treatment groups). Web-based interventions were characterized in terms of approach (standardized, individualized), frequency of intervention delivery, and length of time of delivery. With regard to self-care behavior performed, the type and number of self-care behavior was extracted. These data were used for descriptive purposes.

Source: Fredericks, Martorella, & Catallo (2015, pp. 95–96). Reproduced with permission from SAGE Publications.

Although there is no standard protocol for conducting a systematic review, the general process is to

- specify the research question,
- specify inclusion criteria,
- specify evaluation criteria,
- develop and implement an extensive search strategy,
- screen abstracts and full text to assess eligibility,
- extract and code/score information according to the evaluation criteria, and
- assess and summarize the results.

A key aspect of the process is identifying as many studies that meet the inclusion criteria as possible to provide comprehensive coverage. It is highly recommended to consult a reference librarian to identify appropriate search engines, specify key words/phrases and Medical Subject Headings (MeSH), and identify relevant journals. In addition to conducting electronic searches, the snowball method should be employed to identify studies cited by other reports, especially previously published reviews of relevant literature.

An important limitation of a systematic review is it is not necessarily comprehensive. For example, a search might not identify every relevant study. Other times, inclusion criteria may restrict study eligibility, such as to studies that were completed during a certain time period or were published in a peer-reviewed professional journal. The latter criterion typically is applied to include studies that have been independently evaluated as having employed appropriate research methods, and were reported in a clear and unbiased manner. Nevertheless, being published in a peer-reviewed professional journal does not guarantee either condition. Moreover, such a criterion may introduce *publication bias*, which may occur, for example, if publication preference is given to reports of statistically significant (Chapter 15) results. Reports of null results have been most likely to be published if they are derived from a large, complex study. However, results from well-designed and conducted studies that do not find statistically significant results are just as important as ones that do. Fortunately, publication bias appears to be declining as journal editors and peer reviewers have become increasingly aware of and concerned about the issue. Another source of publication bias is a search might not include the so-called *gray literature*, which comprises research reports that are not disseminated through high-profile channels, such as peer-reviewed journals or academic books. Examples include theses and dissertations, government and nongovernmental organization reports, and conference proceedings.

Meta-analysis

While narrative and systematic reviews may be conducted with qualitative or quantitative data, separately or combined, meta-analysis is a statistical method for synthesizing quantitative results from several similar studies. Most often, meta-analysis is applied to results of studies that used an experimental design. However, the method also may be applied to correlations from observational studies. It treats each study, rather than individuals, as the unit of analysis. Each study's outcome, usually a treatment effect, is the corresponding data. For example, if a meta-analysis includes 26 studies, the number of observations would be 26, not the sum of the individuals in those studies, and the data would be 26 treatment effects. Meta-analysis takes into account the number of individuals in each study by applying weights to each study's treatment effect before calculating a pooled summary statistic to generalize results across studies. Also, it pools results from both studies that did and studies that did not produce a statistically significant difference as compared with a control condition. In contrast, even when reviewing studies that yielded quantitative results, results from narrative and systematic reviews are not presented as a pooled summary statistic. Typically, results from those types of review, expressed in terms such as "some," "most," or "*n* of *N* studies," found a particular treatment did or did not produce a statistically significant difference as compared with a control condition.

Similar to a systematic review, a meta-analysis starts with a search for studies that meet prespecified criteria. However, the inclusion criteria typically are more restrictive than for a systematic review because a meta-analysis requires that each study used the same or very similar

- target population,
- research design,

- treatment/intervention,
- control condition, and
- outcome measure.

In general, limitations of a meta-analysis are the same as for a systematic review. However, a meta-analysis is more likely than a systematic review not to include some studies because of the more stringent inclusion criteria that typically apply for a meta-analysis. If a search identifies only a few studies that meet the inclusion criteria, then instead of a meta-analysis, a systematic review might be done by relaxing the inclusion criteria somewhat.

Assuming an experimental design with two groups, treatment and control, the basic meta-analysis statistic is the average effect size. First, a standardized effect size is calculated for each study by subtracting the control mean from the treatment mean, and dividing by the control group standard deviation or the pooled standard deviation for the two groups combined. Then, the average effect size is calculated by weighting each standardized effect size by the study's sample size. Depending on the nature of the studies to be synthesized, meta-analysis may involve sophisticated statistical methods. Therefore, it is recommended to consult a statistician who is experienced in performing meta-analyses. Box 14.6 presents an example of a published meta-analysis.

BOX 14.6: META-ANALYSIS OF LIFESTYLE INTERVENTIONS IN PRESCHOOL CHILDREN

Ling, Robbins, Wen, and Zhang (2017) conducted a meta-analysis to estimate the effects of lifestyle interventions on body mass index (BMI) among preschool children to encourage maintaining a long-term healthy weight. They followed the Preferred Reporting Items for Systematic Reviews and Meta-Analyses (PRISMA) statement guidelines to conduct the literature search, data coding, and reporting of results. Using a two-phase search strategy, they searched six electronic literature databases and then examined the references cited in articles to identify additional studies to consider for inclusion. They identified 52 articles that met their study eligibility requirements, which were that the study

- used a randomized controlled trial;
- primarily targeted children aged 2–5 years or included children whose average age was ← 6 years;
- evaluated an intervention targeting sedentary activity, screen time, physical activity, or nutrition; and
- used BMI as the outcome measure.

They calculated weighted standardized mean differences for BMI to estimate effect sizes separately for prevention interventions and treatment interventions. They found statistically significant effect sizes for both types of interventions. They found greater effects for interventions that included parenting skill training and behavioral change strategies, and ones that included general health and nutrition education for children. The authors concluded that their findings indicate that such intervention strategies are promising for achieving both immediate and sustained effects of lifestyle on BMI among preschool children.

CHECK YOUR UNDERSTANDING 14.4

- What are the *strengths* and *limitations* of each of the three methods for synthesizing results from multiple studies?
    - Narrative review
    - Systematic review
    - Meta-analysis

Key Points

Basic Concepts for Secondary Data Analysis

- Secondary data analysis is the analysis of data previously collected and analyzed by others.
- The term *secondary* should not be interpreted as implying that the result from a secondary data analysis is less valuable than a primary analysis result.

The Secondary Data Analysis Process

Secondary data analysis is a process, the main features of which are

- specifying the research question and conceptual approach;
- specifying a research design, a target population, key variables, and measurement and data collection strategies;
- searching for and accessing a suitable data set;
- preparing data for analysis; and
- conducting the analysis.

Advantages of Secondary Data Analysis

- Data already are available.
- A large, representative sample is available.
- There is a large number of variables.
- Data quality is high.
- Longitudinal data may be available.

Limitations of Secondary Data Analysis

- It might not cover the desired population.
- Key variables might not be included.
- Key variables might not be measured in an acceptable format.
- Data might not be current.

Ethical Aspects of Secondary Data Analysis

- A secondary data analyst still is responsible for protecting the privacy of the individuals who provided the data.
- Whenever possible, the best practice is to request a copy of the data set that does not include any individual identifiers.
- Secondary analysts must comply with any requirements of their own institutional review board regarding their data access and analysis plans.

Secondary Data Sources

- The most frequently used sources for secondary data analysis are large-scale surveys conducted by academic, commercial, and government organizations.
- Many data sets may be searched and accessed over the internet at data repositories, data archives, and portals.
- Other data sets are available from individual study or organizational websites, or by contacting the original researcher(s) directly.
- Most data available for secondary data analysis are quantitative.
- Documents and records typically are neither designed nor maintained for analysis by external investigators, and it typically is more challenging to access them.
- Big data are generated organically and may be captured from a wide variety of electronic sources, such as social media and retail purchase records. Such data are vulnerable to several sources of bias.

Synthesizing Results From Multiple Studies

- **Narrative review** describes each study individually and summarizes the main points of agreement, disagreement, strengths, limitations, and gaps; it is vulnerable to reviewer selection bias.
- **Systematic review** assesses and summarizes results from studies identified through an extensive search using explicit, prespecified inclusion criteria.
- **Meta-analysis** is a statistical method for synthesizing quantitative results from studies identified through an extensive search using explicit, prespecified inclusion criteria; each study is treated as the unit of analysis.

Review and Apply

1. Review the research plan you developed in the "Review and Apply" sections of the previous chapters. Follow the secondary data analysis process described in this chapter and conduct an online search for possible data sets for a secondary data analysis to address your research problem. Start your search by visiting one or both of the following websites:

   - Inter-university Consortium for Political and Social Research (ICPSR), University of Michigan: www.icpsr.umich.edu/icpsrweb/
   - National Center for Health Statistics (NCHS), Centers for Disease Control and Prevention (CDC): www.cdc.gov/nchs/nchs_for_you/researchers.htm

   OPTION: Instead, do this activity for another health-related problem that interests you.

2. After exploring one or both of the two websites above on your own, make an appointment to consult with a reference librarian to conduct a more extensive search for appropriate secondary data sets.

3. Select one data set that might be appropriate to address your research problem and obtain as much information about it as possible—see the suggestions in this chapter.

4. Make a list of the main advantages, limitations, and ethical aspects of using the data set to address your research problem.

5. Search for a systematic review or meta-analysis of studies related to your research problem. Compare it to at least one narrative review related to your research problem, such as may be found in one of the first sections of a published journal article. Write a brief description of how they differ. Which one do you regard as more valid and reliable? Explain why.

Study Further

Daas, P. J. H., & Puts, M. J. H. (2014). Big data as a source of statistical information. *The Survey Statistician*, 69(January), 22–31.

MacInnes, J. (2017). *An introduction to secondary data analysis with IBM SPSS Statistics*. Thousand Oaks, CA: Sage.

MIT Critical Data. (2016). *Secondary analysis of electronic health records*. Cham, Switzerland: Springer International. Retrieved from https://www.springer.com/us/book/9783319437408

Moher, D., Shamseer, L., Clarke, M., Ghersi, D., Liberati, A., Petticrew, M., . . . PRISMA-P Group. (2015). Preferred reporting items for systematic review and meta-analysis protocols (PRISMA-P) 2015 statement. *Systematic Reviews*, 4(1). Retrieved from https://systematicreviewsjournal.biomedcentral.com/articles/10.1186/2046-4053-4-1Tate

Tate, J. A., & Happ, M. B. (2018). Qualitative secondary analysis: A case exemplar. *Journal of Pediatric Health Care*, 32(3), 308–312.

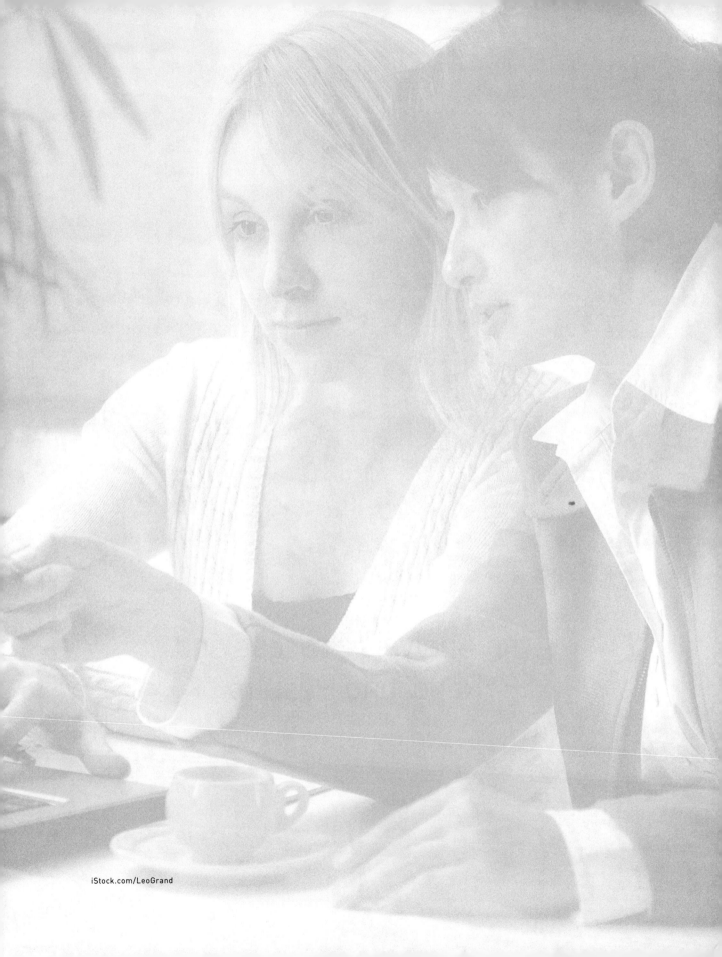

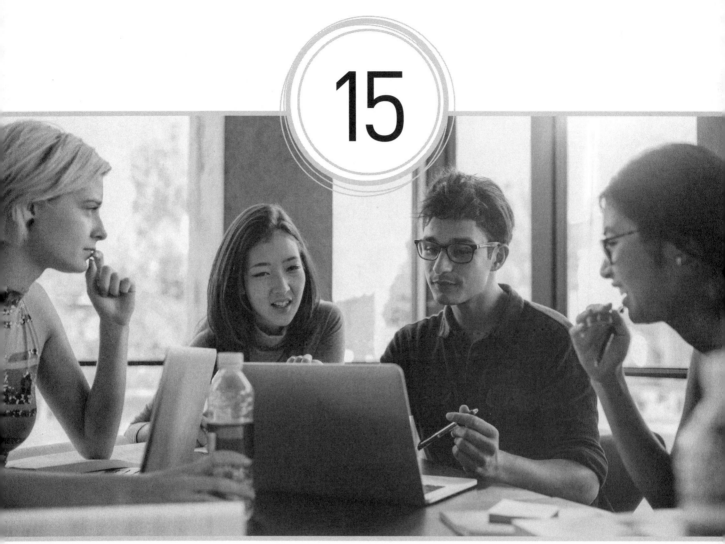

15

The Analysis Process and Reporting Results

Chapter Outline

Overview
Learning Objectives
The Data Analysis Process
    Data Preparation
    Analysis File Preparation
    Modification and Finalization
Overview of Quantitative Data Analysis
    Description
    Contingency
    Correlation
    Regression
    Differences
    Hypothesis Testing
    Validity and Substantive Significance
Overview of Qualitative Data Analysis
    Data Preparation
    Coding
    Themes and Conclusions
    Trustworthiness
Reporting Research Results
    Abstract
    Introduction
    Background/Literature Review
    Methods
    Results/Findings
    Discussion
    References
    Appendix
    Other Components
    Authorship
Key Points

Learning Objectives

After studying Chapter 15, the reader should be able to:

- Implement the data analysis process
- Prepare both quantitative and qualitative data for analysis
- Select data analysis techniques that are appropriate for the research question and type of data
- Prepare a thorough and unbiased research report

Overview

As the final stages of the research process (Chapter 1), data analysis and reporting results constitute a study's ultimate objective. They are the culmination of all the preceding plans, decisions, and activities. As emphasized in Chapter 1 and reinforced in subsequent chapters, it is essential to take data analysis and reporting results into consideration throughout the research process. Scientific research results are derived from analyzing and interpreting valid empirical observations (data) in a systematic and unbiased manner. Analytic procedures should be employed that are expected to yield the same conclusion regardless of who performs the analysis. With quantitative data, an analysis may draw upon a variety of well-established statistical methods. Qualitative data analysis involves a more subjective approach owing to the largely unstructured nature of qualitative research methods and the types of data they collect (Chapter 13). Regardless of the method and type of data, results must be reported clearly, thoroughly, and objectively.

The Data Analysis Process

After data are collected, the next step is *not* immediately to conduct the planned analysis and derive an answer to a study's research question. Data analysis is a process, depicted in Figure 15.1, comprising a logical sequence of several activities. Jumping ahead in the sequence is unproductive and inefficient because it results only in returning to the deviation point. Most of the following discussion assumes analyzing the types of data that constitute the majority of research measurements, which primarily are quantitative (ordinal or interval/ratio level), or simple nominal-level measurements, such as response choices to a survey question, for which it is considered appropriate to assign numerical codes.

> **Key Concept**
>
> Data analysis is a process comprising a logical sequence of several activities.

FIGURE 15.1 • The Data Analysis Process

Data Preparation → Analysis File Preparation → Modification and Finalization → Analysis

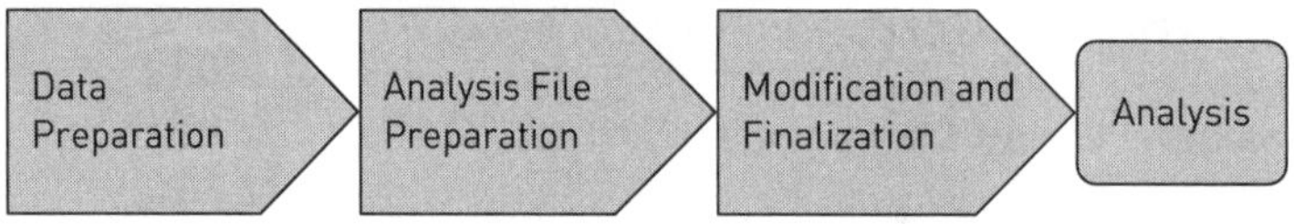

Data Preparation

After data are collected, they must be prepared for entry into a computer analysis file. In survey research, this activity commonly is called *data reduction*. The first data preparation activity is *editing* data records to carefully check for completeness and clarity. This should be done as soon as possible so research participants are contacted promptly to resolve issues such as illegibility, unclear meanings, contradictory responses, and missing observations. It is not reliable to ask interviewers or observers to guess what a response might have been to a question they did not ask, or recall a response or event they did not record. Each record must be checked for any instances where information was not recorded for one or more variables that are applicable to a participant or observation situation. For example, interviewers might not have asked a question that applied, or they might not have recorded a response to a question they asked. Also, each recorded response/observation must be checked for information that is not clear, owing to being either illegible or uninterpretable. Instances should be flagged where multiple responses or observations are recorded but only a single response/observation is appropriate. Also, information that is out of the acceptable or logical range should be flagged.

Next, **coding** involves assigning a numerical code for every measurement for every variable so it may be entered in a data analysis file. The original data source always should be preserved so it may be consulted in the event of a coding error. For quality control, the editing and coding work for precoded variables should be verified by independently **check-coding** a random sample of 10%–15% of each coder's completed cases, although as much as 100% may be check-coded in situations such as when coding is done by inexperienced staff or to maximize coding accuracy. As described in Chapter 11, the response choices for most questions on a structured questionnaire, and data fields for other instruments using a structured or semistructured format (e.g., records extraction and semistructured observation), are precoded. Nevertheless, codes must be assigned to responses that are not in the precoded scheme, such as ones in an "other" category and open-ended question responses. Moreover, all unstructured observations must be coded for entry into a computer analysis file. A list should be compiled of such responses or observations. Then codes may be assigned to categories developed based on major themes that are identified among them. For quality control, the coding of such responses should be assessed by interrater reliability as described in Chapter 8. Coders must be trained regarding procedures such as where and how to enter codes, standard codes such as for "don't know" or "refused," and how to flag problems. Examples should be presented that illustrate correct and incorrect procedures for dealing with issues coders are most likely to encounter. Finally, they must complete training in protecting human research subjects by treating all information about research participants confidentially (Chapter 2).

Analysis File Preparation

Data entry

Data entry is the first activity to prepare a computer data analysis file. Data must be entered for each individual record. Typically, the first element entered is the subject's study-specific identification code (Chapter 2). Thereafter, assuming data were collected using a structured questionnaire, for example, codes are entered for all responses the subject provided in the order they appear in the questionnaire. When a computer-assisted or online data collection method is employed (Chapter 12), data for precoded responses are entered as part of the data collection process. However, codes developed for responses in an "other" category or to an open-ended question must be entered subsequently. For quality control, data entry should be verified by independent reentry of a random sample of at least 10%–15% of each data entry operator's cases. As much as 100% may be verified in situations such as when data entry is done by inexperienced staff or to maximize accuracy. Most computer analysis programs include a data entry verification function to compare entries and flag discrepancies. Data entry and verification should be done on a rolling basis over the course of a large study.

Data cleaning

Following data entry, **data cleaning** identifies and corrects problems in three areas: legal entries, contingencies, and consistency. It is not efficient to perform data cleaning for each individual data record. Instead, it should be done either after all data are entered, or in batches for a large study. Although data cleaning software is available, data cleaning for a small number of variables may be done by reviewing preliminary frequency distributions. When a computer-assisted or online data collection method is employed (Chapter 12), the data collection software may be programmed to perform cleaning as data are collected and entered in an analysis file.

Legal entries. Code values within the specified range for a variable are considered "legal" entries. For example, for a question that asks for a "yes" (1) or "no" (2) response, a code of 3 would not be a legal entry. Data cleaning should flag the problem, and the original data record (e.g., questionnaire) should be checked to enter the correct code. When an illegal code is entered using a computer-assisted or online data collection method, the software may be programmed to flag the error immediately and require a legal code to be entered before proceeding to the next variable. However, having entered a legal code does not guarantee it was entered accurately. For example, if a response to a yes/no question is entered as 1 (*yes*) instead of 2 (*no*), a check for legal entries will not detect the error. However, it might be detected by data reentry or by checking for the two other data cleaning conditions.

Contingencies. In this context, contingency refers to whether a data record conforms to an expected pattern. The most notable condition in which contingency checks are essential is when data are entered from a structured questionnaire or similar instrument that includes one or more skip patterns (Chapter 10). For example, if respondents answered "No" to a filter question such as "Have you ever been told by a doctor or other health professional that you have cancer?" then they should have skipped follow-up questions about a cancer diagnosis. There should be no response codes entered for those questions, which are *contingent* on having answered "Yes" to the filter question.

Consistency. Consistency checks actually seek to identify logical *inconsistencies* in a data record. For example, if a woman reports having two children of school age living in her household, then the number of children she reports regarding other variables, such as how many of the children ever were taken to an emergency room to treat an injury, should not exceed two.

Names and labels

Performing data analysis and interpreting its output is facilitated greatly by entering variable names, variable labels, and value labels in an analysis file. *Variable names* reference variables by recognizable names instead of numbers. For example, analyzing a cross tabulation of "Diagnosis" by "Sex" is more convenient than "Variable 023" by "Variable 078." *Variable labels* are longer descriptions of variables that appear on analysis output. For example, "Diagnosis" might be labeled "Ever been diagnosed with any type of cancer." *Value labels* may be assigned to code numbers to facilitate interpretation. For example, instead of a cross tabulation of "Diagnosis" by "Sex" displaying codes 1 and 2 for each variable, the output may display categories labeled "Yes" (1) and "No" (2) for "Diagnosis," and "Female" (1) and "Male" (2) for "Sex."

Modification and Finalization
Recoding and computing variables

After an analysis file is prepared, the next activity is to recode variables and compute variables, as appropriate (Chapter 9). The coding for the original version of a variable never should be changed because if there is an error in the recoding, or a different recoding strategy subsequently is considered, the original data record will have to be retrieved to reenter the data. Moreover, if the original data record cannot be retrieved, then the data for the erroneously recoded variable might not be usable as intended. The best practice is to create a copy of an original variable (e.g., "Diagnosis") and recode the copy (e.g., "Diagnosis-2"), leaving the original version still available.

Reverse-coding. Sometimes the original version of a variable, such as an ordinal scale, is coded in a way that may confuse its interpretation. For example, suppose a sample of men is asked the following question on a self-administered questionnaire:

If a man about your age engages in physical exercise regularly, how likely do you think it is he ever will get heart disease?

Very Likely	Most Likely	Somewhat Likely	Slightly Likely	Not Likely
1	2	3	4	5

Contrary to what might be expected, the *lower* the score for this unipolar scale, the *more likely* a participant is to perceive that regular physical exercise reduces heart disease risk. Interpretation would be rendered straightforward by **reverse-coding** the scale scores for a copy of the original variable as follows:

Very Likely	Most Likely	Somewhat Likely	Slightly Likely	Not Likely
5	4	3	2	1

Now the *lower* the scale score, the *less likely* a participant is to perceive that regular physical exercise reduces heart disease risk.

Combining categories. In general, it is best to obtain as much detail in measurements as possible. However, for simplicity of interpreting and presenting results, it may be advantageous to combine or collapse a variable's categories. For example, at the nominal level, responses to a person's birthplace might be combined into countries, states, or regions. At the ordinal level, responses to a 10-point single-item scale might be combined into three levels: low = 1–3, medium = 4–7, and high = 8–10. At the interval/ratio level, age might be combined in various ways, such as 18–29, 30–44, 45–64, and 65 or older. Combining categories, especially at the ordinal or interval/ratio level, involves a compromise between simplicity and loss of detail. For example, collapsing a 10-point scale into three levels, as described above, loses the distinction among responses in the "medium" category that are below the midpoint (4 and 5) and those above it (6 and 7). When combining categories, it is essential to consider how the combined categories will be responsive to the research question and relevant for guiding policy and practice applications. For instance, specifying age categories might consider ability to compare a study's results with other studies, and specifying income categories might consider their relevance to eligibility for certain assistance programs.

Dummy coding. Sometimes, especially for certain multiple regression techniques, it facilitates an analysis to recode a variable using the values 0 and 1, which is called dummy coding. The simplest situation for this type of coding is when a variable already is measured as a dichotomy. For example, suppose "Sex" is coded as 1 = "Female" and 2 = "Male." Dummy coding a copy ("Sex-2") of the original variable would keep the original code of 1 for "Female" and recode "Male" as 0. Subsequently, the dummy-coded version of "Sex" would be interpreted as "Female" (1) versus "Not Female" (0). For a polychotomous variable with three or more nominal categories, a value of 1 would be assigned to one category, and the others would be combined into a single category coded as 0. For example, suppose cigarette smoking status is classified as "Never smoked," "Former smoker," and "Current smoker." If the analysis plan is to compare people who "Never smoked" with those who "Ever smoked," then the "Former smoker" and "Current smoker" categories would be combined and labeled "Ever smoked." Dummy coding would assign values as "Never smoked" = 0 and "Ever smoked" = 1. Alternatively, if the analysis plan is to compare people who are not smoking currently with those who are smoking, then the "Never smoked" and "Former smoker" categories would be combined into "Nonsmoker" (0), versus "Current smoker" (1). When it is anticipated that dummy coding will be employed, it is most convenient to assign a code of 1 to the primary category so only the secondary category must be recoded.

Computing variables. Sometimes, a "new" variable must be computed using the data that were collected. For example, age might be computed using date of birth, or map coordinates might be used to compute a household's distance to the nearest urgent care source. Another common situation is to compute scores for a multiple-item scale (Chapter 9). For ordinal- and interval-/ratio-level items, the scale score typically is expressed as the mean (arithmetic average) of the item scores. For dichotomous items (e.g., "Yes" or "No"), the scale score typically is the number of items that are "endorsed" (i.e., "Yes" responses).

Imputation. **Imputation** is a strategy for estimating a valid value for a missing value so a case may be included in an analysis. Imputation maintains the analytical power that is available if all cases are included, and it preserves the representativeness of the analysis units. For example, suppose 30 respondents are asked a series of seven items using a 5-point scale, with the intention of computing a multiple-item scale. Typically, a "don't know" response is treated as a "missing value" and would not be included in the computation. The common default procedure, called *listwise deletion* of missing cases, would not include any respondent who has a missing value for any of the seven items. As an extreme example, suppose *different* respondents answer "don't know" to *different* items. As illustrated in Table 15.1, the consequence of excluding any respondent with a missing value on any of the seven items would be devastating. Eighteen respondents would be excluded, leaving only 12 (40%) of the original 30 respondents in the analysis. Moreover, if the respondents included in the analysis differ systematically from those who are excluded,

TABLE 15.1 ● Respondents With a Missing Value ("Don't know" = 8) for Seven 5-Point Scale Items

Item 1	Item 2	Item 3	Item 4	Item 5	Item 6	Item 7
R7	R3	R17	R1	R22	R5	R2
R9	R10		R12		R13	R19
R18			R26			R24
R21						R30
R29						

the representativeness of the sample will be compromised. For instance, if only the 12 oldest respondents answered all seven items within the scale range, the analysis would not be representative of the full range of ages in the target population.

Many imputation methods have been and continue to be developed (Allison, 2010; Groves et al., 2009), most of which are quite sophisticated and beyond the scope of this presentation. They should be employed in collaboration with a qualified statistician, and the impact of imputation should be assessed by conducting a *sensitivity analysis* comparing results with and without imputation. There is no consensus about which imputation method is best, the conditions for which imputation is appropriate, or whether imputation ever should be employed. Basic imputation methods are to replace a missing value with the

- mean for the items an individual answered within the scale range,
- scale midpoint,
- mean of similar respondents (e.g., age, education, or sex) for the missing item, or
- value of an item predicted from a regression analysis.

Intent-to-treat. The **intent-to-treat (ITT)** strategy, which may be employed to address an attrition threat to internal validity when analyzing a randomized controlled trial (Chapter 6), is related closely to imputation. The outcome for individual participants is analyzed within the study condition to which they are assigned (Gross & Fogg, 2004; Lachin, 2000; Little et al., 2012). Accordingly, the outcome for a participant assigned to a treatment condition who does not complete the treatment, or is lost to follow-up, is coded as a treatment *failure*. For example, in a smoking cessation program evaluation, a treatment participant who does not complete the program or is lost to follow-up is considered as not having stopped smoking. Thus, the intent-to-treat strategy provides a conservative estimate of a treatment's effect. It also is relevant for guiding policy decisions because in a typical "uncontrolled" practice setting, some participants do not complete a program.

Reliability and validity

After an analysis file is prepared, the next activity is to assess the reliability and validity of key variables. There is no point to analyzing measurements of variables that are not reliable and valid. Variables that are not acceptably reliable and valid should either be measured again using more trustworthy methods, if feasible, or not be included in the analysis. Methods for assessing measurement reliability and validity are described in Chapter 8.

Weighting

Next, as appropriate, cases must be weighted to adjust for selection probabilities and nonresponse/nonparticipation.

Selection probabilities. As described in Chapter 7, it is necessary to weight a random sample with unequal probabilities of selection. For example, a stratified random sample with disproportionate allocation must be weighted to adjust for oversampling some strata and undersampling others. Also, a cluster sample must be weighted to adjust for the design effect.

Nonresponse/Nonparticipation. Weighting also may be applied to adjust for unit nonresponse/nonparticipation. That is especially important when such outcomes are not random events, such that sample members with certain characteristics are more likely than others not to participate. The goal and procedure for this type of weighting is similar to that for a stratified random sample with disproportionate allocation (Chapter 7).

Final frequencies

At this point in the process, an analysis file should be ready for reviewing final frequencies output for each original, recoded, and computed variable. This provides a final check that the activities described in the preceding sections have been completed and are correct.

Documentation

Finally, analysis file documentation should be prepared to provide a record of how the file was prepared and guidance for analyzing it. As appropriate, it should include

- standard coding rules,
- additional codes developed for "other" categories and unstructured observations,
- how any variables were recoded,
- how any variables were computed,
- imputation methods, and
- weighting methods.

A **codebook** is a key documentation component. It is an index to an analysis file's structure and content, and includes a profile for each variable. There is no standard codebook format. Box 15.1 presents an example of basic information from a codebook for the first series of questions from a self-administered questionnaire completed by focus group participants (men who were current cigarette smokers). Depending on the analysis software and the information desired, additional parameters may be included.

Another useful documentation component is summary descriptive statistics for every variable in an analysis file. Box 15.2 presents an example for the variables included in the codebook output displayed in Box 15.1.

In addition, cross-reference variable lists arranged by question/variable number and variable name facilitate navigating from a data collection instrument to an analysis file, and vice versa. Box 15.3 presents examples of such cross-reference variable lists for the current smokers' focus groups questionnaire.

Another convenient cross-reference is to annotate the data collection instrument/questionnaire by adding variable labels (not for viewing by data collectors or participants) alongside the corresponding variables/questions. For instance, this component provides convenient access to the exact wording and structure for each question and response choice in a structured questionnaire.

Other components that may be included in analysis file documentation are descriptions of the

- research problem and question,
- conceptual framework,
- research design,
- sampling design,
- measurement strategies for key variables,
- reliability and validity assessments for key variables,
- data collection protocol and time schedule, and
- unanticipated problems and how they were addressed.

BOX 15.1: CODEBOOK EXAMPLE

File Information

Number of Cases	Unweighted	32
	Weighted	32

selfhs

		Value	Count	Percent
Standard Attributes	Label	Q.1: General health status		
Valid Values	1	Very poor	1	3.1%
	2	Poor	11	34.4%
	3	Good	19	59.4%
	4	Very good	1	3.1%

comphs

		Value	Count	Percent
Standard Attributes	Label	Q.2: Health compared to those my age		
Valid Values	1	Worse than average	7	21.9%
	2	About average	18	56.3%
	3	Better than average	6	18.8%
Missing Values	9	Missing	1	3.1%

avecig

		Value	Count	Percent
Standard Attributes	Label	Q.3: Avg #cigarettes per day		
N		Valid	31	
		Missing	1	
Central Tendency and Dispersion		Mean	14.13	
		Standard Deviation	9.366	
Labeled Values	999	Missing	1	3.1%

concern

		Value	Count	Percent
Standard Attributes	Label	Q.4: Concern about health effects of smoking		
Valid Values	1	Not concerned at all	3	9.4%
	2	Somewhat concerned	18	56.3%
	3	Very concerned	11	34.4%

Source: Produced using IBM SPSS Statistics version 22.

Information about such aspects is derived from a study's proposed research plan and maintaining a careful record of how issues encountered while conducting a study are addressed.

BOX 15.2: SUMMARY DESCRIPTIVE STATISTICS EXAMPLE

Descriptive Statistics

	N	Range	Minimum	Maximum	Mean		Std. Deviation	Variance
	Statistic	Statistic	Statistic	Statistic	Statistic	Std. Error	Statistic	Statistic
Q.1: General health status	32	3	1	4	2.63	.108	.609	.371
Q.2: Health compared to those my age	31	2	1	3	1.97	.118	.657	.432
Q.3: Avg #cigarettes per day	31	44	1	45	14.13	1.682	9.366	87.716
Q.4: Concern about health effects of smoking	32	2	1	3	2.25	.110	.622	.387
Valid N (listwise)	31							

Source: Produced using IBM SPSS Statistics version 22.

BOX 15.3: EXAMPLE OF VARIABLE CROSS-REFERENCE LISTS

By Question Number		By Variable Name	
Q.1	selfhs	avecig	Q.3
Q.2	comphs	comphs	Q.2
Q.3	avecig	concern	Q.4
Q.4	concern	selfhs	Q.1

CHECK YOUR UNDERSTANDING 15.1

- Describe the major stages in the data analysis process.
- Describe the purpose and process of "data cleaning."
- List some reasons for recoding an original variable.
- List three methods for addressing "missing values."
- Describe the key documentation components for an analysis file.

Overview of Quantitative Data Analysis

Description

As with other components of the research process, quantitative data analysis involves a progressive series of activities. Typically, the first step is to describe study participants' background characteristics, which is an important component of considering to whom a study's results may be generalized. In particular, when data are available for the target population's background characteristics, they may be compared with those of study participants to assess how well they represent the population. In a pretest–posttest design or a panel study (Chapter 6), change in participants' background characteristics is an indicator of the nature and extent of potential attrition bias.

Tables

It is most effective to present quantitative results using a visual format, such as a table, graph, or chart. Most often, participants' background characteristics are presented in tabular format, as illustrated in Table 15.2 for male participants in three separate focus groups. A table should have a clear title describing what variables are presented and to whom the data refer. A table's "body" is arranged in columns and rows that should be labeled clearly. There is no rule about what types of information should be arrayed down columns or across rows, which generally is determined by how the information may be presented most efficiently. In most situations, the best practice is to label variables using an abbreviated format. For example, instead of presenting the complete wording of each question, Table 15.2 uses labels that conveniently convey the type of data being reported. However, sometimes it is important to report a question's exact wording, especially for ones about attitudes, knowledge, and behavior. If the exact wording is too long to include in a table, abbreviated labels may be used, and the exact wording may be presented in accompanying text or an appendix.

TABLE 15.2 ● Background Characteristics: Male Focus Group Participants ($N = 32$)

Characteristic	Statistic
Age	mean: 57.5
	sd: 11.22
Marital status	
Married or living with a partner	73.4%
Not married or living with a partner	26.7%
Education (highest level)	
< High school	32.3%
High school graduate	22.6%
Some college	25.8%
College graduate	19.4%
Employed full-time	
Yes	41.4%
No	58.6%

Table 15.3 illustrates a more efficient format for presenting the information in Table 15.2. It presents only one value for each variable instead of a value for every category of every variable. The percentages in categories not displayed may be determined by subtracting the displayed value from 100%. However, that format may result in a loss of detail for some

variables. For example, the four original education categories in Table 15.2 were combined into a dichotomy (high school or less, and more than high school).

TABLE 15.3 Background Characteristics: Male Focus Group Participants ($N = 32$)	
Characteristic	Statistic
Age	mean: 57.5
	sd: 11.22
Married or living with a partner	73.4%
High school or less education	54.9%
Employed full-time	41.4%

Percentages

It is most effective to present data for variables measured at the nominal or ordinal levels in terms of percentages, which standardize frequencies on a scale from 0% to 100% and facilitate comparisons across groups or conditions with different numbers of cases. For example, Table 15.4 presents the frequency counts for each of the three focus groups across categories of their general health status. In contrast, Table 15.5 presents those results in terms of percentages. It is much easier to make comparisons across groups using percentages than to do so using frequency counts. Moreover, when desired, the number of cases in a category may be calculated by converting a percentage to a decimal and multiplying by the number of cases.

TABLE 15.4 General Health Status: Male Focus Group Participants				
Characteristic	Group A $N = 12$	Group B $N = 13$	Group C $N = 7$	Total $N = 32$
General health status				
Very poor	0	0	1	1
Poor	2	8	1	11
Good	9	5	5	19
Very good	1	0	0	1

TABLE 15.5 General Health Status: Male Focus Group Participants				
Characteristic	Group A $N = 12$	Group B $N = 13$	Group C $N = 7$	Total $N = 32$
General health status				
Very poor	0.0%	0.0%	14.3%	3.1%
Poor	16.7%	61.5%	14.3%	34.4%
Good	75.0%	38.5%	71.4%	59.4%
Very good	8.3%	0.0%	0.0%	3.1%

Central tendency

Measures of **central tendency** summarize the distribution of results for an individual variable in terms of *location*. There are three basic central tendency measures: mode, median, and mean.

Mode. The **mode** indicates the most frequently occurring observation or value. It is used most often with nominal- and ordinal-level measurements. In Table 15.2, the mode for education is "< High school," which is the answer received from 32.3% of the focus group participants. As illustrated in this example, the mode is not necessarily the majority response (i.e., > 50%).

Median. The **median** indicates the point in a distribution of interval-/ratio-level measurements where half the observations are located above and half are below. It is not necessarily the midpoint of the scale range. The median is especially useful when a distribution is highly *skewed*, such that most of the observations are located near one end of the range of possible values. The mean value, which is discussed in the next section, for a highly skewed (asymmetrical) distribution will not be representative of the "typical" values because it will be drawn toward the extreme values.

Mean. The **mean** ($\overline{X}$) is the arithmetic average for a set of interval-/ratio-level measurements. It is calculated as the sum of the observed values (X_i) divided by the number of observations (N), expressed by the formula $\overline{X} = \Sigma X_i / N$, where Σ is the summation symbol. The mean is the preferred central tendency measure in most analyses of interval-/ratio-level measurements because it incorporates every observation's value.

Dispersion

Measures of **dispersion** indicate how broadly observations are distributed across an ordinal- or interval-/ratio-level measurement scale.

Range. The **range** is the distance between the *observed* minimum and maximum values: maximum − minimum. It does not refer to a measurement scale's lowest and highest possible values. For example, if the minimum and maximum observed scores for a 10-point ordinal scale measuring perceived lung cancer risk are 3 and 9, respectively, the range is 9 − 3 = 6. It is not 10, or 10 − 1 = 9. In addition to reporting the size of the range, it is helpful also to report the observed minimum and maximum values.

Variance and standard deviation. With interval-/ratio-level measurements, the variance and standard deviation typically are preferred over the range, which takes into consideration the value of only two observations, the minimum and maximum. The variance and standard deviation are based on the average of distances, called *deviations*, between each observation and the mean ($X_i - \overline{X}$). The variance is calculated first, and the standard deviation is derived from it. The sum of deviations for values below the mean always equals the sum of deviations for values above the mean. Therefore, their sum always will equal zero. That problem is addressed by squaring the deviations ($X_i - \overline{X}$)^2 so they all are expressed as positive values. The **variance** (σ^2) is the arithmetic average (mean) of the squared deviations: $\sigma^2 = \Sigma(X_i - \overline{X})^2 / N$. The **standard deviation** (σ) is the square root of the variance: $\sigma = \sqrt{\sigma^2}$. When the variance and standard deviation are computed for data collected from a random sample, they are designated as s^2 and s, respectively. Technically, the denominator for the variance of a sample is $n - 1$, which is an adjustment to obtain an unbiased estimate of the population variance (for an illustrated explanation, see Kahn Academy, 2018). However, the $n - 1$ adjustment is negligible for large sample sizes. For instance, it will make little difference if a sum of squared deviations is divided by 400 or 399.

The variance is a key element in many statistical analysis techniques, such as regression, and analysis of variance (ANOVA). The standard deviation is used to convert observed values into standard scores (z scores) that designate points in the normal distribution (Chapter 7). It also is used to estimate the standard error for a population parameter estimate based on data from a random sample. For example, the standard error is used to calculate a confidence interval (Chapter 7).

Contingency

Chapter 3 introduced the concept of contingency to assess whether an observation in a particular category of one variable is contingent on, or associated with, the category in which that observation occurs for another variable. A contingency analysis is conducted by casting data in a contingency table (also called a "cross-classification table," a "cross-tabulation," or "crosstabs"), as displayed in Table 15.6 for focus group participants. Although the data were collected using an observational design, it is reasonable to posit that whether smokers attempted to quit during the past 12 months is contingent on whether they saw a doctor during that time period. For instance, a doctor might have advised them to quit and/or discussed the relationship between certain symptoms and smoking. Therefore, percentages in Table 15.6 were calculated *within* categories of having seen a doctor (independent variable) to compare them *across* categories of attempting to quit (dependent variable). As the table shows, smokers who saw a doctor during the past 12 months were more likely to have tried to quit (52.2%) during that period than those who did not see a doctor (22.2%).

TABLE 15.6 ● Tried to Quit in Past 12 Months by Saw a Doctor in Past 12 Months

Tried to Quit	Saw a Doctor	
	No ($N = 9$)	Yes ($N = 23$)
No	77.8%	47.8%
Yes	22.2%	52.2%

Correlation

Chapter 3 introduced the concept of correlation, which refers to how reliably the amount of change in one variable may be predicted when another variable changes by a certain amount. Pearson's product moment correlation coefficient (r), which also is referred to as **Pearson's r**, or simply r, assesses the linear correlation between two interval-/ratio-level measurements. It indicates the direction and strength of a correlation, ranging from -1.00 to $+1.00$, with ± 1.00 indicating perfect correlation and zero indicating no correlation. There is no standard interpretation for a correlation's strength. In general, a correlation is stronger the closer it is to ± 1.00. A practical method for assessing strength is to compare correlations across different pairs of variables, populations, or conditions.

The *squared correlation coefficient* (r^2) ranges from 0 to $+1.00$. If a causal order is assumed, r^2 may be interpreted as the proportion of the variance for one variable (B) accounted for or "explained" by change in another variable (A). However, because correlations are symmetrical, r^2 also may be interpreted as the proportion of the variance for variable A accounted for or "explained" by change in variable B. Thus, unless data are collected using an appropriate research design, such as a randomized controlled trial (Chapter 6), r^2 alone is not sufficient to indicate a causal relationship. Pearson's r and the analysis methods described in the following sections are readily available in virtually all data analysis software, and detailed descriptions are available in virtually every introductory statistics text. Therefore, details about their calculation are not presented here.

Spearman's rank-order coefficient, also called "Spearman's rho (ρ)," may be used for ordinal-level measurements, such as smokers' rating of their concern about the health effects of smoking cigarettes and their general health status rating. It also may be used to assess the correlation between one ordinal- and one interval-/ratio-level measurement, such as smokers' rating of their concern about the health effects of smoking cigarettes and number of quit attempts in the past 12 months. Like Pearson's r, values range from –1.00 to + 1.00, with zero indicating no correlation.

Regression

Regression analysis is a method for assessing how well values for a dependent variable may be predicted using information about one or more independent variables. *Bivariate regression* includes one independent variable; *multiple regression* includes two or more independent variables. Depending on the nature of the data and the research question, several regression models are available. The least-squares model and the logistic model are employed most often. An advantage of the logistic model is it may be employed when the dependent variable is a dichotomy, such as whether participants in a smoking cessation intervention did or did not stop smoking. Also, it typically is the preferred approach for an epidemiological analysis to identify the main risk factors that account for whether individuals do or do not experience an adverse health outcome.

When there are multiple independent variables or potential risk factors, instead of conducting several bivariate regressions, it is more efficient and effective to conduct a single multiple regression analysis. Moreover, multiple regression assesses the extent to which each independent variable or risk factor accounts for variation in the dependent variable while controlling for potential moderator variables.

Differences

There are two basic methods for assessing differences in outcomes measured as means, such as between groups in an experimental research design. The *t* test assesses differences in the means for two groups, such as treatment and control. Analysis of variance (ANOVA) assesses differences in means across three or more groups, such as no treatment, a standard treatment, and an experimental treatment. Both tests are calculated differently depending on whether the groups are *independent* or *related* samples. For a pretest–posttest control group design (Chapter 6), the independent samples approach would be appropriate to test for posttest differences across groups. The related samples, also called repeated measures, approach should be used to test pretest–posttest differences within groups because those differences will be dependent on the same group's pretest status.

Hypothesis Testing

Hypotheses

A **hypothesis** posits whether it is likely there is or is not a relationship between certain variables or a difference across groups and/or time. It may be based on a study's conceptual approach, goal, and/or prior research results. A **research hypothesis (H_1)** posits there *is* a relationship or difference. For example, prior to constructing Table 15.6, it might have been hypothesized that the proportion (percent) of smokers who tried to quit during the past 12 months would be larger among those who saw a doctor than among those who did not see a doctor during that period. A null hypothesis (H_0) posits there is *no* relationship or difference. It comprises all results that do not comport with the research hypothesis. In this example, the research hypothesis is *directional*, indicating which group of smokers will be most likely to have tried to quit. Therefore, the null hypothesis includes both: (1) There is *no difference* in the proportion of smokers who tried to quit, whether they did or did not see a doctor, and (2) the proportion of smokers who tried to quit is larger among those who did *not* see a doctor than among those who did see a doctor. If the research hypothesis were *nondirectional*, it would posit that there is a difference between the two groups such that *either* group of smokers might be more likely to quit than the other group. Then the null hypothesis would be that there is *no difference* in the proportion of smokers who tried to quit, whether they did or did not see a doctor.

A research hypothesis should be specified *prior* to collecting data. Basing it on potential relationships or differences detected during data processing and analysis will bias the result in favor of supporting it. Also, that approach may lead to not testing hypotheses that appear unlikely to be supported by the data. If an unanticipated relationship or difference is identified, it is best to report such serendipitous results as exploratory, describe how they were discovered, and recommend they be replicated in subsequent independent investigations.

Most often, a study's conceptual approach and/or goal denotes a directional hypothesis. For instance, there is no point in conducting a randomized controlled trial if it is expected an experimental treatment condition will not yield an outcome more favorable than that for a control condition. However, an exploratory study might posit a nondirectional research hypothesis, such as that the prevalence of having gotten a mammogram during the past 12 months is different among African Americans and Asian Americans, without specifying among which group prevalence is higher. The corresponding null hypothesis would be that there is no difference in the proportions of African American and Asian American women who have gotten a mammogram during the past 12 months.

Process

In virtually all research, the true status of a population is not known; otherwise, there would be no need to collect data from a sample. Unfortunately, random samples might display relationships or differences by chance even when there are no such relationships or differences in a population (Chapter 7). In other words, a research hypothesis might *appear* to be true when in fact the corresponding null hypothesis (H_0) is true. A **hypothesis test** assesses the probability of observing a particular result by chance *if the null hypothesis is true*. If an observed relationship is so strong, or a difference is so large, that the probability of observing that result by chance is low, then the null hypothesis should be rejected. Consequently, the research hypothesis should be accepted and deemed *statistically significant*. Conversely, if the probability of observing a particular result by chance is high, then the null hypothesis should be accepted, and the research hypothesis should be rejected and deemed *not* statistically significant.

Key Concept

A hypothesis test assesses the probability of observing a particular result by chance if the null hypothesis is true.

The outcome of a hypothesis test, called the ***p* value**, is the probability of obtaining an observed result by chance under the assumption the null hypothesis is true. The way a *p* value is determined depends on which statistical test is employed. In the past, *p* values were determined by referencing tables in the appendices of statistical textbooks. However, now *p* values are calculated by statistical analysis software. By convention, most often the **critical value** for designating **statistical significance**, called **alpha** (α), is set at .05, whereby the probability that an observed result may be attributed to chance is .05 (5%) or less.

Hypothesis tests do not test a research hypothesis directly. Instead, they assess whether a corresponding null hypothesis should be accepted or rejected. Then an inference is made regarding whether to accept or reject the research hypothesis, which sometimes is called the alternative hypothesis (H_A). Moreover, the hypothesis testing process is structured in favor of accepting the null hypothesis, whereby the alpha criterion is specified such that rejecting the null hypothesis requires a result that is quite unlikely (e.g., ≤ .05) to be attributable to chance. Deciding to accept or reject the null hypothesis by comparing the *p* value and alpha assigns the opposite disposition to the research hypothesis. Table 15.7 depicts decisions for the null and research hypotheses when α = .05.

TABLE 15.7 ● **Hypothesis Testing Decisions: α = .05**

Hypothesis	*p* > .05	*p* ≤ .05	Direction of Decision
Null (H_0)	Accept	Reject	↓
Research (H_1)	Reject (not statistically significant)	Accept (statistically significant)	

Different statistical methods are employed to test hypotheses depending on factors such as the research question, research design, sampling design, and level of measurement. For Table 15.6, which presents data in nominal categories, it would be appropriate to apply the chi-square test (χ^2) for independence. Without going into detail, it assesses the difference between the *observed* distribution of cases and their *expected* distribution if they were distributed randomly, that is, by chance. Panel A of Table 15.8 reproduces the observed distribution from Table 15.6; panel B presents the expected chance distribution. The test result is: $\chi^2 = 2.36$ (*df* = 1) and *p* = .1246, where *df* is the degrees of freedom. It is not statistically significant because the *p* value is greater than α (.05), indicating the result is likely to have occurred by chance. Thus, the null hypothesis is accepted, and the research hypothesis is rejected.

This result might be surprising considering the size of the observed difference (panel A) between smokers who tried to quit depending on whether they saw a doctor. The explanation is the number of observations

> **Key Concept**
>
> *Different statistical methods are employed to test hypotheses depending on factors such as the research question, research design, sampling design, and level of measurement.*

TABLE 15.8 ● **Tried to Quit in Past 12 Months by Saw a Doctor in Past 12 Months**

	A. Observed		B. Expected	
	Saw a Doctor		Saw a Doctor	
Tried to Quit	No (*N* = 9)	Yes (*N* = 23)	No (*N* = 9)	Yes (*N* = 23)
No (*N* = 18)	77.8% (*N* = 7)	47.8% (*N* = 11)	55.6% (*N* = 5)	56.5% (*N* = 13)
Yes (*N* = 14)	22.2% (*N* = 2)	52.2% (*N* = 12)	44.2% (*N* = 4)	43.5% (*N* = 10)

is small ($N = 32$) and distributions of small numbers are not stable. As stated in Chapter 7, the larger the number of cases, the greater is the statistical power, which is the probability of rejecting the null hypothesis when it is not true. Statistical power for this analysis is low. That is demonstrated by a simulation in which each case is multiplied by 10, artificially increasing the total to 320 cases. The observed and expected percentage distributions would remain exactly the same as in Table 15.8. However, the chi-square value would increase by a factor of 10, from 2.36 to 23.6, for which the p value would be $< .00001$. The probability of obtaining the observed distribution by chance then would be much smaller than the $\alpha \leq .05$ criterion. Therefore, the chi-square test would be statistically significant, and the null hypothesis would be rejected. That result reflects the principle that the more observations on which a particular result is based, the more likely it is reliable.

Decision errors

A hypothesis test does not prove whether a hypothesis is true or not true. It is not possible to know if an inferential decision is correct because that requires knowing the true status of the population under study. Table 15.9 depicts the relationship between inferential decisions and two types of potential error. A **type I error**, also called an **alpha error** (α), is committed when a null hypothesis is true but is rejected. Consequently, the corresponding research hypothesis incorrectly is accepted and deemed statistically significant. A **type II error**, also called a **beta error** (β), is committed when a null hypothesis is not true but is accepted. Consequently, the research hypothesis incorrectly is rejected and deemed not statistically significant.

TABLE 15.9 • Inference Decisions and Potential Errors

Decision	H_0 True	H_0 Not True
Reject H_0 (Accept H_1)	Type I Error (α)	Correct Decision
Accept H_0 (Reject H_1)	Correct Decision	Type II Error (β)

Committing a type I error might lead to implementing an ineffective or even potentially harmful treatment or policy in practice, and discouraging further research to develop a truly effective treatment or policy. The maximum probability of committing a type I error is alpha. Thus, setting alpha at .05 means an analyst is willing to accept as much as a 5% chance of incorrectly rejecting the null hypothesis. The type I error risk may be reduced by setting alpha lower, such as at .01 or .001. Whenever a p value is smaller than alpha, the null hypothesis should be rejected. However, the actual probability of committing a type I error is the p value, not alpha. For example, if $\alpha \leq .05$ and the p value for a hypothesis test is .024, the type I error probability is .024.

Committing a type II error might lead to not investigating a relationship or difference further, which may result in missing an opportunity to develop and implement a potentially effective treatment or policy. That is a concern particularly when conducting a pilot study with a small sample, which provides low statistical power. The type II error risk may be reduced by setting alpha higher, such as .10 instead of .05, to make it more likely to reject the null hypothesis if it is not true and correctly accept the research hypothesis. Whenever possible, the best strategy to reduce the type II error risk is to select a large sample to increase statistical power to reject a null hypothesis when it is not true.

There is a trade-off in setting alpha lower or higher. A lower alpha reduces type I error risk but increases type II error risk. Conversely, a higher alpha reduces type II error risk but increases type I error risk. Typically, this issue should be addressed by considering a study's purpose and context in terms of whether the "cost" of committing one type of error is substantially greater than that for the other type.

Validity and Substantive Significance

If a hypothesis test rejects the null hypothesis and concludes a result is statistically significant, that does not necessarily mean the result is valid. As discussed throughout the preceding chapters, research validity is based on a holistic assessment of all aspects of a study: research design, sample, measurement, data collection, and analysis. Moreover, a statistically significant result is not necessarily *substantively significant*, such that it should or can be incorporated into practice. Moreover, as illustrated in the discussion about Table 15.8, with a sufficiently large sample, even a small difference or weak relationship may be statistically significant. There are no standard tests or formats for assessing **substantive significance**. It is based on weighing the potential benefits of implementing a treatment or policy against its feasibility and potential costs, including factors such as materials, equipment, space, administration, staffing, training, and risks to and receptivity by clients/patients. Although the published research literature focuses heavily on statistical significance, substantive significance determines whether a result is incorporated into practice.

> **Key Concept**
>
> A statistically significant result is not necessarily substantively significant.

CHECK YOUR UNDERSTANDING 15.2

- In your own words, describe the hypothesis testing process. Be sure to include each of the following aspects:
    - Research hypothesis
    - Null hypothesis
    - Alpha
    - *p* value
    - Types of decision errors
    - Strategies for minimizing each type of decision error

Overview of Qualitative Data Analysis

As described in Chapter 13, qualitative data may include a variety of formats. However, most qualitative analysis is performed with text in participants' own words that most often is obtained from interviews. Therefore, this overview focuses on analyzing textual data. Qualitative data do not lend themselves to hypothesis testing methods as do quantitative data. Moreover, by design, the qualitative analysis process primarily is inductive, rather than deductive (Chapter 1). It involves discerning major themes, categories, patterns, and relationships. The goal of qualitative data analysis is to gain a holistic and context-specific

> **Key Concept**
>
> Qualitative data do not lend themselves to hypothesis testing.

understanding of participants' experiences and interpretations of them within their real-life context. Social scientists call this an *emic* approach, as opposed to an *etic* approach, which characterizes most quantitative analysis, in which an external perspective guides classifying and interpreting differences and relationships. Indeed, analysis is integral to the iterative qualitative data collection process, whereby information continually is assessed to identify topics to explore in greater depth, emergent topics to explore further, and topics not worth pursuing further (Chapter 13).

Data Preparation

After qualitative data are collected, they must be prepared for analysis. If data are not already in a textual format, such as audio or video recording, they must be transcribed. All transcriptions should be *verbatim* to capture participants' exact words and sentence structure; they should not be a paraphrase or summary. Transcription may be done as recordings become available. Accurately transcribing hours of recordings is an arduous task that typically takes several times longer than the recordings. When feasible, it is best for transcription to be done independently by a professional transcriber. When appropriate, additional allowance must be made to translate records from other languages (Chapter 9). Lines of text should be numbered. Participants' confidentiality should be protected by referring to them only by a study-specific code number or pseudonym (e.g., see Box 13.4). In addition to spoken words, a transcript should include notations of other information, such as laughter, crying, shouting, lengthy pauses, body language, facial expressions, and contextual aspects such as interruption by an unexpected loud noise. Also, a transcript should include notations about any words or statements that are unintelligible. When an initial transcript draft is prepared, it should be reviewed independently for accuracy and completeness by comparing it directly to the source. Then a final draft that includes revisions should be prepared. Multiple copies of each data record and transcription should be stored separately and securely.

Coding

Codes must be assigned to each significant thread of text. In addition to reviewing transcripts, consulting field notes often is helpful in developing and assigning codes to qualitative data. Coding should be done by at least two independent coders, whose performance is assessed using interrater reliability methods described in Chapter 8. Although codes may be entered by hand in the margins of a transcript hard copy, it is most effective and efficient to use a qualitative research software package (e.g., ATLAS.ti or NVivo) that also facilitates searching and compiling coded text segments to catalog major themes. Qualitative data codes may be letters, words, or phrases instead of or in addition to numerical ones. Moreover, more than one code may be assigned to a text segment. Qualitative coding schemes are specific to a study's participants, context, and purpose. For example, consider the focus group excerpts from Box 13.4 that are reproduced in Box 15.4. The following ideas may be extracted from the participants' comments:

- Others say smoking is bad for health.
- A healthy constitution protects against health effects from smoking.

- Participants are not worried about smoking.
- Whether smoking is bad for health depends on physical condition/constitution.
- Whether smoking is bad for health depends on environment.
- Others say to quit.
- Nonsmokers die of lung cancer.
- The media says smoking is bad for health.
- Participants don't know a smoker who died from smoking.
- Smokers die from causes other than smoking.
- Smoking is not related to health.

> ### BOX 15.4: FOCUS GROUP EXCERPTS: PERCEPTIONS ABOUT SMOKING-RELATED SYMPTOMS AMONG MALE KOREAN AMERICAN CIGARETTE SMOKERS
>
> M: Some people say that some symptoms might be caused by smoking. What do you think about that?
>
> A2: Generally, many say smoking is bad. I have such a healthy constitution that I don't have to worry about it. It depends on an individual's physical condition.
>
> A7: As A2 said, it depends not only on an individual's physical constitution, but also on one's environment. If you sleep in a room with dry or dusty air, even a healthy person will cough as you get up in the morning. In my opinion, this is not related with smoking problem.
>
> A5: People close to me say smoking is bad for my health.
>
> A7: Generally smoking is known to be bad for health, so they say, "quit, quit."
>
> A3: I don't have anybody telling me, "You seem to have this or that symptom because of smoking." One of my close friends died of lung cancer five years ago. He never smoked in his entire life, but he suddenly died of lung cancer.
>
> A5: TV and newspapers constantly say smoking is bad, but I've never heard of anybody who died of smoking. I heard a lot of death from drinking. I discuss with other people about this a lot. I don't know if it is because I am very healthy even if I am smoking.
>
> A2: Two of my friends who hadn't smoked are already dead. Rather than having problems, those friends who smoke are alive and well. Certainly, as I told you before, you cannot relate health with smoking.
>
> M = moderator; A = participants

Themes and Conclusions

Codes must be synthesized into major themes that characterize the main issues expressed in qualitative data. For example, after analyzing transcripts from focus groups with Korean American males who were current smokers, Kviz et al. (2003) identified three major themes:

- Smoking is not related to health.

  Example 1: "Two of my friends who hadn't smoked are already dead. Rather than having problems, those friends who smoke are alive and well. Certainly, as I told you before, you cannot relate health with smoking."

  Example 2: "Friends who like to drink and smoke are all healthy. They look healthy. People who don't smoke or drink make me think that they don't do so because they have some health problems. Indeed, there are my friends who cannot smoke because of health problems. Many people have problems like feeling chest pain among those who do not smoke."

- Symptoms may be attributed to causes other than smoking.

  Example 3: "[I]t depends not only on an individual's physical constitution, but also on one's environment. If you sleep in a room with dry or dusty air, even a healthy person will cough as you get up in the morning. In my opinion, this is not related with smoking problem."

  Example 4: "People with high blood pressure would have these problems such as short breath, chest pain. So smoking has nothing to do with these symptoms."

- A person's physical constitution affects smoking and health.

  Example 5: "Generally, many say smoking is bad. I have such a healthy constitution that I don't have to worry about it. It depends on an individual's physical condition."

It is helpful to create a **conceptual map** of key relationships qualitative data reveal. For example, Figure 15.2 facilitates concluding the focus group smokers

- attributed symptoms to conditions other than smoking cigarettes,
- perceived a person's physical constitution is related to experiencing symptoms,

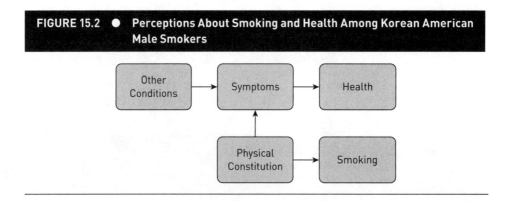

FIGURE 15.2 • Perceptions About Smoking and Health Among Korean American Male Smokers

- perceived a person's physical constitution is related to smoking, and
- believed smoking is not related to health.

Based on these conclusions, it was recommended that for Korean American men who smoke cigarettes, interventions should be developed that address their perceptions about the meaning of health, the relationship between smoking and health, and a physical constitution that protects against smoking's health effects.

Trustworthiness

Qualitative analysis is largely subjective, which makes it potentially more vulnerable than quantitative analysis to influences that may bias results. Qualitative data cannot be analyzed using mathematical methods as can quantitative data. Therefore, results often are assessed in terms of their *trustworthiness*, which comprises four components (Guba, 1981; Lincoln & Guba, 1985). Detailed descriptions of strategies for assessing each component are presented in Guba (1981) and Shenton (2004).

Credibility

Credibility is the degree of confidence that may be attributed to a qualitative result as being "true." It is approximately parallel to internal validity in a quantitative analysis. Frequently used strategies to assess credibility are triangulation with other data sources and member checks, whereby target population members independently review results and conclusions.

Transferability

Transferability is the degree to which a qualitative result may be generalized to other contexts, such as similar situations, populations, and phenomena. It is approximately parallel to external validity in a quantitative analysis. Advocating the transferability of qualitative results is challenging because of the iterative, responsive, and context-specific approach to collecting and analyzing qualitative data. It is assessed by reviewing data collection and analysis procedures, and appraising the extent to which a result might apply to other contexts.

Dependability

Dependability is the extent to which a qualitative result is consistent and repeatable. As with transferability, advocating the dependability of qualitative results is challenging because of the naturalistic qualitative research approach to collecting and analyzing data. It is assessed by independent peer review of data collection and analysis procedures and replication by other researchers.

Confirmability

Confirmability is the degree to which a qualitative result is shaped by participants and conditions, rather than a researcher's expectations and perspective. One strategy for assessing confirmability is an independent audit of data collection and analysis procedures. Another strategy is researcher reflexivity, which is self-awareness throughout conducting a qualitative study of one's motivations, expectations, and perceptions that may influence a result. Accordingly, researchers strive to maintain neutrality and assess the extent to which their predisposition may have influenced a result.

CHECK YOUR UNDERSTANDING 15.3

- Describe how the qualitative data analysis process is *similar* to the quantitative data analysis process.
- Describe how the qualitative data analysis process is *different* from the quantitative data analysis process.
- Describe the following four components of the trustworthiness of a qualitative result and identify at least one strategy for assessing each component.
    - Credibility
    - Transferability
    - Dependability
    - Confirmability

Reporting Research Results

The final activity in the research process is reporting how a completed study contributes to the body of scientific knowledge about the research problem. A report should describe a study's purpose, context, research design, methods and procedures, results, and conclusions. There are several formats for presenting a report that vary depending on the audience and venue. These include

- an article published in a professional journal,
- a book or book chapter,
- a written final report to a funding agency,
- a written report and/or oral presentation to a client,
- an oral presentation at a professional association meeting/conference,
- a written report and/or oral presentation for a class,
- a master's degree thesis or doctoral degree dissertation,
- an oral presentation in defense of a master's thesis or doctoral dissertation,
- an oral presentation as part of an employment interview, and
- a written report and/or oral presentation to a collaborating agency, such as a community-based organization or health clinic.

In some situations, a specified format must be followed rigorously (e.g., a journal manuscript or a doctoral degree dissertation) while in others the format may be flexible (e.g., a report to a client or collaborating agency). Manuscript preparation specifications vary somewhat across journals. Therefore, it is essential to review carefully the instructions to authors, which typically may be accessed at a journal's website. Also, the format for a master's thesis or doctoral dissertation may vary by institution. The following sections assume a format that generally is required for a professional journal article, which is familiar to most audiences and may be adapted to other types of reports/presentations.

The general report format follows a logical organization with the following sections that are identified by major headings and may include subheadings to facilitate accessing specific information:

- Abstract
- Introduction
- Background/Literature Review
- Method(s)
- Results/Findings
- Discussion
- References
- Appendix

Abstract

An **abstract** is a brief overview and summary of a report. Professional journals specify various word limits for an abstract, generally ranging from about 150 to 250 words. The format may be unstructured or structured, but in either case, it should describe a study's purpose, method, results, and conclusion. A structured abstract, which often is required by a professional journal, includes subheadings to aid readers to access information quickly. Box 15.5 presents an example of a structured abstract presented by Buller et al. (2018). Guidelines for preparing and submitting a manuscript, including an abstract, to the *American Journal of Health Promotion* in which the article was published may be accessed at https://mc.manuscriptcentral.com/societyimages/ajhp/2017_InstructionstoAuthors_AJHP.pdf.

BOX 15.5: EXAMPLE OF AN ABSTRACT

Abstract

Purpose: To evaluate an intervention promoting adoption of occupational sun protection policies by employers in a randomized trial.

Design: A randomized pretest–posttest controlled design with 2-year follow-up was conducted in 2010 to 2013.

Setting: Local government organizations in Colorado who had outdoor workers in public works, public safety, and/or parks and recreation.

Participants: Ninety-eight local government organizations ($n = 51$ municipalities, 10 counties, and 37 special districts).

Intervention: Organizations were randomly assigned to receive a policy and education intervention comprised of personal contacts and theory-based training and materials or to an attention control group.

(Continued)

> (Continued)
>
> **Measures:** Occupational policy documents were coded for sun safety content by a trained research assistant blind to condition.
>
> **Analysis:** Policy scores were analyzed with logistic and Poisson regression models using imputation.
>
> **Results:** At posttest, more organizations in the intervention group had a sun protection policy than in the control group (odds ratio [OR] = 4.91, $P < .05$; intent to treat: OR = 5.95, $P < .05$) and policies were more extensive ($\chi^2 = 31.29$, $P < .01$; intent to treat: $\chi^2 = 73.79$, $P < .01$) and stronger ($\chi^2 = 24.50$, $P < .01$; intent to treat: $\chi^2 = 51.95$, $P < .01$). Policy adoption was higher when the number of contacts and trainings increased ($P < .05$).
>
> **Conclusion:** The intervention had a large effect on adoption of formal sun protection policies, perhaps because of its fit with legal requirements to maintain safe workplaces. Personal contacts with managers were influential on adoption of occupational policy even in this age of communication technology and social media.
>
> *Source:* Buller et al. (2018). Reproduced with permission from Sage Publications.

A lengthy report, such as one issued by a governmental agency, often includes an **executive summary** instead of an abstract. The purpose of an executive summary is similar to an abstract. However, it typically is longer, such as three to six or more pages. It may include elements that are not normally included in an abstract, such as tables, charts, graphs, and reference citations. Examples are the executive summaries for the *Healthy People 2020 Leading Health Indicators: Progress Update*, available at www.healthypeople.gov/sites/default/files/LHI-ProgressReport-ExecSum_0.pdf (accessed July 25, 2018), and the U.S. Surgeon General's report on *E-Cigarette Use Among Youth and Young Adults*, available at https://e-cigarettes.surgeongeneral.gov/documents/2016_SGR_Exec_Summ_508.pdf (accessed November 13, 2018).

Introduction

The introduction presents a study's objectives. Sometimes the heading is not required; other times it may be titled differently, such as *Purpose* or *Objective*. It should include a statement of the research problem, justification for its importance, and the study's potential to advance scientific understanding of the problem. Also, it should specify the research question(s) investigated and/or hypothesis(es) tested. It also may describe the study's scope by identifying the key variables, target population, setting, research design, and analytic approach.

Background/Literature Review

The purpose of a background or literature review section is to describe a study's context in terms of the current state of knowledge, policy, and practice regarding the research problem. Sometimes that information may be included in the introduction instead of a separate section. The presentation should address only the most relevant background information rather than a comprehensive review. It should present an up-to-date and balanced overview of issues, points of agreement and disagreement, limitations, and gaps in the literature to establish the need for the study and its potential contribution. All sources used to develop this section must be appropriately cited in the body of the text and in a "References" or "Bibliography" section.

Methods

The methods section describes how a study was conducted. A variety of subsections may be included, but the main ones generally are as follows:

- Research design
- Subjects/participants
- Measurements/instrumentation
- Data collection
- Analysis

Sometimes, especially for a large and complex study, a previously published report may be referenced that presents details of a methodological aspect, such as the sampling design or instrument development. Nevertheless, all aspects of a study should be described sufficiently in the present report so a reader may know the essential aspects about how a study was conducted and be able to assess the validity of its results without accessing one or more other reports.

Research design

In addition to describing the research design, the rationale for choosing it should be presented. When appropriate, a design diagram should be included (Chapter 6). If the design involves an experimental intervention, a report should describe how it was developed, the nature and theory of the intervention, and how exposure to it was controlled. Sometimes that information may be presented under a *Procedures* subheading. Virtually all professional journals require that reports of randomized controlled trials conform to CONSORT (2010) reporting guidelines (CONSORT stands for *Consolidated Standards of Reporting Trials*). It is good practice to follow those guidelines even when not required.

Subjects/participants

The description of the subjects/participants (only one heading is used depending on requirements or preference) typically includes the following aspects, which may be presented under separate subheadings:

- Target population—including why it was chosen
- Sampling design, sampling frame, and selection method
- Sample size and how it was determined
- Inclusion/exclusion criteria—including rationale and how subjects were screened
- Recruitment—including how subjects were approached, informed consent, and whether any incentives were provided
- Assignment to study groups/conditions, when relevant
- CONSORT flow diagram, when relevant (www.consort-statement.org)

Measurements/instrumentation

The description of the measurements/instrumentation (only one heading is used depending on requirements or preference) typically includes the following aspects, which may be presented under separate subheadings:

- Key variables—including the conceptual constructs and operational definitions
- Sources of preexisting instruments—including how and why they were modified, when relevant
- Procedures and rationale for developing new instruments
- Evidence supporting reliability and validity—both from previous studies, when relevant, and for the current study
- Procedure for coding/scoring an instrument's results

Data collection

The description of data collection methods typically includes the following aspects:

- Data collection mode, rationale, and protocol
- Setting and location
- Times data collection started and ended
- Who collected the data—including training and supervision
- Number of participants—including cooperation/response rate and how it was calculated

Analysis

The final methods subsection is a description of the analysis procedure(s). This section should include the rationale for choosing the procedure(s), any special codes that were developed, and the statistical analysis software that was used. Also, as appropriate, it should describe the rationale and procedures for missing data imputation, subgroup breakdowns, comparisons across time or conditions, and comparisons with benchmark data such as national health statistics.

Results/Findings

This section reports what the analysis revealed. Typically, it starts with a profile of the participants' background characteristics. How well participants represent the target population should be assessed by taking into account factors such as the sampling frame, inclusion/exclusion criteria, availability, and cooperation. Also, as is feasible, participants' background characteristics should be compared with those for the target population and nonparticipants to assess potential noncoverage and nonparticipation bias, respectively. Sometimes that information may be presented in the subjects/participants subsection of methods instead of the results section.

It is essential to focus on addressing the research question and avoid issues of secondary relevance. Results should be presented objectively, stating *what was found* in the analysis. This section should not interpret results or assess their validity. Both results that are and results that are not statistically significant should be reported. A result that is not statistically significant is important, especially when it means rejecting the research hypothesis on which a study focused. For instance, it is equally important to find an experimental intervention is not effective as it is to find it is effective. Reports of qualitative findings are presented primarily in a narrative format that includes participants' quotes rather than statistical analyses. However, some qualitative findings may be presented in a numeric format, such as the number of times participants mentioned a certain theme (Goldberg & Allen, 2015; Sutton & Austin, 2015).

Discussion

The discussion section presents a study's results in context. It addresses what a study's results contribute to the body of scientific knowledge about the research question in particular, and more broadly, the research problem. It typically addresses the following aspects:

- An interpretation of what the results mean or what was learned about the research question and problem
- An assessment of the plausibility of alternative interpretations
- An assessment of implications for internal and external validity of limitations and potential sources of bias
- A comparison of findings to previous research in terms of points of agreement/ disagreement and gaps
- A conclusion about what the results contribute to understanding the research question and research problem
- Recommendations for next steps for further research, theory development, and practice applications, as appropriate

Sometimes conclusions and/or recommendations may be presented as subsections of the discussion or in a final section with a heading such as *Summary and Conclusions*, *Conclusions*, *Recommendations*, or *Lessons Learned*. Conclusions and recommendations should be specific. They should not be general statements such as "This study contributes to our understanding of how people think about health" or "This study indicates the need for further research about how people think about health."

References

The references section lists literature (articles, books, agency documents, websites, etc.) cited in a report. It should not include literature that is related to the research problem but did not guide planning, conducting, or reporting about the study. Also, except for a report with an educational objective, the references section should not include recommended reading.

Appendix

An appendix may be included to present supplemental information that enhances a report, such as the following:

- Exact wording for key questions, or an entire questionnaire
- Detailed tabular information
- Graphic materials such as photographs, maps, diagrams, or charts
- Detailed coding procedures
- Technical information such as formulae and/or calculations

An appendix should not include information that is essential for a reader to adequately understand and assess a report's main components. To save publication space, readers may be provided online-only access to appendix material.

Other Components

Acknowledgements

Individuals and agencies should be acknowledged who provide support for conducting a study and/or preparing the report. Examples include providing the following:

- Clerical or technical support
- Facilities, equipment, or material
- Language translation services
- Assistance with recruiting participants
- Data collection assistance
- Comments on report drafts
- Copyediting services
- Consultant services

Funding support

Sources of funding support to plan and conduct a study should be cited. Funding agencies may specify exact wording for citing the source and award number. The amount of funding support is not stated. If a study did not receive any external funding support, some journals require a statement to that effect.

Human subjects protection

In addition to describing procedures for protecting human subjects in the methods section, most professional journals require an explicit statement that a study involving human subjects was approved by an institutional review board (IRB). Sometimes the protocol approval number and date are required as well. If not required, including such information is recommended.

Conflict of interest disclosure

Most professional journals require a statement about any real or potential conflicts of interest on the part of any report authors. If there are no conflicts, then a statement to that effect should be included. Guidance for identifying and reporting conflicts of interest are available from the International Committee of Medical Journal Editors (ICMJE) at www.icmje.org/recommendations/browse/roles-and-responsibilities/author-responsibilities--conflicts-of-interest.html#two (accessed July 25, 2018).

Authorship

Most professional journals require all authors to sign a declaration that they meet the criteria specified by the ICMJE (www.icmje.org/recommendations/browse/roles-and-responsibilities/defining-the-role-of-authors-and-contributors.html, accessed July 25, 2018):

- Substantial contributions to the conception or design of the work; or the acquisition, analysis, or interpretation of data for the work; AND

- Drafting the work or revising it critically for important intellectual content; AND

- Final approval of the version to be published; AND

- Agreement to be accountable for all aspects of the work in ensuring that questions related to the accuracy or integrity of any part of the work are appropriately investigated and resolved.

Moreover, a journal may require the specific contribution(s) of each author to the study and report to be described either in a cover letter to the editor or in an authorship form. When not required, subscribing to the ICMJE criteria is recommended in general. The ICMJE specifies meeting all four authorship criteria. Accordingly, examples of individuals who might not qualify as an author but instead might be cited in an acknowledgement are the following:

- Department head
- Thesis or dissertation advisor or committee member
- Community-based organization director or staff member
- Clerical or technical assistant
- Language translator
- Interviewer or focus group moderator
- Consultant
- Draft reviewer

CHECK YOUR UNDERSTANDING 15.4

- Identify the major sections of a research report.
- Briefly describe the purpose and general content for each major report section.

Key Points

The Data Analysis Process

Data analysis is a process comprising a logical sequence as follows:

- Data preparation
- Analysis file preparation
- Modification and finalization
- Analysis

Overview of Quantitative Data Analysis

It is most effective to present quantitative results using a visual format, such as a table, graph, or chart.

It is most effective to present nominal- or ordinal-level data as percentages, which standardize frequencies on a scale from 0% to 100% and facilitate comparisons.

Measures of central tendency summarize a variable's distribution variable in terms of location.

- The mode indicates the most frequently occurring observation or value.
- The median indicates the point in a distribution of interval-/ratio-level measurements where half the observations are located above and half are below.
- The mean is the arithmetic average for a set of interval-/ratio-level measurements.

Measures of dispersion indicate how broadly observations are distributed across an ordinal- or interval-/ratio-level measurement scale.

- The range is the distance between the observed minimum and maximum values.
- The variance is the arithmetic average of the squared deviations from the mean.
- The standard deviation is the square root of the variance.

Contingency assesses whether an observation in a category of one variable is contingent on the category in which that observation occurs for another variable.

Correlation indicates the direction and strength (−1.00 to +1.00) of a relationship between ordinal- and/or interval-/ratio-level measurements.

Regression analysis assesses how well values for a dependent variable may be predicted using information about one or more independent variables.

Differences: The *t* test assesses differences in means for two groups; analysis of variance (ANOVA) assesses differences in means across three or more groups.

Hypothesis testing: A hypothesis test assesses the probability of observing a particular result by chance if the null hypothesis is true.

- A **research hypothesis** posits there is a relationship or difference.
- A **null hypothesis** posits there is no relationship or difference.

- If the null hypothesis is rejected, the research hypothesis is accepted (statistically significant), and vice versa.
- **Type I error:** A null hypothesis is true but is rejected.
- **Type II error:** A null hypothesis is not true but is accepted.
- A statistically significant result is not necessarily substantively significant regarding incorporating it into practice.

Overview of Qualitative Data Analysis

- Most qualitative analysis is performed with text in participants' own words.
- The qualitative analysis process primarily is inductive.
- Qualitative data must be transcribed verbatim.
- Codes are assigned to each significant thread of text.
- It is most effective and efficient to use a qualitative research software package.
- Codes are synthesized into major themes.
- It helps to create a conceptual map of key relationships qualitative data reveal.
- Qualitative results may be assessed in terms of trustworthiness.
  - **Credibility:** the degree of confidence that a result is "true"
  - **Transferability:** the degree to which a result may be generalized
  - **Dependability:** the extent to which a result is consistent
  - **Confirmability:** the degree to which a result is shaped by participants and conditions, rather than a researcher's expectations and perspective

Reporting Research Results

In general, a report should include the following major components:

- The **abstract** presents a brief overview and summary.
- The **introduction** presents a study's objectives.
- The **background/literature review** section describes a study's context in terms of the current state of knowledge, policy, and practice regarding the research problem.
- The **methods** section describes how a study was conducted in terms of
  - research design,
  - subjects/participants,
  - measurements/instrumentation,
  - data collection, and
  - analysis.
- The **results/findings** section describes what the analysis revealed.
- The **discussion** section addresses what the results contribute to scientific knowledge about the research question and problem.

- The **references** section lists literature cited.
- The **appendix** presents supplemental information.
- **Other Components**
    - Acknowledgements
    - Funding support
    - Human subjects protection
    - Conflict of interest disclosure
- **Authorship:** Subscribing to the four criteria recommended by the International Committee of Medical Journal Editors (ICMJE) is required by most professional journals and is recommended in general.

Review and Apply

1. Review the research plan you developed in the "Review and Apply" sections of the previous chapters.
    - Draft an outline of what you would include as documentation for your project.
    - Draft an outline for preparing a report about your project. As appropriate, specify subheadings you would include within the major sections.
2. Select an article relevant to your project or another health-related problem that interests you. Read the article carefully at least twice. Write a critical review of the article assessing the following aspects.
    - Purpose
        - Clarity of the research problem and objectives
        - Presentation of the context, literature, and need for the study
    - Research Design
        - Appropriateness of the research design
        - Internal and external validity threats
    - Subjects/Participants
        - Appropriateness of the target population
        - Procedure(s) for selecting subjects and evaluation of how well they represent the target population
        - Appropriateness of the sample size
    - Data Collection Procedures
        - Appropriateness and effectiveness of data collection procedures
        - Evidence supporting the validity and reliability of measurements
    - Data Analysis and Results
        - Appropriateness of the data analysis procedures (Do not be overly concerned about technical/statistical aspects.)
        - Clarity and thoroughness of presenting results
    - Discussion
        - Appropriateness of the interpretation of the results
        - Limitations and how they were taken into account in interpreting results
        - How the results contribute to scientific knowledge about the research problem
        - Appropriateness of conclusions and recommendations

If you and another student or colleague read the same article, meet to discuss aspects of your evaluations about which you agree and disagree after you complete your reviews independently.

Study Further

Fink, A. (2003). *How to manage, analyze, and interpret survey data* (2nd ed.). Thousand Oaks, CA: Sage.

Miles, M. B., Huberman, A. M., & Saldaña, J. (2014). *Qualitative data analysis: A methods sourcebook* (3rd ed.). Los Angeles, CA: Sage.

Wasserstein, R. L., & Lazar, N. A. (2016). The ASA's statement on *p*-values: Context, process, and purpose. *The American Statistician, 70*(2), 129–133.

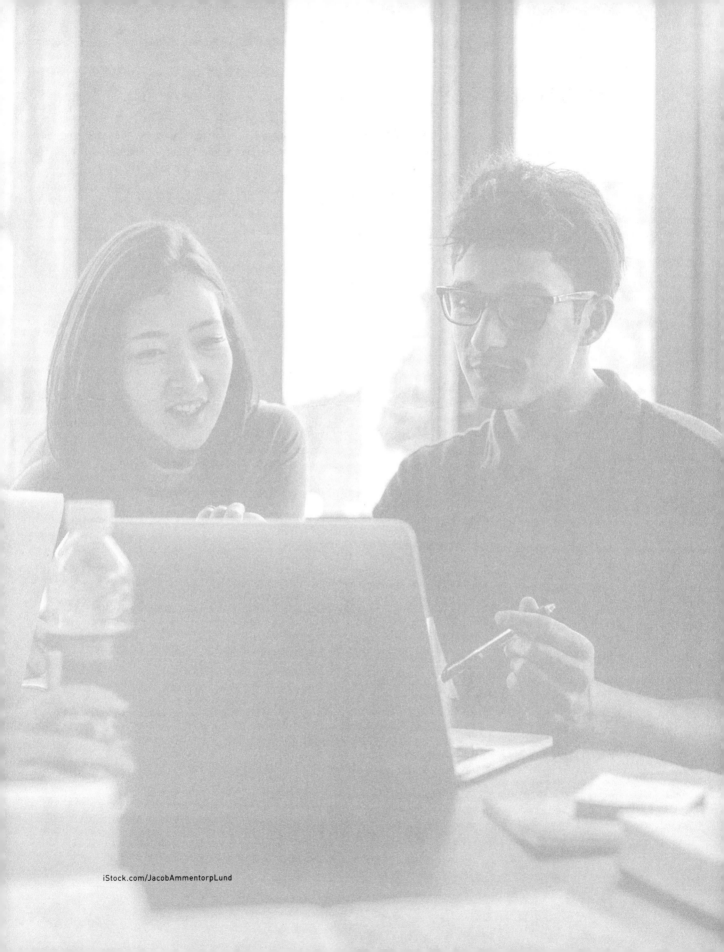

• Glossary •

Abstract: A brief overview and summary of a research report.

Acquiescence bias: Survey participants who are eager to please others select a response choice that is more positive than their true status or agree with statements that do not reflect their true opinion.

Address-based sampling (ABS): A sample is selected by a licensed vendor from the U.S. Postal Service (USPS) Delivery Sequence File (DSF), which contains all delivery-point addresses serviced by the USPS.

Advisory panel: A group of professional and/or lay experts that reviews plans and progress according to a predetermined protocol and schedule.

Alpha: See *critical value*.

Alpha error (α): See *type I error*.

Alternate forms reliability: See *parallel forms reliability*.

Anonymity: It is not possible for anyone, including researchers, to identify individual research participants.

Attention placebo: A control condition where participants receive attention or information that simulates the basic features of a treatment/intervention. Also called an "informational control."

Attrition: Loss of research participants from one observation to a subsequent one.

Attrition bias: An internal validity threat presented by a difference in a dependent variable that is a result of a systematic loss of participants across groups or within a group over time.

Atypical case sample: A nonprobability sample that selects units (cases) to focus on ones that deviate from the average or normative condition. Also called a "deviant case sample," "special case sample," "extreme case sample," or "outlier sample."

Audio computer-assisted self-interview (ACASI): An in-person survey interviewer provides the respondent a device with which to self-complete a programmed questionnaire. The respondent listens to a synchronized voice recording of an interviewer reading aloud instructions, questions, and response choices.

Back translation: An instrument is translated from the source language into a second language, and then is independently translated from the second language back into the source language. Predominantly has been replaced by committee translation.

Basic random selection: Numbers from 1 through N are assigned to all elements in a sampling frame, a random number source is used to select n unique numbers, and an element whose number is selected is included in the sample.

Behavior coding: Observing, coding, and assessing interaction between respondents and interviewers for a field pretest of an interview survey.

***Belmont Report*:** A report by the National Commission for the Protection of Human Subjects of Biomedical and Behavioral Research that delineates ethical principles (respect for persons, beneficence, and justice) for conducting research with human subjects.

Beneficence: An ethical principal in the *Belmont Report* that possible benefits should be maximized and possible harms should be minimized.

Beta error (β): See *type II error*.

Big data: Extremely large data sets derived from electronic formats for communication, data capture, and data storage, such as internet usage and retail purchases.

Bipolar scale: Measures ordinal levels in opposite (negative and positive) directions.

Blinding: Researchers and/or participants are not aware of which participants are assigned to which study condition/group.

Block randomization: Participants within subgroups, called "blocks," are randomly assigned to conditions/groups as they are recruited.

Case-control design: A nonexperimental design to identify the primary factor(s) that caused one group, called "cases," to experience a particular, usually adverse outcome while a similar group, called "controls," did not experience it.

Causal design: Assesses whether an independent variable (treatment) causes a change in a dependent variable (outcome).

427

Causal relationship: An independent variable accounts for change in a dependent variable.

Cause: A factor that, when it is present or changed, produces the presence or a change in the value of another factor, called its effect.

Central limit theorem: A proposition in probability theory that states if repeated simple random samples of the same size are selected from a large population, the sampling distribution will approach a normal distribution, regardless of the shape of the population distribution.

Central tendency: Measures of central tendency summarize the distribution of results for an individual variable in terms of location.

Certainty cluster: A cluster whose probability of selection in a cluster random sample is 1.00.

Certificate of Confidentiality (CoC): Protects identifiable research information from forced disclosure when potential harm to research subjects is severe, such as a risk of criminal prosecution or civil action. A certificate of confidentiality may be issued by the National Institutes of Health (NIH) and other federal agencies, including the Centers for Disease Control and Prevention (CDC) and the Food and Drug Administration (FDA).

Chain referral sample: A referral sample in which an initial sample of seed cases is interviewed and is asked for referrals to other target population members. Also called a "snowball sample."

Check-coding: Verification of coding accuracy by independently coding a random sample of a coder's completed cases.

Classical test theory (CTT): The predominant theoretical measurement model. Assumes there is a true value for every observation. If a measurement is perfectly accurate, then the observed value will equal the true value; observed values will differ only owing to variation in true values across observation units and/or time. Treats a multiple-item measurement as comprising parallel or equivalent measures of the same construct.

Closed question: A survey question for which the response choices are presented in a closed-response format.

Closed-response format: Questions for which a respondent is asked to select from a predetermined set of response choices.

Cluster random sampling: Randomly selects elements within a randomly selected sample of preexisting population subgroups, called clusters.

Cluster size: In cluster random sampling, the number of elements within a cluster.

Clusters: Preexisting population subgroups selected in cluster random sampling.

Codebook: An index to an analysis file's structure and content.

Coding: Assigning a numerical code for every measurement for every variable so it may be entered in a data analysis file.

Cognitive interview: A method for assessing questions in a structured questionnaire to gain insight into how respondents understand key questions, search their memory for relevant information, form judgments, and edit their responses.

Cohort: A group or population that shares an event-based common characteristic that usually is anchored at some time point, such as being born in the same year (called a "birth cohort").

Committee translation: An instrument is translated from the source language into a second by a team of three or more translators who work both independently and collaboratively to determine the most appropriate terminology, grammar, and syntax.

Common cause: A variable that affects two variables simultaneously, causing them to be correlated. May lead to a false conclusion that there is a causal relationship between the two variables.

Common Rule: A U.S. Department of Health and Human Services regulation (45 CFR part 46, subpart A) that specifies basic protections for human subjects in biomedical and behavioral research. It also specifies institutional review board (IRB) requirements.

Comparison group: See *control group*.

Compensatory equalization: A nondesign internal validity threat presented by a third party providing control participants an alternative treatment/intervention.

Compensatory rivalry: A nondesign internal validity threat presented by control participants striving to achieve positive outcomes despite not receiving a treatment/intervention.

Complete mediation: A mediated causal relationship in which all of an independent variable's effect on a dependent variable is expressed through a mediator variable. In this condition, the independent variable has only an indirect effect on the dependent variable, through the mediator.

Complete participant: An observer who is fully engaged in the activities of a group he or she is observing.

Component cause: A causal factor that is part of a group of causal factors that when combined constitute a sufficient causal condition.

Compound question: A question that includes more than one concept. Also called a "double-barreled" question.

Computer-assisted in-person interview (CAPI): An in-person survey interviewer reads aloud questions and response choices displayed on a screen by software and records responses as code numbers via a keyboard or mouse clicks.

Computer-assisted self-interview (CASI): An in-person survey interviewer provides the respondent a device with which to self-complete a programmed questionnaire.

Computer-assisted telephone interview (CATI): A telephone survey interviewer reads aloud questions and response choices displayed on a screen by software and records responses as code numbers via a keyboard or mouse clicks.

Conceptual approach: See *theory*.

Conceptual definition: Describes a construct in the context of a theory or conceptual model.

Conceptual framework: See *theory*.

Conceptual map: A diagram of key relationships revealed by an analysis of qualitative data.

Conceptualization: Specifying a definition for an abstract construct in theoretical terms.

Concurrent criterion validity: Assesses agreement with another measurement of the same construct, the criterion, at the same time.

Confidence interval (CI): In random sampling, an interval calculated around a point estimate of a population parameter to account for sampling error. General structure is CI = statistic ± confidence level × standard error.

Confidence level: In random sampling, the degree of confidence that a particular confidence interval is one that includes the population parameter being estimated. It is indicated by a standard score (z) from the normal distribution.

Confidentiality: Although researchers are able to identify individual research participants, they do not disclose their identity outside the research context.

Confirmability: The degree to which a qualitative result is shaped by participants and conditions, rather than a researcher's expectations and perspective.

Confounder variable: See *extraneous variable*.

Construct: An abstract factor that is not observable directly.

Construct-specific scale: See *item-specific scale*.

Construct validity: Assesses whether a measurement relates to measurements of other constructs in a way that is consistent with theoretical expectations.

Contact log: A record of dates, times, and outcomes when attempts are made to contact survey respondents.

Content validity: Assesses whether a measurement appears to represent a construct's content domain.

Contingency analysis: An assessment of whether the occurrence of an observation in a particular category of one variable is contingent on the category in which that observation occurs for another variable.

Contingency table: A table that simultaneously classifies observations in categories of two or more variables, to assess whether observations in categories of one variable are contingent on the categories in another variable. Also called a "cross-classification table," a "cross-tabulation," or "crosstabs."

Continuous variable: A variable that may be measured in terms of an infinite number of possible values.

Control: Managing the conditions under which a study is conducted and employing systematic protocols throughout the research process to enhance the comparability of results across individuals, groups, populations, settings, and time.

Control condition: In general, the prevailing conditions individuals normally would experience during a study period. Also may be an alternative treatment.

Control group: Research participants who are not exposed to a treatment/intervention.

Control group contamination: See *treatment diffusion*.

Control group model: A research design that simulates the counterfactual model by comparing a control group to a treatment group.

Convenience sample: A nonprobability sample in which units are selected because they are conveniently accessible.

Convergent validity: Assesses whether measures of the same construct are correlated with each other.

Correlation coefficient: A measure of the direction and strength of a relationship between two variables. Values typically range from 0 (no relationship) to 1.00 (a perfect relationship); direction is indicated by a coefficient's sign (+/−).

Counterbalancing: Equal numbers of treatment participants are randomly assigned to receive treatment/intervention components in a different order.

Counterfactual condition: The hypothetical status of research participants when they are not exposed to an experimental treatment at the same time as they are exposed to it.

Counterfactual model: A hypothetical research design in which research participants are simultaneously exposed and not exposed to an experimental treatment.

Covariation: A pattern of concordant change in two variables in terms of amount and direction; an essential condition for a causal relationship.

Coverage: The extent to which a sampling frame includes all population elements.

Covert observation: Observation is conducted without people being aware they are being observed.

Credibility: The degree of confidence that may be attributed to a qualitative result as being true.

Critical value: A hypothesis test result that indicates whether the probability that an observed result may be attributed to chance. See also *alpha*.

Cronbach's coefficient alpha: A measure of reliability that estimates the average split-half correlation for all possible random splits of items.

Cross-sectional design: Observations of one or more populations are made under prevailing conditions at one observation point. There is no manipulation of any variable(s).

Data cleaning: Identifying and correcting problems after data are entered into an analysis file.

Data collection: The process of collecting observations from or about research participants/study units.

Deductive disclosure: Occurs in research when others who are familiar with subjects might be able to identify them from their data.

Deductive reasoning: Reasoning that proceeds from empirical observations of specific instances to general conclusions.

Deferred-treatment condition: Control group participants are provided the experimental treatment/intervention at the end of a study.

De-identification: Removal of individual research participant identifiers before a data set is provided to a third party; typically done for secondary data analysis.

Demoralization: A nondesign internal validity threat presented by control participants' performance and outcomes being reduced by disappointment at not receiving a treatment/intervention.

Dependability: The extent to which a qualitative result is consistent and repeatable.

Dependent variable: A variable whose values change in response to change in another variable (the independent variable).

Descriptive notes: A factual and comprehensive account of what is observed.

Design effect (deff): In cluster random sampling, the ratio of the variance of the sampling distribution for a cluster sample (VAR_C) to the variance of the sampling distribution for a simple random sample (VAR_{SRS}) of the same size. Used to adjust sample size for within-cluster homogeneity.

Dichotomous classification: Distinguishes between observations in terms of two categories, indicating whether a particular characteristic is present or not.

Difference-in-differences analysis: An assessment of within-group change for a treatment group relative to within-group change for a control group.

Direct effect: An independent variable's effect on a dependent variable without an influence from a mediator variable.

Direction of a relationship: An indication of whether values for one variable change in a predictable way when values for another variable change.

Disclosure by association: Might result from being observed participating in research by others who are familiar with the subjects.

Discrete variable: A variable that may be measured only in terms of particular units.

Discriminant validity: Assesses whether measures of different constructs are not correlated or are weakly correlated.

Dispersion: Measures of dispersion indicate how broadly observations are distributed across an ordinal- or interval-/ratio-level measurement scale.

Disproportionate allocation: In stratified random sampling, the sample is allocated to strata to ensure that the number of elements selected from each stratum is adequate to conduct a meaningful analysis within a stratum and/or to compare results across strata.

Distal outcome: A long-term treatment result.

Double-barreled question: See *compound question*.

Double blind: Both researchers and research participants are blinded to which study condition/group participants are assigned.

Dual frame sample: A random sample that is selected from a sampling formed by merging information from two or more sources.

Ecological fallacy: A logical error that results from interpreting aggregate-level results at the individual level.

Effect: A factor whose presence or value is determined by the presence or a change in another factor, called its cause.

Effectiveness: A treatment's beneficial effect when it is delivered under optimum conditions.

Effectiveness trial: A causal study that emphasizes external validity.

Efficacy: A treatment's beneficial effect when it is delivered under optimum conditions.

Efficacy trial: A causal study that emphasizes internal validity.

Element: An individual population entity.

Email survey: A questionnaire is sent embedded in or attached to an email message to respondents, who complete and return it by email.

Endogenous variable: A variable whose value is determined by other variables in a causal model.

EPSEM design: A sampling design for which each element has the same selection probability. EPSEM = Equal Probability Selection Method.

Equal Probability Selection Method: See *EPSEM design*.

Equivalent groups: Groups that do not differ, especially in terms of their status on a dependent variable, by more than would be expected by random chance.

Exclusion criteria: Characteristics that disqualify target population members from participating in a particular study.

Executive summary: An overview and summary of a research report that is longer than an abstract and may include elements that are not normally included in an abstract, such as tables, charts, graphs, and reference citations.

Exogenous variable: A variable whose value is determined by factors outside the context of a causal model.

Expected value: In random sampling, the value of the population parameter being estimated.

Experimental design: Research participants are randomly assigned to at least one treatment/intervention group and at least one control group.

Experimental research: Research whereby subjects are assigned to two or more comparison groups, such as treatment and control.

Explanatory variable: An extraneous variable that explains a spurious relationship.

Exploratory study: A research study investigating a new problem about which little is known to gain a basic understanding of the problem's nature and scope.

External validity: The extent to which there is confidence that a study's result may be generalized to hold over variations in populations, settings, treatments, and outcomes.

Extraneous variable: A third variable that accounts for a spurious relationship (also see *spurious relationship*). Also called a "confounder variable."

Face validity: Assesses whether a measurement appears to represent a particular construct.

Factorial design: Ensures that all possible conditions are considered for inclusion in a multiple-component evaluation. The design is derived by cross-classifying all categories or levels for all treatment components, called factors.

False negative: An erroneous conclusion that an experimental treatment/intervention did not produce a desirable outcome.

False positive: An erroneous conclusion that an experimental treatment/intervention produced a desirable outcome.

Field notes: Notes recorded by an observer about what they observe.

Field pretest: A small-scale trial run to assess an instrument and procedures for administering it under study conditions before conducting the main study.

Field sample size (FSS): A sample size that is adjusted by increasing the initial sample size to account for contingencies that may be encountered during data collection, such as contact, eligibility, and cooperation rates.

Fill-in-the-blank format: A question response format where respondents are asked to write in their response in a blank space.

Filter question: A question that determines which of two or more subsequent questions is appropriate for a respondent to answer.

Finite population correction (fpc): A sample size adjustment to account for the population size when a random sample will be selected from a relatively small population.

Focus group: A moderator uses a semistructured guide and encourages a small group of participants to interactively respond to questions about a narrowly defined topic.

Forced-choice: Rating scale response choices that do not include a midpoint.

Frequency matching: A matching procedure that yields groups with similar frequency distributions on one or more particular characteristics.

Full blind: Researchers are not aware of which participants are assigned to which study condition/group from the time of assignment through analyzing results.

Full disclosure: Reporting research results with all aspects of how a study was designed and conducted so others may evaluate its validity and replicate it.

Funnel sequence: Respondents are asked to provide an overall rating before being asked to rate individual components of their overall rating.

Grounded theory: Theory derived from interpreting empirical observations, rather than having been generated by speculation.

Heterogeneous sample: A nonprobability sample that selects units to capture diversity.

History effect: An internal validity threat presented by one or more events that affect the dependent variable occurring concurrently with a treatment/intervention.

Homogeneous sample: A nonprobability sample that selects units to focus on ones that are similar.

Human subject: Defined by the Common Rule as "[a] living individual about whom an investigator (whether professional or student) conducting research obtains (1) Data through intervention or interaction with the individual, or (2) Identifiable private information."

Hypothesis: A proposition about whether it is likely there is or is not a relationship between certain variables or a difference across groups and/or time.

Hypothesis test: A statistical procedure for assessing the probability of observing a particular result by chance if the null hypothesis is true.

Identifier: Information about an individual research participant that enables identifying them either directly or indirectly. Examples of identifiers are a participant's address, telephone number, email address, Social Security number, medical record code, employee identification number, and student identification number.

Imputation: A strategy for estimating a valid value for a missing value so a case may be included in an analysis.

Inadvertent disclosure: Occurs in research when individuals who are not members of the research staff become privy to a subject's data.

Inclusion criteria: Characteristics target population members must meet to be eligible to participate in a particular study.

Independent monitoring: A strategy for minimizing researcher bias whereby a third party provides oversight for how a study is planned, conducted, and reported.

Independent variable: A variable that causes change in another variable (the dependent variable).

In-depth interview: See *unstructured interview*.

Indirect effect: An independent variable's effect on a dependent variable that is influenced by a mediator variable.

Inductive reasoning: Reasoning that proceeds from empirical observations of specific instances to general conclusions.

Inference process: A sample's characteristics (statistics) are used to estimate a population's characteristics (parameters).

Informational control: See *attention placebo*.

Informed consent: Individuals have a right to decide whether to participate in research. They must be provided a clear and complete understanding about their participation in research, and they must be competent to consent voluntarily.

In-person interview survey: An interviewer reads questions aloud in-person and records responses on a questionnaire. Also called a "face-to-face" and "personal" interview survey.

Institutional review board (IRB): A board that is required at each institution where research is conducted that is subject to the Common Rule (DHHS regulation 45 CFR part 46, subpart A) that must review and approve all protocols for conducting research with human subjects before the research may be initiated. An IRB also conducts continuing review of approved research.

Instrument: A method for collecting and recording observations.

Instrumentation: Specifying procedures for observing and recording empirical indicators of the variables.

Instrumentation bias/effect: An internal validity threat presented by different dependent variable measurements within or across groups.

Intact group: A preexisting, naturally occurring group, such as students in the same classroom or employees in the same department.

Intent-to-treat (ITT): When analyzing a randomized controlled trial, the outcome for all participants is analyzed within the study condition to which they are assigned, regardless of whether they changed conditions.

Interaction effect: The combined effect of an independent and a moderator variable.

Intercoder reliability: See *interrater reliability*.

Intermediate outcome: A change in a mediator variable.

Internal validity: The extent to which plausible alternative explanations may be ruled out that a change in a dependent variable is not caused by the independent variable.

Internet survey: See *web survey*.

Interobserver reliability: See *interrater reliability*.

Interrater reliability: Assesses agreement between independent concurrent observations of the same individual(s) using the same procedure. Also called "interobserver reliability" or "intercoder reliability." Also see *Kappa coefficient*.

Interval-/ratio-level measurement: Distinguishes between observations in terms of the amount in standard units.

Interview guide: A list of topics in prospective order that ensures addressing all topics.

Interviewer variance: Differences in how interviewers administer the same survey questionnaire.

Interviewer/staff debriefing: Asking survey field pretest interviewers to discuss their experience administering the questionnaire.

Inverted funnel sequence: Respondents are asked to provide ratings about individual components before being asked to provide their overall rating.

Interviewer bias: Differences in how a survey respondent answers questions resulting from differences in how interviewers ask questions, probe answers, and/or record answers.

IRB: See *institutional review board*.

Item nonresponse: Survey participants do not respond to a question that applies to them.

Item response theory (IRT): A measurement theory that treats items in a multiple-item measurement as assessing levels of difficulty for providing a correct answer.

Item-specific scale: A unipolar scale focused directly on the underlying construct to be measured. Also called a "construct-specific scale."

Judgment-based validity: Assesses whether a measurement appears to measure the construct it is intended to measure.

Judgmental sample: See *purposive sample*.

Justice: An ethical principle in the *Belmont Report* that the burdens and benefits of participating in research should be distributed fairly.

Kappa coefficient: A measure of interrater reliability that adjusts for chance agreements.

Key informants sample: A nonprobability sample in which individuals are selected because they have special insight about a research problem.

Key personnel: Individuals involved in the design or conduct of human subjects research.

Levels of measurement: Measurements are classified in a series of levels (nominal, ordinal, interval/ratio) according to the nature and amount of information they capture.

Likert scale: A bipolar scale that asks participants to respond to a statement about a topic by choosing among ordinal options ranging from the most negative to the most positive. A typical Likert scale presents five ordered points indicating two degrees each of agreement and disagreement, plus a neutral midpoint.

Limited participant: An observer who is fully engaged in the activities of a group he or she is observing except in certain situations, such as engaging in illegal behavior.

Linear relationship: A data pattern tends toward describing a straight line.

Literature review: An examination and assessment of existing research reports related to a particular research problem.

Longitudinal design: Observations are collected from the same individuals or the same population, typically under prevailing conditions, at multiple observation points called "waves."

Look-back: Referring to a response to a previous question in a multiple-page questionnaire.

Mail survey: A paper questionnaire is sent by standard mail to respondents, who complete and return it by standard mail.

Manipulated conditions: Conditions that researchers create entirely or existing conditions that researchers modify to address a study's purpose.

Manipulation: Researchers control whether, when, and how participants are exposed to a treatment.

Margin of error (MOE): The width of a confidence interval when calculating sample size or reporting a point estimate.

Matched pairs: See *pairwise matching*.

Matching: A procedure for assigning participants to conditions/groups to ensure they are similar in terms of one or more particular characteristics. Typically used when participants are very diverse and their number is small.

Maturation threat: An internal validity threat presented by a time-related change in participants that affects the dependent variable.

Mean: The arithmetic average for a set of interval-/ratio-level measurements.

Measure of size (MOS): See *cluster size*.

Measurement: The process of systematically assigning labels and/or numbers to differentiate observations in terms of quality or quantity, across units and/or time.

Measurement accuracy: The degree to which a measurement is free of error or bias.

Measurement bias: Error whereby the observed value always is lower or higher than its true value.

Measurement levels: See *levels of measurement*.

Measurement precision: The degree of detail at which at measurement is made.

Measurement reliability: The extent to which a measurement is free of random error and thus obtains consistent outcomes when the true value is constant.

Measurement validity: The extent to which a measurement accurately measures the construct it is intended to measure. A valid measurement is free of both random and systematic error.

Median: The point in a distribution of interval-/ratio-level measurements where half the observations are located above and half are below.

Mediated effect: An independent variable's effect through its influence on a mediator variable.

Mediated relationship: An independent variable affects a dependent variable through its effect on another variable (also see *mediator variable*).

Mediator variable: A variable that is affected by an independent variable and then has an effect on a dependent variable (also called an "intervening variable").

Meta-analysis: A statistical method for synthesizing quantitative results from several similar studies, treating each study as the unit of analysis.

Minimal risk: According to the Common Rule, "the probability and magnitude of harm or discomfort anticipated in the research are not greater in and of themselves than those ordinarily encountered in daily life or during the performance of routine physical or psychological examinations or tests."

Missing data: Information about a research participant is not available owing to factors such as not responding to one or more questions or not being available for follow-up observations, such as in a pretest–posttest design or a longitudinal design.

Mixed methods research design: A research design that uses at least one qualitative and one quantitative method that may be implemented concurrently or sequentially.

Mixed-mode survey: A survey plan that employs two or more data collection modes.

Mock interviews: A trainer plays the respondent role and provides feedback to an interviewer.

Mode: The most frequently occurring observation or value.

Mode effect: Differences in response to the same survey question depending on the data collection mode employed.

Moderated effect: An independent variable's effect when influenced by a moderator variable.

Moderated causal relationship: A variable modifies the strength and/or direction of an independent variable's effect on a dependent variable (also see *moderator variable*).

Moderator variable: A variable that modifies the strength and/or direction of an independent variable's effect on a dependent variable.

Monitored self-administered questionnaire: A paper questionnaire is distributed by staff to respondents who complete and return it to staff.

Multiple-item scale: An ordinal rating scale derived by combining responses to several single-item rating scales that measure different facets of a construct.

Multiple response: A respondent may select more than one response choice for a question. Also called "check/mark all that apply."

Narrative review: A summary of completed studies selected by the reviewer that summarizes the main points of agreement, disagreement, strengths, limitations, and gaps.

Necessary condition: A dependent variable changes only if the independent variable changes.

Negative relationship: Two variables change in opposite directions.

Nominal-level measurement: Distinguishes between observations in terms of kind or quality.

Noncoverage bias: Systematic exclusion of certain population elements from a sampling frame.

Nondifferentiation bias: A survey respondent selects the same scale point for each item in a multiple-item rating scale.

Nondisclosure: Research staff should not share information that might disclose a participant's identity outside the research context.

Nonequivalent groups: An internal validity threat presented by a systematic preexisting difference across groups.

Nonexperimental design: Does not include a control group, or includes a control group without random assignment and a pretest observation point.

Nonlinear relationship: A data pattern changes over the range of two variables.

Nonparticipant observation: The observer is an outsider, or spectator, who does not interact with the people he or she observes.

Nonrandom sample: A sample selected based on judgment. Also called a "nonprobabiity sample.'"

Nonrandom sampling: The process for selecting a nonrandom sample.

Nonresponse bias: Nonrespondents differ from respondents systematically in a way that might influence a survey's results.

Normal distribution: A distribution of observations that resemble a bell-shaped curve, called a "normal curve."

No-treatment control condition: A control condition in which participants are exposed neither to an experimental treatment nor to an alternative treatment.

Null hypothesis (H_0): A hypothesis that posits there is no relationship or difference between certain variables or a difference across groups and/or time. It comprises all results that do not comport with the research hypothesis.

Objectivity: Throughout the research process, researchers should maintain an impartial posture to prevent researcher bias influencing results.

Observational design: Observations of one or more populations are made under prevailing conditions at one or more observation points. There is no manipulation of any variable(s).

Observation points: Times in a research design when measurements will be made.

Observed value: The value of a variable that is observed and recorded during data collection.

Open question: A survey question for which the response choices are presented in an open-response format.

Open-response format: Questions for which respondents are asked to respond in their own words. Also called "open-ended."

Operational definition: Describes how a construct may be observable through collecting information about one or more variables.

Operationalization: A process of identifying observable variables that represent a construct.

Optimizing: A survey respondent carefully and completely performs each cognitive task in the response process to provide a response that is as accurate and unbiased as possible.

Ordinal-level measurement: Distinguishes between observations in terms of relative amount.

Pairwise matching: A matching procedure that identifies pairs of participants who are similar on one or more particular characteristics and then randomly assigns pair members to different conditions/groups.

Panel: Research participants who are measured in a longitudinal design.

Panel conditioning: Panel participants are influenced by a "testing effect."

Panel design: One group of research participants, called the "panel," is measured at multiple observation points.

Panel maintenance: Refreshing a panel by selecting supplemental samples to update the panel's representativeness and maintain analytical power.

Parallel forms reliability: Assesses the correlation between equivalent, concurrent measurements of the same construct, with the same individual(s). Also called "alternate forms reliability."

Parameter: A population characteristic, designated by a capital Roman or Greek character.

Partial blind: Researchers are not aware of which participants are assigned to which study condition/group during one or more parts of a study.

Partial mediation: An independent variable affects a dependent variable both directly and through a mediator variable.

Participant observation: The observer becomes, or already is, a member of a group being observed to gain an insider's perspective.

Participant reactivity: A nondesign internal validity threat presented by a change in participants' performance in response to being aware they are being studied.

Participating observer: An observer who gains access to a setting, but collects data primarily as an outsider, perhaps because he or she is not qualified to participate fully, or to enable him or her to record observations objectively.

Path: An element in a path diagram that indicates a relationship between two variables.

Path diagram: A diagram that indicates the pathways through which variables influence other variables.

Pearson's r: A correlation coefficient commonly applied to two interval-/ratio-level measurements. Also called "Pearson's product moment correlation coefficient."

Peer review: Independent researchers review a study proposal and/or reports of research results.

Performance-based validity: Compares empirical outcomes for a measurement with those of other measures with which it is or is not expected to be correlated.

Periodicity bias: In systematic random sampling, a bias that may result if the sampling frame is arranged in a cyclical, periodic pattern that coincides with the selection interval.

Pilot study: A small-scale, developmental study conducted to assess the feasibility of and plan a larger study.

Placebo control: Control group participants receive a bogus "treatment" that is an inactive agent.

Point estimate: A sample estimate of a population parameter that is expressed as a single value, such as a mean or proportion.

Polychotomous classification: Assigns observations to three or more nominal-level categories.

Population: The total set of entities targeted for a study.

Population size: The number of population elements, N.

Positive relationship: Two variables change in the same direction.

Posttest observation: A measurement of research participants after implementing a treatment/intervention to assess change in a dependent variable and other key variables.

Precoded: A numeric code value is assigned to each closed question response choice in advance of administering a questionnaire.

Predictive criterion validity: Assesses agreement with a future measurement with which a measurement is expected to be correlated.

Prenotification: Providing information about a study to participants in advance.

Pretest observation: A measurement of research participants before implementing a treatment/intervention to assess their baseline status on a dependent variable and other key variables. Also may be done as a randomization check.

Pretest–posttest control group design: An experimental design in which participants are randomly assigned to a treatment or control group condition. Both groups are measured before (pretest) and after (posttest) the treatment group is exposed to a treatment/intervention. Also called a "randomized controlled trial."

Prevailing conditions: Conditions that already exist at the time a study is conducted and over which researchers do not exercise any control.

Primacy response effect: Survey respondents select the first response choice presented, regardless of their true response.

Principal investigator: The lead researcher, who is responsible for all aspects of a study, from planning to reporting results.

Privacy Rule: A section of the Health Insurance Portability and Accountability Act of 1996 (HIPAA) and the Family Educational Rights and Privacy Act of 1974 (FERPA) that established federal policies for protecting the privacy of individually identifiable information for research that requires access to medical and school administrative records.

Private information: Defined by the Common Rule as "[I]nformation about behavior that occurs in a context in which an individual can reasonably expect that no observation or recording is taking place, and information which has been provided for specific purposes by an individual and which the individual can reasonably expect will not be made public (for example, a medical record)."

Probabilities proportionate to size (PPS): In cluster random sampling, a procedure that takes cluster size into account by adjusting each cluster's selection probability to be proportionate to its size.

Probability theory: A mathematical/statistical theory that describes how randomly selected elements are expected to be distributed.

Probing: A method of asking follow-up questions in an interview to encourage a response, clarify a response, or obtain a complete response.

Problem statement: A general statement of the problem addressed by a research study.

Process evaluation: An assessment of how a study is implemented, especially for a design that includes a treatment condition.

Proportionate allocation: In stratified random sampling, the sample is allocated to strata in proportion to their size in the population.

Proximal outcome: A treatment result that is observed immediately or shortly after a treatment is completed.

Purposeful sample: See *purposive sample*.

Purposive sample: A nonprobability sample selected based on factors that lead to an expectation they will provide the type of information that will serve a study's purpose. Also called "purposeful sample" or "judgmental sample."

***p* value:** The probability of obtaining an observed result by chance under the assumption the null hypothesis is true.

Qualitative data: Observations that are not recorded in a numerical format.

Qualitative methods: Data collection methods that use unstructured, context-specific techniques in natural settings to primarily collect qualitative information from the participant's perspective. They use an inductive, iterative approach to develop an in-depth understanding of a problem's nature and scope.

Quantitative data: Observations that are recorded in a numerical format.

Quasi-experimental design: Assesses causality when it is not feasible to employ random assignment or include a control group by using other strategies to address internal validity threats.

Questionnaire: See *structured questionnaire*.

Quota sample: A nonprobability sample that selects units to reflect similar proportions as the target population regarding key variables.

Random assignment: A random process is used to assign research participants to conditions/groups.

Random-digit dialing (RDD): A sampling method for telephone surveys that enables including respondents with unlisted numbers and cell phone users.

Random error: In classical test theory, an unsystematic deviation of an observed value from its true value.

Random number selection: A procedure for selecting a random sample using a random number source, such as a random number table, a random number generator, or random selection software.

Random sample: A sample selected using a random process where each population element has an independent chance of selection that is greater than zero, and the selection probability for each element is known or may be calculated. Also called a "probability sample."

Random sampling: The process for selecting a random sample.

Random starting point: In systematic random sampling, the point randomly selected within the first selection interval from which all subsequent elements are selected.

Randomization: See *random assignment*.

Randomization check: A comparison of randomly assigned groups to assess their comparability before implementing a treatment/intervention.

Randomized controlled trial (RCT): See *pretest–posttest control group design*.

Range: The distance between the observed minimum and maximum values: maximum − minimum.

Ranking: Classification of observations in a hierarchical order.

Rating: Classification of observations along an ordinal-level continuum.

Rating scale: Asks participants to locate themselves along an ordinal continuum.

Recall error: A respondent is unable to recall an event or certain details about it.

Recency response effect: Survey respondents select the last response choice presented, regardless of their true response.

Reciprocal causality: Two variables appear to affect and be caused by each other virtually simultaneously.

Referral sample: A nonprobability sample that selects units by referral from others.

Reflective notes: An account of the observation process, and insights about the potential meaning and significance of what is observed.

Refusal conversion: Survey interview nonrespondents are contacted in an attempt to complete interviews with them.

Regression analysis: A method for assessing how well values for a dependent variable may be predicted using information about one or more independent variables. Bivariate regression includes one independent variable; multiple regression includes two or more independent variables.

Regression toward the norm: An internal validity threat presented by studying participants who are at an atypical pretest status on the dependent variable regressing (returning) to or toward their normal status at posttest.

Repeated-measures design: Data are collected from the same research participants at two or more observation points.

Replication: Assessing whether consistent results are obtained from two or more studies using a design and procedures that are as similar as possible.

Research: Defined by the Common Rule as "a systematic investigation, including research development, testing and evaluation, designed to develop or contribute to generalizable knowledge."

Research design: The pattern for how to conduct a particular study.

Research design diagram: A graphic device for developing a design, assessing potential threats to validity, implementing a research plan, and guiding analyzing and interpreting results.

Research hypothesis (H_1): A hypothesis that posits there is a relationship or difference between certain variables or a difference across groups and/or time.

Research process: A cyclical approach to building a valid body of scientific evidence about a particular problem.

Research question: A statement of the purpose and focus of a study. It guides all aspects of a study, from planning to reporting results.

Research Randomizer: Free access online software for random selection and random assignment. Available from www.randomizer.org.

Research validity: The extent to which there is confidence in drawing conclusions based on research results.

Researcher bias: A researcher's personal values and/or expectations influence how he or she conducts a study and/or interprets its results.

Researcher blind: Researchers are not aware of which participants are assigned to which study condition/group.

Respect for persons: An ethical principle in the *Belmont Report* that individuals should be treated as autonomous agents, and persons with diminished autonomy should be protected.

Respondent: An individual who answers questions in a survey.

Respondent debriefing: Asking survey field pretest respondents to discuss their experience responding to the questionnaire.

Respondent-driven sample (RDS): A variation of chain referral sampling in which after a sample of seed cases is interviewed, the participants are asked to recruit, rather than make referrals to, other target population members.

Response heaping: Respondents use only a few familiar points when asked to respond in terms of percentages using a fill-in-the-blank format.

Response process: Responding to a question typically requires a respondent to perform a series of four cognitive tasks: question comprehension, information retrieval, judgment formation, and response editing.

Response review: An examination of responses to questions in a field pretest questionnaire to detect potential problems.

Reverse-coding: Reversing the scale scores for an ordinal scale so higher values indicate a higher rating.

Risk factor: An independent variable that is neither a necessary nor a sufficient cause of change in another variable. In epidemiology, a risk factor is a variable that increases the probability of incurring a particular adverse health outcome.

Rostering: A questionnaire complexity aspect that asks respondents to identify by first name or relationship certain other individuals, such as household members or coworkers. Then they are asked to answer a series of questions about each individual on that roster.

Sample: A subgroup selected to represent a target population.

Sample size: The number of sampling units, n, in a sample.

Sampling distribution: The distribution of a sample statistic for all possible random samples of size n from a population of size N.

Sampling error: The difference between a sample statistic from one random sample and its corresponding population parameter.

Sampling fraction: A population element's probability of selection (f), also called the "sampling rate," where $f = n/N$.

Sampling frame: A source that identifies population elements and is a vehicle from which a sample may be selected.

Sampling unit: The type of population element that may be selected in a sample.

Satisficing: A survey respondent does not perform each cognitive task in the response process carefully and completely, which may result in an inaccurate or biased response.

Satisficing theory: A theory that addresses how survey respondents go through the response process.

Saturation point: In qualitative research, the point at which data collection is stopped when it appears that it is not likely to yield substantial new information.

Scientific approach: Research seeks to derive valid conclusions by systematically following certain principles throughout the research process, including objectivity, control, and replication.

Secondary data analysis: The analysis of data previously collected and analyzed by others.

Selection bias: When research participants are not selected randomly, decisions of researchers or potential participants may cause a sample to be unrepresentative of the target population.

Selection interval: See *systematic random sample*.

Self-administered questionnaire (SAQ): A respondent completes the questionnaire with no or minimal assistance from staff.

Self-assignment: Research participants select their study group/condition. May introduce self-selection bias.

Self-monitoring: A strategy for minimizing researcher bias by routinely conducting self-reflective checks.

Self-selection bias: When research participants select their study group/condition, individual preferences may result in a nonequivalent groups threat to internal validity.

Semistructured interview: An interviewer uses an interview guide that lists topics in prospective order.

Sensitive topic: A topic that may cause a respondent to feel uncomfortable, embarrassed, or threatened.

Silent probe: Technique in which an interviewer allows time for a respondent to process their response to a question.

Simple random assignment: A random determination is made for assigning each individual participant to a condition/group.

Simple random sampling (SRS): The basic random sampling design, whereby each population element is selected individually and all population elements have the same probability of selection. All possible combinations of n elements from a population of size N have the same chance to be selected.

Simple random sampling with replacement: When an element is randomly selected, it is returned to the population before making the next selection. An element may be selected more than once.

Simple random sampling without replacement: When an element is randomly selected, it is not returned to the population before making the next selection. Each element may be selected only once.

Single blind: Only researchers or research participants are blinded to which study condition/group participants are assigned.

Single-item scale: A rating scale that asks participants to respond to a single item. Used when a construct is regarded as unidimensional, to assess a participant's overall rating for a multidimensional construct, or to measure a particular facet of a multidimensional construct to develop a multiple-item scale.

Skip pattern: A branching sequence in a structured questionnaire that routes respondents to the next appropriate question according to their response to a filter question.

Social desirability bias: Interview participants respond in ways they expect are socially acceptable.

Spearman's rank-order coefficient: A correlation coefficient commonly applied to two ordinal-level measurements. Also called "Spearman's rho (ρ)."

Split-half reliability: The correlation between parallel forms of a multiple-item measurement created by randomly dividing the items into halves. Also see *Cronbach's coefficient alpha*.

Spurious relationship: A noncausal relationship that may appear to be causal but is explained by the influence of a third variable.

Standard deviation: The square root of the variance.

Standard error (SE): In random sampling, the standard deviation of a sampling distribution: $\sigma/\sqrt{n}$.

Standard-treatment control condition: Control participants receive the current standard treatment.

Statistic: A sample characteristic that is used to estimate a corresponding population parameter, designated by a lowercase Roman character.

Statistical power: The probability that a statistical test will reject the null hypothesis when it is not true.

Statistical significance: A statistical conclusion that the probability of observing a particular result by chance is so low that the null hypothesis should be rejected and the research hypothesis should be accepted.

Statistically equivalent groups: If a test of statistical significance is applied after random assignment, it would find no significant difference across groups on the dependent variable or any other variable.

Statistically significant: An observed outcome that is not likely to have been obtained by random chance.

Straight, single-headed arrow: An element in a path diagram that indicates the path from a cause (independent variable) to an effect (dependent variable).

Stratified random assignment: Equal numbers of participants from each stratum are assigned to each condition/group.

Stratified random sampling: A population is divided into subgroups, called strata, and a random sample is selected from each stratum.

Stratum: A population subgroup in a stratified random sample. *Strata* is plural.

Stratum weight: In stratified random sampling with disproportionate allocation, a weight that adjusts the number of elements in each stratum to reflect the stratum's proportion in the population.

Strength of a relationship: An indication of how reliably the amount of change in one variable may be predicted given the amount of change in another variable.

Structured open-ended interview: An interviewer uses an interview guide with open-ended questions.

Structured questionnaire: The measurement instrument used primarily to conduct a survey. For each respondent, the following aspects are the same: wording of each question, response choices for each question, and the order in which questions are presented.

Study-specific codes: Alphabetical and/or numeric codes assigned to individual research participants to protect their identity.

Subject: A research participant. Also see *human subject*.

Subject blind: Research participants are not aware of which study condition/group they are assigned.

Subsample: A random sample of an initial sample or pool of subjects.

Substantive significance: A determination that a result is sufficiently trustworthy and important to incorporate into practice.

Sufficient condition: A dependent variable changes whenever the independent variable changes.

Survey: A method for systematically collecting self-reported information using a structured questionnaire.

Survey plan: The protocol for conducting a survey.

Systematic error: In classical test theory, a consistent deviation of an observed value from its true value that results in measurement bias, whereby the observed value always is lower or higher than its true value.

Systematic random sample: Population elements are selected using a fixed selection interval (k) from a random starting point in a sampling frame, where $k = N/n$.

Systematic review: A summary and assessment of completed studies that meet explicit prespecified inclusion criteria.

Target population: See *population*.

Telephone interview survey: An interviewer reads questions aloud on a telephone and records responses on a questionnaire.

Temporal precedence: Change in an independent variable must precede change in a dependent variable as an essential condition for a causal relationship.

Testing effect: An internal validity threat presented by repeated administration of a measurement instrument affecting subsequent measurement outcomes.

Test–retest reliability: Assesses the correlation between repeated measurements of the same individuals, under the same conditions, by the same observer, and using the same procedure.

Theory: A conceptual model, sometimes called a conceptual framework, that identifies and defines key factors and describes relationships among them.

Time frame: The period that typically starts with selecting and recruiting participants, and ends when all observations are completed.

Timing: The points in a research design when group assignment, observations, and group conditions will be implemented.

Total effect: An independent variable's effect on a dependent variable is the sum of its indirect effect and direct effects.

Transferability: The degree to which a qualitative result may be generalized to other contexts, such as similar situations, populations, and phenomena.

Treatment: An experimental intervention that is hypothesized to produce a positive outcome.

Treatment condition: A change in an independent variable manipulated by researchers.

Treatment diffusion: A non-design internal validity threat presented by control group participants being unintentionally exposed to part or all of a treatment/intervention. The same as "control group contamination."

Treatment group: Research participants who are exposed to a treatment/intervention.

Treatment imitation: A nondesign internal validity threat presented by control participants independently adopting the same or a similar treatment as the experimental treatment/intervention.

Trend study: A series of cross-sectional studies with separate samples selected from the same population at each observation point. Also called a "sequential cross-sectional design."

True value: The actual value of a variable at the time when the variable is observed during data collection.

Two-headed curved arrow: An element in a path diagram that indicates two variables are correlated in a noncausal relationship.

Type I error: A statistical inferential error committed when a null hypothesis is true but is rejected. Also called an "alpha error."

Type II error: A statistical inferential error committed when a null hypothesis is not true but is accepted. Also called a "beta error."

Typical case sample: A nonprobability sample that selects units (cases) to focus on ones that represent the average or normative condition.

Unbiased sample: Sampling error overall, computed as the sum of sampling errors for all possible random samples of size n selected from a population of size N, equals zero. A sample statistic's mean value derived from all possible random samples equals the population parameter being estimated, which is its expected value.

Unipolar scale: Measures ordinal levels in one direction (negative or positive) from a null or zero point to a maximum end point.

Unit response rate: The proportion of sample members who are known or assumed to meet a survey's eligibility criteria from whom a completed questionnaire is collected.

Units of study: The target population entities from or about which data will be collected and analyzed.

Unobtrusive measurement: A measurement procedure that does not involve interacting with participants.

Unrepresentative outcome: An external validity threat presented by not being able to observe the outcome similarly outside the research context.

Unrepresentative setting: An external validity threat presented by the setting differing from the setting to which results will be generalized.

Unrepresentative treatment: An external validity threat presented by it not being feasible to implement an experimental treatment similarly outside the research context.

Unrepresentative units: An external validity threat presented by the units of study not representing the units of generalization.

Unstructured interview: A guided conversation that proceeds naturally and interactively to explore relevant topics from the participant's perspective. Also called an "in-depth interview."

Variable: An attribute of an observation whose quality or quantity may change (vary) from one observation to another, either across observation units and/or within units across time.

Variable chart: Specifies the mode, timing, and measurement protocol for each variable.

Variable list: Specifies the independent, dependent, moderator, and mediator variables, as appropriate.

Variance: A measure of dispersion computed as the arithmetic average of the squared deviations from the mean.

Vulnerable population: Individuals who are vulnerable to manipulation owing to reasons such as diminished cognitive capacity, a power differential, or a lack of resources. The Common Rule specifies that special protections should be provided for such individuals.

Wait-list control condition: If an experimental treatment/intervention demonstrates a positive outcome it subsequently is provided to the control group participants.

Wave: An observation point in a longitudinal research design.

Web survey: Respondents are provided a link to a website to complete and submit the questionnaire online. Also called an "internet survey."

Within-cluster homogeneity: In cluster random sampling, the degree of similarity among elements within a cluster. Also see *design effect*.

• References •

AAPOR Big Data Task Force. (2015). *AAPOR report: Big data*. American Association for Public Opinion Research. Retrieved from https://www.aapor.org/Education-Resources/Reports/Big-Data.aspx

Ajzen, I. (1991). The theory of planned behavior. *Organizational Behavior and Human Decision Processes, 50*, 179–211.

Allison, P. D. (2010). Missing data. In P. V. Marsden & J. D. Wright (Eds.), *Handbook of survey research* (2nd ed., pp. 631–657). Bingley, UK: Emerald Group.

American Association for Public Opinion Research. (2016). *Standard definitions: Final dispositions of case codes and outcome rates for surveys* (9th ed.). Retrieved from http://www.aapor.org/AAPOR_Main/media/publications/Standard-Definitions20169theditionfinal.pdf

Baker, F. B. (2001). *The basics of item response theory*. College Park, MD: ERIC Clearinghouse on Assessment and Evaluation. Retrieved from http://echo.edres.org:8080/irt/baker/final.pdf

Bandura, A. (2001). Social cognitive theory: An agentic perspective. *Annual Review of Psychology, 52*, 1–26.

Bao, Y., Bertoia, M. L., Lenart, E. B., Stampfer, M. J., Willett, W. C., Speizer, F. E., & Chavarro, J. E. (2016). Origin, methods, and evolution of the three Nurses' Health Studies. *American Journal of Public Health, 106*(9), 1573–1581.

Barber-Parker, E. D. (2002). Integrating patient teaching into bedside patient care: A participant-observation study of hospital nurses. *Patient Education and Counseling, 48*, 107–113.

Barbour, R. (2014). *Introducing qualitative research: A student's guide* (2nd ed.). Thousand Oaks, CA: Sage.

Baron, R. M., & Kenny, D. A. (1986). The moderator-mediator variable distinction in social psychological research: Conceptual, strategic, and statistical considerations. *Journal of Personality and Social Psychology, 5*(6), 1173–1182.

Beatty, P. C., & Willis, G. B. (2007). Research synthesis: The practice of cognitive interviewing. *Public Opinion Quarterly, 71*, 287–311.

Bell, B. A., Onwuegbuzie, A. J., Ferron, J. M., Jiao, Q. G., Hibbard, S. T., & Kromrev, J. D. (2012). Use of design effects and sample weights in complex health survey data: A review of published articles using data from 3 commonly used adolescent health surveys. *American Journal of Public Health, 102*(7), 1399–1405.

Bernard, H. R. (2000). *Social research methods: Qualitative and quantitative approaches*. Thousand Oaks, CA: Sage.

Blair, J., Czaja, R. F., & Blair, E. A. (2014). *Designing surveys: A guide to decisions and procedures*. Los Angeles, CA: Sage.

Blumberg, S. J., & Luke, J. V. (2017, December). *Wireless substitution: Early release of estimates from the National Health Interview Survey, January–June 2017*. National Center for Health Statistics. Retrieved from https://www.cdc.gov/nchs/data/nhis/earlyrelease/wireless201712.pdf

Bollen, K. (1989). *Structural equations with latent variables*. New York, NY: Wiley.

Bollen, K. A., & Barb, K. H. (1981). Pearson's r and coarsely categorized measures. *American Sociological Review, 46*(2), 232–239.

Booth, J., Davidson, I., Winstanley, J., & Waters, K. (2001). Observing washing and dressing of stroke patients: Nursing intervention compared with occupational therapists. What is the difference? *Journal of Advanced Nursing, 33*(1), 98–105.

Bradburn, N. M., Sudman, S., & Wansink, B. (2004). *Asking questions*. San Francisco, CA: Jossey-Bass.

Bruening, M., Adams, M. A., Ohri-Vachaspati, P., & Hurley, J. (2018). Prevalence and implementation practices of school salad bars across grade levels. *American Journal of Health Promotion, 32*(6), 1375–1382.

Buller, D. B., Walkosz, B. J., Buller, M. K., Wallis, A., Andersen, P. A., Scott, M. D., . . . Cutter, G. (2018). Results of a randomized trial on an intervention promoting adoption of occupational sun protection policies. *American Journal of Health Promotion, 32*(4), 1042–1053.

Butler, D. (2013). When Google got flu wrong. *Nature, 494*(February 14), 155–156.

Campbell, D. T., & Stanley, J. C. (1963). *Experimental and quasi-experimental designs for research.* Chicago, IL: Rand McNally.

Cannell, C. F., Fowler, F. J., & Marquis, K. H. (1968). The influence of interviewer and respondent psychological and behavioral variables on the reporting of household interviews. National Center for Health Statistics. Vital and Health Statistics, Series 2, No. 26.

Caraballo, R. S., Giovino, G. A., Pechacek, T. F., & Mowery, P. D. (2001). Factors associated with discrepancies between self-reports on cigarette smoking and measured serum cotinine levels among persons aged 17 years or older: Third National Health and Nutrition Examination Survey, 1988–1994. *American Journal of Epidemiology, 153*(8), 807–814.

Centers for Disease Control and Prevention. (2012). Cancer screening—United States, 2010. *MMWR, 61*(3), 41–45.

Centers for Disease Control and Prevention. (2015). *Community health assessments & health improvement plans.* Retrieved from https://www.cdc.gov/stltpublichealth/cha/plan.html

Centers for Disease Control and Prevention. (2016). *Behavioral Risk Factor Surveillance System (BRFSS) questionnaire.* Retrieved from https://www.cdc.gov/brfss/questionnaires/pdf-ques/2016brfss_questionnaire_10_14_15.pdf

Centers for Disease Control and Prevention. (2018a). *Behavioral Risk Factor Surveillance System.* Retrieved from https://www.cdc.gov/brfss/index.html

Centers for Disease Control and Prevention. (2018b). *BRFSS: Graph of current binge drinking among adults.* Retrieved from https://chronicdata.cdc.gov/Behavioral-Risk-Factors/BRFSS-Graph-of-Current-Binge-Drinking-among-adults/xnuv-rv9p

Centers for Disease Control and Prevention. (2018c). *BRFSS questionnaires.* Retrieved from https://www.cdc.gov/brfss/questionnaires/index.htm

Centers for Disease Control and Prevention. (2018d). *Longitudinal studies of aging.* National Center for Health Statistics and National Institute on Aging. Retrieved from https://www.cdc.gov/nchs/lsoa/index.htm

Centers for Disease Control and Prevention. (2018e). *National Health Interview Survey.* Retrieved from https://www.cdc.gov/nchs/nhis/index.htm

Centers for Disease Control and Prevention. (2018f). *National Health Interview Survey: NHIS data, questionnaires and related documentation.* Retrieved from https://www.cdc.gov/nchs/nhis/data-questionnaires-documentation.htm

Centers for Disease Control and Prevention. (2018g). *National Health and Nutrition Examination Survey.* Retrieved from https://www.cdc.gov/nchs/nhanes/index.htm

Champion, V. L. (1999). Revised susceptibility, benefits, and barriers scale for mammography screening. *Research in Nursing & Health, 22*, 341–348.

Cochran, W. G. (1963). *Sampling techniques.* New York, NY: Wiley.

Cohen, J. (1960). A coefficient of agreement for nominal scales. *Educational and Psychological Measurement, 20*(1), 37–46.

Cohen, J. (1988). *Statistical power analysis for the behavioral sciences.* Hillsdale, NJ: Erlbaum.

Cohen, J. (1992). A power primer. *Psychological Bulletin, 112*(1), 155–159.

Community Commons. (2016). *Community Health Needs Assessment.* Retrieved from https://www.communitycommons.org/chna/

Cook, T. D., & Campbell, D. T. (1979). *Quasi-experimentation: Design and analysis issues for field settings.* Boston, MA: Houghton Mifflin.

CONSORT. (2010). *The CONSORT statement.* Retrieved from http://www.consort-statement.org/

Couper, M. P. (2008). *Designing effective web surveys.* Cambridge, UK: Cambridge University Press.

Couper, M. P. (2013). Is the sky falling? New technology, changing media, and the future of surveys. *Survey Research Methods, 7*(3), 145–156.

Cox, E. P. (1980). The optimal number of response alternatives for a scale: A review. *Journal of Marketing Research, 17*(4), 407–422.

Cranford, J. A., McCabe, S. E., & Boyd, C. J. (2006). A new measure of binge drinking: Prevalence and correlates in a probability sample of undergraduates. *Alcoholism Clinical & Experimental Research, 30*(11), 1896–1905.

Creswell, J. W. (2015). *A concise introduction to mixed methods research.* Thousand Oaks, CA: Sage.

Creswell, J. W, & Plano Clark, V. L. (2011). *Designing and conducting mixed methods research* (2nd ed.). Thousand Oaks, CA: Sage.

CUBIT: Demographic data nerds. (2018). Retrieved from https://www.cubitplanning.com/data/quick-reports

Daas, P. J. H., & Puts, M. J. H. (2014). Big data as a source of statistical information. *The Survey Statistician, 69*(January), 22–31.

de Leeuw, E. D. (2005). To mix or not to mix data collection modes in surveys. *Journal of Official Statistics*, *21*(2), 233–255.

Dillman, D. A., Smyth, J. D., & Christian, L. M. (2014). *Internet, phone, mail, and mixed-mode surveys: The tailored design method.* Hoboken, NJ: Wiley.

Edwards, B. (2015). Cross-cultural considerations in health surveys. In T. P. Johnson (Ed.), *Handbook of health survey methods* (pp. 243–274). Hoboken, NJ: Wiley.

Federal Interagency Working Group on Improving Measurement of Sexual Orientation and Gender Identity in Federal Surveys. (2016). *Current measures of sexual orientation and gender identity in federal surveys.* Retrieved from https://s3.amazonaws.com/sitesusa/wp-content/uploads/sites/242/2014/04/WorkingGroupPaper1_CurrentMeasures_08-16.pdf

Flay, B. R. (1986). Efficacy and effectiveness trials (and other phases of research) in the development of health promotion programs. *Preventive Medicine*, *15*, 451–474.

Flay, B. R., Biglan, A., Boruch, R. F., Castro, F. G., Gottfredson, D., Kellam, S., . . . Ji, P. (2005). Standards of evidence: Criteria for efficacy, effectiveness and dissemination. *Prevention Science*, *6*(3), 151–175.

Forrestal, S. G., Issel, L. M., Kviz, F. J., & Chávez, N. (2008). Validating a children's self-report plate waste questionnaire. *Journal of Child Nutrition & Management*, *32*(2), 1–12.

Fredericks, S., Martorella, G., & Catallo, C. (2015). A systematic review of web-based educational interventions. *Clinical Nursing Research*, *24*(1), 91–113.

Glaser, B. G., & Strauss, A. L. (1967). *The discovery of grounded theory: Strategies for qualitative research.* Chicago, IL: Aldine.

Goldberg, A. E., & Allen, K. R. (2015). Communicating qualitative research: Some practical guideposts for scholars. *Journal of Marriage and Family*, *77*, 3–22.

Google Flu Trends. (2018). Accessed May 28, 2018 at: https://www.google.org/flutrends/about/.

Google Search Statistics. (2018). Retrieved from http://www.internetlivestats.com/google-search-statistics/

Greenberg-Seth, J., Hemenway, D., Gallagher, S. S., Ross, J. B., & Lissy, K. S. (2004). Evaluation of a community-based intervention to promote rear seating for children. *American Journal of Public Health*, *94*, 1009–1013.

Greifinger, R., St. Louis, G., Lunstead, J., Malik, N., & Vibbert, M. (2013). Participant observation at a youth HIV conference. *Qualitative Social Work*, *13*(2), 237–254.

Grivios-Shah, R., Gonzalez, J. R., Khandekar, S. P., Howerter, A. L., O'Connor, P. A., & Edwards, B. A. (2018). Impact of healthy vending machine options in a large community health organization. *American Journal of Health Promotion*, *32*(6), 1425–1430.

Gross, D., & Fogg, L. (2004). A critical analysis of the intent-to-treat principle in prevention research. *The Journal of Primary Prevention*, *25*(4), 475–489.

Groves, R. M. (2011). Three eras of survey research. *Public Opinion Quarterly*, *75*(5), 861–871.

Groves, R. M., Fowler, F. J., Jr., Couper, M. P., Lepkowski, J. M., Singer, E., & Tourangeau, R. (2009). *Survey methodology* (2nd ed.). Hoboken, NJ: Wiley.

Guba, E. G. (1981). Criteria for assessing the trustworthiness of naturalistic inquiries. *Educational Communication and Technology*, *29*(2), 75–91.

Guthrie, B., Auerback, G., & Bindman, A. B. (2010). Health plan competition for Medicaid enrollees based on performance does not improve quality of care. *Health Affairs*, *29*(8), 1507–1516.

Hanson, T. (2015). Comparing agreement and item-specific response scales: Results from an experiment. *Social Research Practice*, *1*, 17–25.

Harkness, J. A., Braun, M., Edwards, B., Johnson, T. P., Lyberg, L. E., Mohler, P., . . . Smith, T. W. (2010). Comparative survey methodology. In J. A. Harkness et al. (Eds.), *Survey methods in multinational, multiregional, and multicultural contexts* (pp. 3–16). Hoboken, NJ: Wiley.

Harkness, J. A., Pennell, B.-E., & Schoua-Glusberg, A. (2004). Survey questionnaire translation and assessment. In S. Presser et al. (Eds.), *Methods for testing and evaluating survey questionnaires* (pp. 453–473). Hoboken, NJ: Wiley.

Hayes, A. F. (2009). Beyond Baron and Kenny: Statistical mediation analysis in the new millennium. *Communication Monographs*, *76*(4), 408–420.

Health and Psychosocial Instruments (HaPI). (2018). Retrieved from https://www.ebscohost.com/academic/health-and-psychosocial-instruments-hapi

Heckathorn, D. D. (1997). Respondent-driven sampling: A new approach to the study of hidden populations. *Social Problems*, *44*(2), 174–199.

Heckathorn, D. D. (2002). Respondent-driven sampling II: Deriving valid population estimates from chain-referral samples of hidden populations. *Social Problems*, *49*(1), 11–34.

Hill, A. B. (1965). The environment and disease: Association or causation? *Proceedings of the Royal Society of Medicine, 58*(5), 295–300.

Holbrook, A. L., Krosnick, J. A., Carson, R. T., & Mitchell, R. C. (2000). Violating conversational conventions disrupts cognitive processing of attitude questions. *Journal of Experimental Social Psychology, 36*, 465–494.

Holland, P. W. (1986). Statistics and causal inference. *Journal of the American Statistical Association, 81*(396), 945–960.

Hoyle, R. H., Harris, M. J., & Judd, C. M. (2002). *Research methods in social relations* (7th ed.). Belmont, CA: Wadsworth Thomson Learning.

Hsu, C. C., & Sandford, B. A. (2007). The Delphi technique: Making sense of consensus. *Practical Assessment, Research & Evaluation, 12*(10), 1–8.

Iannacchione, V. G. (2011). Research synthesis: The changing role of address-based sampling in survey research. *Public Opinion Quarterly, 75*, 556–575.

Iannacchione, V. G., Staab, J. M., & Redden, D. T. (2003). Evaluating the use of residential mailing addresses in a metropolitan household survey. *Public Opinion Quarterly, 67*, 202–210.

International Committee of Medical Journal Editors. (2018a). *Author responsibilities—Conflicts of interest*. Retrieved from http://www.icmje.org/recommendations/browse/roles-and-responsibilities/author-responsibilities-conflicts-of-interest.html#two

International Committee of Medical Journal Editors. (2018b). *Defining the role of authors and contributors*. Retrieved from http://www.icmje.org/recommendations/browse/roles-and-responsibilities/defining-the-role-of-authors-and-contributors.html

Janz, N. K., & Becker, M. H. (1984). The Health Belief Model: A decade later. *Health Education Quarterly, 11*(1), 1–47.

Johnson, R. B., & Onwuegbuzie, A. J. (2004). Mixed methods research: A research paradigm whose time has come. *Educational Researcher, 33*(7), 14–26.

Johnson, R. B., Onwuegbuzie, A. J., & Turner, L. A. (2007). Toward a definition of mixed methods research. *Journal of Mixed Methods Research, 1*(2), 112–133.

Jones, S. R. G. (1992). Was there a Hawthorne effect? *American Journal of Sociology, 98*(3), 451–468.

Kahn Academy. (2018). *Why we divide by $n-1$ in variance*. Retrieved from https://www.khanacademy.org/math/ap-statistics/summarizing-quantitative-data-ap/more-standard-deviation/v/another-simulation-giving-evidence-that-n-1-gives-us-an-unbiased-estimate-of-variance

Kish, L. (1965). *Survey sampling*. New York, NY: Wiley.

Krosnick, J. A. (1991). Response strategies for coping with the cognitive demands of attitude measures in surveys. *Applied Cognitive Psychology, 5*, 213–236.

Krosnick, J. A. (1999). Survey research. *Annual Review of Psychology, 50*, 537–567.

Krosnick, J. A., & Fabrigar, L. R. (1997). Designing rating scales for effective measurement in surveys. In L. Lyberg et al. (Eds.), *Survey measurement and process quality* (pp. 141–164). New York, NY: Wiley.

Krosnick, J. A., & Presser, S. (2010). Question and questionnaire design. In P. V. Marsden & J. D. Wright (Eds.), *Handbook of survey research* (2nd ed., pp. 263–313). Bingley, UK: Emerald Group.

Krueger, R. A., & Casey, M. A. (2015). *Focus groups: A practical guide for applied research* (5th ed.). x Thousand Oaks, CA: Sage.

Kviz, F. J. (1977). Toward a standard definition of response rate. *Public Opinion Quarterly, 41*, 265–267.

Kviz, F. J., Cho, Y. I., Johnson, T. P., Willgerodt, M. A., Clark, M. A., Chavez, N., . . . Freels, S. (2003). Korean American men's perceptions about smoking-related symptomatology: Implications for intervention. *Korean and Korean American Studies Bulletin, 13*, 71–83.

Lachin, J. M. (2000). Statistical considerations in the intent-to-treat principle. *Controlled Clinical Trials, 21*, 167–189.

Lavrakas, P. J. (2008). Surveys by telephone. In W. Donsbach & M. W. Traugott (Eds.), *The Sage handbook of survey research* (pp. 249–261). Los Angeles, CA: Sage.

Lavrakas, P. J. (2010). Telephone surveys. In P. V. Marsden & J. D. Wright (Eds.), *Handbook of survey research* (2nd ed., pp. 471–498). Bingley, UK: Emerald Group.

Lazer, D. M., Kennedy, R., King, G., & Vespignani, A. (2014). The parable of Google flu: Traps in big data analysis. *Science, 343*(6176), 1203–1205.

Lee, E., Menon, U., Nandy, K., Szalacha, L., Kviz, F., Cho, Y., . . . Park, H. (2014). The effect of a couples intervention to increase breast cancer screening among Korean Americans. *Oncology Nursing Forum, 41*(3), E185–E193.

Leung, B., Lauche, R., Leach, M., Zhang, Y., Cramer, H., & Sibbritt, D. (2018). Special diets in modern America: Analysis of the 2012 National Health Interview Survey data. *Nutrition and Health, 24*(1), 11–18.

Levine, B., & Harter, R. (2015). Optimal allocation of cell-phone and landline respondents in dual-frame surveys. *Public Opinion Quarterly, 79,* 91–104.

Likert, R. (1932). A technique for the measurement of attitudes. *Archives of Psychology, 22*(140), 3–55.

Lincoln, Y. S., & Guba, E. G. (1985). *Naturalistic inquiry.* Beverly Hills, CA: Sage.

Lippold, M. A., Greenberg, M. T., Graham, J. W., & Feinberg, M. E. (2014). Unpacking the effect of parental monitoring on early adolescent problem behavior: Mediation by parental knowledge and moderation by parent–youth warmth. *Journal of Family Issues, 35*(13), 1800–1823.

Little, R. J., D'Agostino, R., Cohen, M. L., Dickersin, K., Emerson, S. S., Farrar, J. T., . . . Stern, H. (2012). The prevention and treatment of missing data in clinical trials. *New England Journal of Medicine, 367*(14), 1355–1360.

Liu, M., & Keusch, F. (2017). Effects of scale direction on response style of ordinal rating scales. *Journal of Official Statistics, 33*(1), 137–154.

Magnani, R., Sabin, K., Saidel, T., & Heckathorn, D. (2005). Review of sampling hard-to-reach and hidden populations for HIV surveillance. *AIDS, 19*(suppl. 2), S67–S72.

Malhotra, N., Krosnick, J. A., & Thomas, R. K. (2009). Optimal design of branching questions to measure bipolar constructs. *Public Opinion Quarterly, 73*(2), 304–324.

Marshall, G. N., & Hays, R. D. (1994). *The patient satisfaction questionnaire short form* (PSQ-18). P-7865. Sana Monica, CA: RAND.

Mayoh, J., Bond, C. S., & Todres, L. (2012). An innovative mixed methods approach to studying the online health information seeking experiences of adults with chronic health conditions. *Journal of Mixed Methods Research, 6*(1) 21–33.

McDowell, I. (2006). *Measuring health: A guide to rating scales and questionnaires* (3rd ed.). New York, NY: Oxford University Press.

McDowell, I., & Newell, C. (1996). *Measuring health: A guide to rating scales and questionnaires* (2nd ed.). New York, NY: Oxford University Press.

McLeroy, K. R., Bibeau, D., Steckler, A., & Glanz, K. (1988). An ecological perspective on health promotion programs. *Health Education Quarterly, 15*(4), 351–377.

Measurement Instrument Database for the Social Sciences (MIDSS). (n.d.). Retrieved from http://www.midss.org/

Mercer, S. L., De Vinney, B. L., Fine, L. J., Green, L. W., & Dougherty, D. (2007). Study designs for effectiveness and translation research: Identifying trade-offs. *American Journal of Preventive Medicine, 33*(2), 139–154.

Miller, G. A. (1956). The magical number seven, plus or minus two: Some limits on our capacity for processing information. *The Psychological Review, 63*(2), 81–97.

Moher, D., Shamseer, L., Clarke, M., Ghersi, D., Liberati, A., Petticrew, M., . . . PRISMA-P Group. (2015). Preferred reporting items for systematic review and meta-analysis protocols (PRISMA-P) 2015 statement. *Systematic Reviews, 4*(1). Retrieved from https://systematicreviewsjournal.biomedcentral.com/articles/10.1186/2046-4053-4-1

Morera, O. F., & Stokes, S. M. (2016). Coefficient α as a measure of test score reliability: Review of 3 popular misconceptions. *American Journal of Public Health, 106*(3), 458–461.

Morgan, D. L. (1998). Practical strategies for combining qualitative and quantitative methods: Applications to health research. *Qualitative Health Research, 8*(3), 362–376.

Morse, J. M. (1991). Approaches to qualitative-quantitative methodological triangulation. *Nursing Research, 40*(1), 120–123.

Muller, D., Judd, C. M., & Yzerbyt, V. Y. (2005). When moderation is mediated and mediation is moderated. *Journal of Personality and Social Psychology, 89*(6), 852–863.

National Cancer Institute. (2018). *Breast cancer prevention.* Retrieved from https://www.cancer.gov/types/breast/hp/breast-prevention-pdq#section/_1

National Commission for the Protection of Human Subjects of Biomedical and Behavioral Research. (1979). *The Belmont Report: Ethical principles and guidelines for the protection of human subjects of research.* Washington, DC: US Government Printing Office. Retrieved from http://www.hhs.gov/ohrp/humansubjects/guidance/belmont.html

National Health Information Center. (2018). *2018 national health observances.* Retrieved from https://healthfinder.gov/NHO/nho.aspx

National Institute on Alcohol Abuse and Alcoholism. (2004). NIAAA council approves definition of binge drinking. *NIAAA Newsletter,* No. 3. Bethesda, MD: Author.

National Institute on Alcohol Abuse and Alcoholism. (2007, January). Alcohol and tobacco. *Alcohol Alert,* No. 71. Retrieved from https://pubs.niaaa.nih.gov/publications/AA71/AA71.htm

National Longitudinal Study of Adolescent to Adult Health. (n.d.). *Study design.* Retrieved from http://www.cpc.unc.edu/projects/addhealth/design

Nicolaas, G., Campanelli, P., Hope, S., Jäckle, A., & Lynn, P. (2015). Revisiting "yes/no" versus "check all that apply": Results from a mixed modes experiment. *Survey Research Methods*, *9*(3), 189–204.

Nicolaas, G., Smith, P., & Pickering, I. (2015). Increasing response rates in postal surveys while controlling costs: An experimental investigation. *Social Research Practice*, *1*, 3–16.

Nurses' Health Study. (2018). Retrieved from http://www.nurseshealthstudy.org/

Ongena, Y. P., & Dijkstra, W. (2006). Methods of behavior coding of survey interviews. *Journal of Official Statistics*, *22*(3), 419–451.

Partin, M. R., Grill, J., Noorbaloochi, S., Powell, A. A., Burgess, D. J., Vernon, S. W., . . . Fisher, D. A. (2008). Validation of self-reported colorectal cancer screening behavior from a mixed-mode survey of veterans. *Cancer Epidemiology Biomarkers & Prevention*, *17*(4), 768–776.

Patton, M. Q. (2015). *Qualitative research & evaluation methods: Integrating theory and practice* (4th ed.). Thousand Oaks, CA: Sage.

Payne, S. L. (1951). *The art of asking questions*. Princeton, NJ: Princeton University Press.

The RAND Corporation. (2001). *A million random digits with 100,000 normal deviates*. Retrieved from http://www.rand.org/pubs/monograph_reports/MR1418.html

RAND Health. (n.d.). *Patient satisfaction questionnaire from RAND Health*. Retrieved from https://www.rand.org/health/surveys_tools/psq.html

Rasinski, K. A., Mingay, D., & Bradburn, N. M. (1994). Do respondents really "mark all that apply" on self-administered questions? *Public Opinion Quarterly*, *58*(3), 400–408.

Rebagliato, M. (2002). Validation of self reported smoking. *Journal of Epidemiology & Community Health*, *56*(3), 163–164.

Research Randomizer. (2018). Retrieved from https://www.randomizer.org

Revilla, M. A., Saris, W. E., & Krosnick, J. A. (2014). Choosing the number of categories in agree–disagree scales. *Sociological Methods & Research*, *43*(1), 73–97.

Robinson, W. S. (1950). Ecological correlations and the behavior of individuals. *American Sociological Review*, *15*(3), 351–357.

Roethlisberger, F. J., & Dickson, W. J. (1939) *Management and the worker*. Cambridge, MA: Harvard University Press.

Rosenstock, I. M., Strecher, V. J., & Becker, M. H. (1988). Social learning theory and the health belief model. *Health Education Quarterly*, *15*(2), 175–183.

Rothman, K. J. (1976). Reviews and commentary: Causes. *American Journal of Epidemiology*, *104*(6), 587–592.

Saldaña, J., & Omasta, M. (2018). *Qualitative research: Analyzing life*. Thousand Oaks, CA: Sage.

Saris, W. E., Revilla, M., Krosnick, J. A., & Shaeffer, E. M. (2010). Comparing questions with agree/disagree response options to questions with item-specific response options. *Survey Research Methods*, *4*(1), 61–79.

Savage, M., & Burrows, R. (2007). The coming crisis of empirical sociology. *Sociology*, *41*(5), 885–899.

Schaeffer, N. C., & Presser, S. (2003). The science of asking questions. *Annual Review of Sociology*, *29*, 65–88.

Schuman, H., & Presser, S. (1977). Question wording as an independent variable in survey analysis. *Sociological Methods & Research*, *6*(2), 151–170.

Schwarz, N. (1999). Self-reports: How the questions shape the answers. *American Psychologist*, *54*(2), 93–105.

Schwarz, N., Knauper, B., Hippler, H. J., Noelle-Neumann, E., & Clark, L. (1991). Rating scales: Numeric values may change the meaning of scale labels. *Public Opinion Quarterly*, *55*(4), 570–582.

Shadish, W. R., Cook, T. D., & Campbell, D. T. (2002). *Experimental and quasi-experimental designs for generalized causal inference*. Boston, MA: Houghton Mifflin.

Shenton, A. K. (2004). Strategies for ensuring trustworthiness in qualitative research projects. *Education for Information*, *22*, 63–75.

Simons, H. R., Unger, Z. D., Lopez, P. M., & Kohn, J. E. (2015). Predictors of human papillomavirus vaccine completion among female and male vaccine initiators in family planning centers. *American Journal of Public Health*, *105*(12):2541–2548.

Singer, E. A., & Ye, C. (2013). The use and effects of incentives in surveys. *The ANNALS of the American Academy of Political and Social Science*, *645*(January), 112–141.

Small, M. L. (2011). How to conduct a mixed methods study: Recent trends in a rapidly growing literature. *Annual Review of Sociology*, *37*, 57–86.

SRNT Subcommittee on Biochemical Verification. (2002). Biochemical verification of tobacco use and cessation. *Nicotine & Tobacco Research*, *4*(2), 149–159.

Stafford, F. P. (2010). Panel surveys: Conducting surveys over time. In P. V. Marsden & J. D. Wright (Eds.), *Handbook of survey research* (pp. 765–193). Bingley, UK: Emerald.

Steckler, A., & McLeroy, K. R. (2008). The importance of external validity. *American Journal of Public Health*, *98*(1), 9–10.

Stewart, D. W., & Shamdasani, P. M. (2015). *Focus groups: Theory and practice* (3rd ed.). Thousand Oaks, CA: Sage.

Streiner, D. L., & Norman, G. R. (1995). *Health measurement scales: A practical guide to their development and use.* Oxford, UK: Oxford University Press.

Sudman, S., & Bradburn, N. M. (1982). *Asking questions: A practical guide to questionnaire design.* San Francisco, CA: Jossey Bass.

Susser, M. (1973). *Causal thinking in the health sciences: Concepts and strategies of epidemiology.* New York, NY: Oxford University Press.

Sutton, J., & Austin, Z. (2015). Qualitative research: Data collection, analysis, and management. *The Canadian Journal of Hospital Pharmacy*, *68*(3), 226–231.

Tate, J. A., & Happ, M. B. (2018). Qualitative secondary analysis: A case exemplar. *Journal of Pediatric Health Care*, *32*(3), 308–312.

Teddlie, C., & Tashakkori, A. (2006). A general typology of research designs featuring mixed methods. *Research in the Schools*, *13*(1), 12–28.

Thangaratinam, S., & Redman, W. E. (2005). The Delphi technique. *The Obstetrician & Gynaecologist*, *7*, 120–125.

Tourangeau, R., Rips, L. J., & Rasinski, K. (2000). *The psychology of survey response.* New York, NY: Cambridge University Press.

Tourangeau, R., & Yan, T. (2007). Sensitive questions in surveys. *Psychological Bulletin*, *133*, 859–883.

UK Data Service. (2018). *QualiBank.* Retrieved from https://discover.ukdataservice.ac.uk/QualiBank

U.S. Department of Education. (n.d.). *Family Educational Rights and Privacy Act (FERPA).* Retrieved from https://www2.ed.gov/policy/gen/guid/fpco/ferpa/index.html

U.S. Department of Health and Human Services. (1993). *Institutional review board guidebook, chapter III, section D.* Retrieved from http://wayback.archive-it.org/org-745/20150930182812/http://www.hhs.gov/ohrp/archive/irb/irb_chapter3.htm

U.S. Department of Health and Human Services. (2015). *Health information privacy: The HIPAA Privacy Rule.* Retrieved from http://www.hhs.gov/ocr/privacy/hipaa/administrative/privacyrule

U.S. Department of Health and Human Services, National Institutes of Health. (2000). *Required education in the protection of human research participants.* Retrieved from http://grants.nih.gov/grants/guide/notice-files/NOT-OD-00-039.html

U.S. Department of Health and Human Services, National Institutes of Health. (2017). *Certificates of Confidentiality (CoC).* Retrieved from http://grants.nih.gov/grants/policy/coc/index.htm

U.S. Department of Health and Human Services, Office of Disease Prevention and Health Promotion. (2014, March). *Healthy People 2020 leading health indicators: Progress update.* Retrieved from https://www.healthypeople.gov/sites/default/files/LHI-ProgressReport-ExecSum_0.pdf

U.S. Department of Health and Human Services, Office of Disease Prevention and Health Promotion. (2018). *Healthy People 2020: Tobacco.* Retrieved from http://www.healthypeople.gov/2020/leading-health-indicators/2020-lhi-topics/Tobacco

U.S. Department of Health and Human Services, Office for Human Research Protections. (2017). *NPRM for revisions to the Common Rule.* Retrieved from http://www.hhs.gov/ohrp/humansubjects/regulations/nprmhome.html

U.S. Department of Health and Human Services, Office for Human Research Protections. (2018). *Code of Federal Regulations*, Title 45 Part 46. Retrieved from https://www.hhs.gov/ohrp/regulations-and-policy/regulations/45-cfr-46/index.html

U.S. Department of Health and Human Services, Office of the Surgeon General. (2016). *E-Cigarette Use Among Youth and Young Adults.* Retrieved from https://e-cigarettes.surgeongeneral.gov/documents/2016_SGR_Exec_Summ_508.pdf

U.S. National Library of Medicine. (2018). *Medical Subject Headings (MeSH).* Retrieved from https://www.nlm.nih.gov/mesh/meshhome.html

VanFrank, B. K., Park, S., Foltz, J. L., McGuire, L. C., & Harris, D. M. (2018). Physician characteristics associated with sugar-sweetened beverage counseling practices. *American Journal of Health Promotion*, *32*(6), 1365–1374.

Vartiainen, E., Seppälä, T., Lillsunde, P., & Puska, P. (2002). Validation of self reported smoking. *Journal of Epidemiology & Community Health*, *56*(3), 167–170.

Vasudevan, V., Rimmer, J. H., & Kviz, F. J. (2015). Development of the Barriers to Physical Activity Questionnaire for people with mobility impairments. *Disability and Health Journal*, *8*, 547–556.

Velicer, W. F., Prochaska, J. O., Rossi, J. S., & Snow, M. G. (1992). Assessing outcome in smoking cessation studies. *Psychological Bulletin, 111*(1), 23–41.

Velozo, C. A., Forsyth, K., & Kielhofner, G. (2006). Objective measurement: The influence of item response theory on research and practice. In G. Kielhofner (Ed.), *Research in occupational therapy: Methods of inquiry for enhancing practice* (pp. 177–200). Philadelphia, PA: F. A. Davis.

Wiklander, M., Rydström, L.-L., Ygge, B.-M., Navér, L., Wettergren, L., & Eriksson, L. E. (2013). Psychometric properties of a short version of the HIV stigma scale, adapted for children with HIV infection. *Health and Quality of Life Outcomes, 11*, 195. Retrieved from https://www.ncbi.nlm.nih.gov/pmc/articles/PMC3842678/

Willis, G. B. (2005). *Cognitive interviewing: A tool for improving questionnaire design.* Thousand Oaks, CA: Sage.

Zeller, R. A., & Carmines, E. G. (1980). *Measurement in the social sciences: The link between theory and data.* Cambridge, UK: Cambridge University Press.

Zephoria Digital Marketing. (2018). The top 20 valuable Facebook statistics—updated October 2018. Retrieved from https://zephoria.com/top-15-valuable-facebook-statistics/

Index

Abbreviations (survey questions), 277
Abstract, 415–416
Acquiescence bias, 228
Address-based sampling (ABS), 321
Advisory panel, 4
Alpha, 406
Alpha error, 408–409
Alternate forms reliability, 206–208
American Association for Public Opinion Research (AAPOR), 312
American College of Cardiology, 51
American Journal of Health Promotion, 415
Analytical design, 149
Anonymity:
    collecting identifiers, 40
    data collection evaluation, 41–42
    data linkages, 42
    data verification, 42
    de-identification of data, 40
    ethical research, 39–43
    follow-up contacts, 41
    identifiers, 39–43
    item nonresponse, 42
    missing data recovery, 42
    payment to subjects, 42
    prenotification strategy, 40, 41 (box)
    recording identifiers, 40
    scheduling subjects, 41
    sharing results, 43
    tracking subjects, 42
ATLAS.ti, 340, 410
Attention-placebo condition, 92
Attrition:
    research design diagrams, 96, 98–99
    strategy for, 116–117
    as validity threat, 107 (box), 109–110
Attrition bias, 110
Atypical case sample, 360
Audio computer-assisted self-interview (ACASI), 316

Back-translation technique, 227
Banner Health, 3 (box)
Basic random selection, 165
Behavior coding, 250, 252
Belmont Report, 26, 27, 29, 30–31, 33
Beneficence principle, 26, 27–28

Beta error, 408–409
Biased survey questions, 283–285
Big data, 371–372, 379, 380 (box)
Bipolar scale, 228–229, 230 (box), 236 (box)
Bivariate regression analysis, 405
Blinding strategy, 4–5
Block randomization, 181, 182–183, 184*t*
Branching strategy, 231

Case-control design, 149
Causal design, 104–105, 106 (box), 140–152
Causal relationships, 54–79
Cause, 54–55
Central limit theorem, 162
Central tendency measures, 403
Certainty cluster, 175
Certificate of Confidentiality (CoC), 45
Chain referral sample, 361
Check-coding, 393
Classical experimental design, 143
Classical test theory (CTT), 199
Closed question, 272, 273
Closed-response format, 244
Cluster, 173
Cluster random sampling, 173–177
Cluster size, 174
Codebook, 398, 399 (box), 400
Coding, 393, 394–397, 410–411
Cognitive interview, 247–248, 249 (box)
Cohen's Kappa, 205–206
Cohort study, 149–150
Collaborative Institutional Training Initiative (CITI), 32
Committee translation, 227
Common cause, 57–58
Common Rule, 29–31, 33–35, 38, 39
Compensatory equalization:
    strategy for, 122
    as validity threat, 120
Compensatory rivalry:
    strategy for, 122
    as validity threat, 120
Complementary concurrent design, 364
Completely-mediated causal relationship, 68, 69*f*
Completely open question, 274
Complete participant observation, 352, 353 (box)
Component causes, 56–57

451

Compound question, 281–282, 288–289
Computer-assisted in-person interview (CAPI), 315–316
Computer-assisted self-interview (CASI), 316
Computer-assisted surveys, 315–317
Computer-assisted telephone interview (CATI), 315
Computer software programs:
   ATLAS.ti, 340, 410
   NVivo, 340, 410
   qualitative data analysis, 410
   qualitative research methods, 340
   random sampling, 179
Conceptual approach, 14
Conceptual definition (measurement), 192–193
Conceptual framework, 7–8
Conceptualization (measurement), 192–193
Conceptual map, 412–413
Conclusions of research, 18
Concurrent criterion validity, 212–213
Concurrent mixed methods design, 364, 365 (box)
Conditions (research design), 84–85, 89–95
Confidence interval (CI), 163
Confidence level, 163
Confidentiality:
   Certificate of Confidentiality (CoC), 45
   deductive disclosure, 44
   disclosure by association, 44
   ethical research, 43–45
   inadvertent disclosure, 44
   limitations of, 45
   necessary information, 44–45
   nondisclosure, 44
   security, 43
   study-specific codes, 43
   subject identification codes, 43
Confirmability, 413
Confirmatory/generalizability sequential design, 364 (box), 366
Confounder variable, 59–60
Construct, 192–193
Construct-specific scale, 231–232
Construct validity, 214–215
Contact log, 323–324
Content validity, 211–212
Contingency analysis, 51, 404
Contingency table, 51, 52*t*
Continuous variable, 50–51
Control conditions, 4, 91–93
Control group, 4
Control group contamination, 98, 114, 119, 121
Control group model, 90, 91 (box)
Control of conditions, 6
Convened research, 31–32
Convenience sample, 361–362
Convergent mixed methods design, 364, 365 (box)

Convergent validity, 213–214
Correlation analysis, 404–405
Correlation coefficient, 54
Counterbalancing design, 152
Counterfactual condition, 90
Counterfactual model, 90
Covariation, 61–62
Coverage, 164
Covert observation, 356–357
Credibility, 413
Critical value, 406
Cronbach's coefficient alpha, 207–208
Cross-classification table, 51, 52*t*
Crossover design, 151–152
Cross-sectional design, 87–88, 136–137

Data analysis:
   check-coding process, 393
   codebook, 398, 399 (box), 400
   coding process, 393, 394–397
   combining categories, 395
   computer file preparation, 393–394
   computing variables, 396
   data cleaning, 393–394
   data entry, 393
   data preparation phase, 392–393
   data reduction phase, 392–393
   dummy coding, 395–396
   file documentation, 398, 399 (box), 400
   final frequencies review, 398
   imputation strategy, 396–397
   intent-to-treat strategy, 397
   modification/finalization phase, 394–400
   recoding variables, 394–397
   reliability assessment, 397
   in research process, 18, 392
   in research report, 418
   reverse coding, 395
   study exercise, 400, 424
   validity assessment, 397
   value labels, 394
   variable labels, 394
   variable names, 394
   weighting procedures, 397
   See also Qualitative data analysis; Quantitative data analysis; Research report; Secondary data analysis
Data cleaning, 393–394
Data collection:
   in research process, 17–18
   in research report, 418
Debriefing interview, 250–251
Deductive disclosure, 44
Deductive reasoning, 8–9

Deferred-treatment control condition, 91–92
De-identification of data, 40
Demoralization:
    strategy for, 122
    as validity threat, 120
Dependability, 413
Dependent variable, 54–55
Descriptive notes, 357–359
Design effect, 176–177
Deviant case sample, 360
Dichotomous classification, 195
Dichtomous-choice survey question, 292, 294
Difference-in-differences analysis, 97
Direct comparison, 196
Direct effect, 113
Direction of relationship, 52–53
Direct research benefit, 28
Direct research effect, 66, 69f
Disclosure by association, 44
Discrete variable, 50
Discriminant validity, 213–214
Dispersion measures, 403–404
Disproportionate allocation, 171–173
Distal outcomes, 67–68
Documents, 378
Double-banking format, 260–261
Double-barreled question, 281–282, 288–289
Double blind protocol, 5
Double negative (survey questions), 282
Dual frame sample, 164
Dummy coding, 395–396

E-Cigarette Use Among Youth and Young Adults, 416
Ecological fallacy, 60, 61f
Effect, 54–55
Effectiveness of treatment, 129
Effectiveness trials, 129, 130f
Efficacy of treatment, 129
Efficacy trials, 129, 130f
Element, 9–10, 159 (box)
Email survey, 310
Empirical assessment, 5
Endogenous variable, 56
EPSEM design. *See* Equal Probability Selection Method
Equal allocation, 171–172
Equal Probability Selection Method, 160
Equivalent groups, 107
Ethical research:
    anonymity, 39–43
    Belmont Report, 26, 27, 29, 30–31, 33
    beneficence principle, 26, 27–28
    Common Rule, 29–31, 33–35, 38, 39
    confidentiality, 43–45
    direct benefits, 28
    federal regulations, 29–38
    human subjects, 26–30
    identifiers, 39–43
    inclusion principle, 28–29
    indirect benefits, 28
    informed consent, 27, 33–38
    institutional review board (IRB), 30–32, 33, 34, 35, 38
    Internet resources, 32, 38, 45
    justice, 26, 28–29
    key personnel, 32
    minimal risk, 28
    nondisclosure, 44
    principle investigator, 32
    privacy, 39
    Privacy Rule of HIPPA (1996), 39
    private information, 39
    research, 26, 29–30
    respect for persons, 26–27, 33
    self-determination principle, 26–27
    sensitive topics, 35, 38
    study exercise, 29, 38, 45, 47
    subjects, 28
    training programs, 32
    treatment equality, 29
    vulnerable population, 27
Exclusion criteria, 16, 17 (box)
Executive summary, 416
Exempt research, 31–32
Exogenous variable, 55–56
Expected value, 162
Expedited research, 31–32
Experimental design, 143–146
Experimenter bias, 3–4
Explanatory sequential design, 364 (box), 366
Explanatory variable, 59–60
Exploratory research, 2
Exploratory sequential design, 364 (box), 365
External validity:
    causal design, 105, 106 (box)
    threats to, 123–129
Extraneous variable, 59–60
Extreme case sample, 360

Face validity, 209–211
Factorial design, 94–95
False negative, 93
False positive, 92
Family Educational Rights and Privacy Act (1974), 39
Field notes, 352, 357–359
Field pretest:
    of measurement instrument, 223–224
    of questionnaires, 248–252
Field sample size (FSS), 180
Fill-in-the-blank survey question, 291, 296

Filter question, 253, 266, 267 (box)
Finite population correction, 178
Focus group, 343t, 345–348
Follow-up mode, 314
Forced-choice method, 233
Frequency matching, 183
Full blind strategy, 4
Full disclosure, 5
Funnel sequence, 264–266

Going-native approach, 352–353
Google Dengue Trends, 380 (box)
Google Flu Trends, 380 (box)
G*Power software, 179
Gray literature, 384
Groups (research design), 83–85, 87–89

Hawthorne effect, 120
Health Belief Model, 7–8, 14, 15 (box), 63–64, 71, 74–75, 193, 194t
Health Insurance Portability and Accountability Act (1996), 39
Healthy People 2020 Leading Health Indicators, 416
Heterogeneous sample, 360
History:
    strategy for, 114–115
    as validity threat, 107 (box), 108–109
History effect, 87
Holistic perspective, 9
Homogeneous sample, 360
Human subjects, 26–30
Hypothesis, 405
Hypothesis testing, 405–409

Identifiers, 39–43
Imputation strategy, 396–397
Inadvertent disclosure, 44
Inclusion criteria, 16, 17 (box)
Independent monitoring, 4
Independent variable, 54–55
In-depth interview, 342–343
Indirect research benefit, 28
Indirect research effect, 66, 69f
Inductive reasoning, 8, 9f, 340
Inference process, 9–11
Informational-control condition, 92
Informed consent:
    alterations, 38
    assessment of, 33–34, 35 (box)
    documentation, 35, 36–37 (box), 38
    elements of, 33, 34 (box)
    ethical research, 27, 33–38
    institutional review board (IRB), 33, 34, 35, 38
    process for, 33
    sample form, 36–37 (box)
    waivers, 35, 38
    written consent, 35
In-person interview, 253–258, 310–313, 324–326
Institutional review board (IRB):
    convened research, 31–32
    educational training programs, 32
    ethical research, 30–32, 33, 34, 35, 38
    for ethical research, 376
    exempt research, 31–32
    expedited research, 31–32
    informed consent, 33, 34, 35, 38
    IRB protocol, 30–32
    IRB review, 31–32
Instrumentation:
    strategy for, 118
    as validity threat, 107 (box), 111–112
Instrumentation bias, 111–112
Instrumentation effect, 111–112
Intact groups, 89
Intent-to-treat strategy, 397
Interaction effect, 73
Intercoder reliability, 205–206
Intermediate outcomes, 66–68
Internal validity:
    causal design, 104–105
    control group model, 90
    research design diagrams, 90
    threats to, 106–123
International Committee of Medical Journal Editors (ICMJE), 420–421
Internet questionnaire, 253–258, 262, 263 (box)
Internet resources:
    abstracts, 415
    ethical research, 32, 38, 45
    executive summary, 416
    Google Flu Trends, 380 (box)
    G*Power software, 179
    journal submission guidelines, 415
    National Health Interview Survey (2012), 372 (box)
    qualitative data sources, 378
    random sampling, 165, 179
    Research Randomizer, 165
    research report, 415, 416, 420–421
    secondary data analysis, 372 (box), 377t, 378
    statistical power analysis, 179
    survey methods, 312
    survey response rates, 312
    UK Data Service QualiBank, 378
    variables, 51
Internet survey, 309–313, 322
Interobserver reliability, 205–206
Interrater reliability, 205–206
Interrupted time-series design, 147–149

Inter-university Consortium for Political and Social Research (University of Michigan), 378
Interval estimate, 163
Interval/ratio-level measurement:
    characteristics of, 197–198
    survey questions, 296–299
    variables, 50
Intervening variable, 66
Interviewer/staff debriefing, 250, 251
Interview guide, 343–344
Interviews:
    audio computer-assisted self-interview (ACASI), 316
    cognitive interview, 247–248, 249 (box)
    computer-assisted in-person interview (CAPI), 315–316
    computer-assisted self-interview (CASI), 316
    computer-assisted telephone interview (CATI), 315
    debriefing interview, 250–251
    focus group, 343t, 345–348
    in-person interview, 253–258, 310–313, 324–326
    interviewer bias, 5
    interviewer characteristics, 330, 331 (box)
    interviewer safety, 313–314
    interviewer/staff debriefing, 250, 251
    interviewer supervision, 331–332
    interviewer training, 331
    interviewer variance, 313
    interview guidelines, 326–330
    interviewing techniques, 349–351
    mock interview, 331
    open-response format, 342
    qualitative research, 342–351
    questionnaires, 247–248, 249 (box), 250–251, 253–258
    semistructured interview, 343–344
    structured open-ended interview, 343t, 344, 345 (box)
    survey methods, 310–317, 322–332
    telephone interview, 253–258, 310–313, 322–324
    unstructured interview, 342–343
Inverted funnel sequence, 264–266
Investigator bias, 3–4
Item nonresponse, 42, 310t, 312–313
Item response theory (IRT), 215–217
Item-specific scale, 231–232

Jottings, 359
Judgmental sampling, 359–360
Judgment-based validity, 209–212
Justice, 26, 28–29

Kappa coefficient, 205–206
Key informants sample, 361
Key personnel, 32

Labeling, measurement instrument, 233–236
Language translation techniques, 227

Levels of measurement, 50, 194–199
Likert scale, 228
Limited open survey question, 274
Limited participant observation, 352
Linear relationship, 52, 53f
Literature review, 12–13, 416–417
Longitudinal data, 375
Longitudinal design, 65–66, 137–139
Look-back, 266

Mailed questionnaire, 253–258
Mail survey, 309–313, 317–321
Manipulated conditions, 89
Manipulation of variables, 62
Margin of error (MOE), 178
Matched pairs, 183
Matching strategy, 181, 183
Maturation:
    strategy for, 115–116
    as validity threat, 107 (box), 109
Mean, 403
Measurement:
    classical test theory (CTT), 199
    conceptual definition, 192–193
    conceptualization of, 192–193
    concurrent criterion validity, 212–213
    constructs, 192–193
    construct validity, 214–215
    content validity, 211–212
    convergent validity, 213–214
    Cronbach's coefficient alpha, 207–208
    dichotomous classification, 195
    direct comparison, 196
    discriminant validity, 213–214
    face validity, 209–211
    interrater reliability, 205–206
    interval/ratio-level measurement, 197–198
    item response theory (IRT), 215–217
    judgment-based validity, 209–212
    Kappa coefficient, 205–206
    levels of measurement, 50, 194–199
    measurement accuracy, 198
    measurement bias, 200–201
    measurement precision, 198
    measurement reliability, 200, 202–208, 216 (box)
    measurement theory, 199–202
    measurement validity, 201, 202, 209–215, 216 (box)
    multiple-item scale, 207
    nominal-level measurement, 195
    observed value, 199
    operational definition, 193
    operationalization of, 192, 193
    ordinal-level measurement, 195–197
    parallel forms reliability, 206–208

performance-based validity, 209, 212–215
polychotomous classification, 195
predictive criterion validity, 213
process model, 192f
random error, 199–200
ranking, 197
rating, 197
reference category comparison, 196–197
in research report, 418
split-half reliability, 207
study exercise, 194, 199, 202, 208, 216, 218–219
systematic error, 200–201
test-retest reliability, 204–205
true value, 199
Measurement accuracy, 198
Measurement bias, 200–201
Measurement instrument:
  acquiescence bias, 228
  back-translation technique, 227
  bipolar scale, 228–229, 230 (box), 236 (box)
  branching strategy, 231
  committee translation, 227
  construct-specific scale, 231–232
  defined, 192, 193, 194 (box), 221
  development model, 222f
  development process, 222–225
  drafting phase, 223
  existing instruments, 225–227
  field pretest, 223–224
  forced-choice method, 233
  item-specific scale, 231–232
  labeling, 233–236
  language translation techniques, 227
  Likert scale, 228
  midpoints, 232–233
  multiple-item scale, 236, 237 (box), 238
  number of points, 232
  numeric labels, 233–236
  rating scale, 227–238
  revision phase, 223
  satisficing, 233
  single-item scale, 228–236, 237 (box)
  social desirability bias, 228
  study exercise, 225, 227, 239, 240–241
  unfolding strategy, 231
  unipolar scale, 229–230, 233 (box), 237 (box)
  variable chart, 223, 224t
  variable list, 222, 223t
  verbal labels, 234–236
Measurement precision, 198
Measurement reliability, 200, 202–208, 216 (box)
Measurement theory, 199–202
Measure of size (MOS), 174–175
Median, 403

Mediated causal relationships, 66–71
Mediated effect, 77
Mediated moderation model, 75, 76f, 77
Mediation model, 66–68
Mediator variable, 66
Meta-analysis, 372, 384–385
Midpoints (measurement), 232–233
Minimal risk, 28
Missing data, 312
Mixed methods program, 363
Mixed methods research designs:
  characteristics of, 362–363
  complementary concurrent design, 364
  concurrent designs, 364, 365 (box)
  confirmatory/generalizability sequential design, 364 (box), 366
  explanatory sequential design, 364 (box), 366
  exploratory sequential design, 364 (box), 365
  monomethod design, 366–367
  notation, 364 (box)
  triangulation, 364
Mixed methods study, 363
Mixed-mode survey, 314–315
Mixed multiple mediator model, 72
Mock interview, 331
Mode, 403
Mode effects, 315
Moderated causal relationships, 73–75
Moderated effect, 77
Moderated mediation model, 76, 77
Moderation model, 73–74
Moderator variable, 73
Monitored questionnaire, 253–258
Monitored self-administered questionnaire, 309–313, 321–322
Monitoring research, 4
Monomethod design, 366–367
Multiple causes, 63–64
Multiple-choice survey question, 292, 294, 297–299
Multiple effects, 63–64
Multiple-group cross-sectional design, 136–137
Multiple-group design, 88, 89, 90–95
Multiple independent variable mediation, 72
Multiple-item scale, 207, 236, 237 (box), 238
Multiple mediator models, 71–72
Multiple regression analysis, 405
Multiple-response survey question, 275, 293

Narrative review, 381
National Commission for the Protection of Human Subjects of Biomedical and Behavioral Research, 26
National Health Interview Survey (NHIS), 138 (box), 372–373 (box)
National Institute on Alcohol Abuse and Alcoholism, 51, 52t

National Institutes of Health (NIH), 32, 38, 45
National Research Act, 26
Necessary condition, 56–57
Negative relationship, 52, 53f
Nominal-level measurement:
    characteristics of, 195
    survey questions, 291–294
    variables, 50
Noncausal relationships, 57–61
Noncoverage bias, 164
Nondifferentiation bias, 246
Nondisclosure, 44
Nonequivalent groups:
    defined, 114
    strategy for, 113–114
    as validity threat, 106–108
Nonequivalent-groups posttest-only design, 142
Nonequivalent pretest-posttest control group design, 146–147
Nonexperimental design, 140–142
Nonlinear relationship, 52–53, 54f
Nonparticipant observation, 351, 352t, 354–355, 356 (box)
Nonprobability sampling, 158
Nonrandom sample, 158
Nonrandom sampling, 158
Nonresponse bias, 312
Normal distribution, 162
Notation:
    mixed methods research design, 364 (box)
    random sampling, 159
No-treatment control condition, 85, 91–92
Null hypothesis, 179, 406–408
Numeric labels, 233–236
Nurses' Health Studies (NHS), 139 (box)
NVivo, 340, 410

Objectivity, 3–5
Observation, 351–359
Observational design, 89, 98–99, 104, 136–139
Observation points, 84–85, 95–99, 375
Observed value, 199
Observer drift, 112
One-group cross-sectional design, 136
One-group design, 87–89
One-group posttest-only design, 140–141
One-group pretest-posttest design, 141–142
Open-ended interview, 342, 343t, 344, 345 (box)
Opening questions (questionnaire), 263–264
Open questions (questionnaires), 257–258
Open-response format, 342
Open survey question, 272, 274–275
Operational definition (measurement), 193
Operationalization (measurement), 192, 193

Optimizing behavior, 245–246
Ordinal-level measurement:
    characteristics of, 195–197
    survey questions, 294–296
    variables, 50
Outlier case sample, 360

Pairwise matching, 183
Panel, 88
Panel conditioning, 139
Panel design, 88
Panel maintenance, 139
Panel study, 138–139
Parallel forms reliability, 206–208
Parallel multiple mediator model, 71
Parameter of population, 9–11, 159 (box)
Paraphrasing technique, 248
Partial blind strategy, 4–5
Partially-mediated causal relationship, 68, 69f
Participant observation, 351–353, 354 (box)
Participant reactivity:
    strategy for, 122
    as validity threat, 120
Participating observer, 352–353, 354 (box)
Path, 55
Path diagram, 55–56
Patient Satisfaction Questionnaire, 227
Pearson's r, 404
Peer review, 5
Performance-based validity, 209, 212–215
Periodicity, 167–168
Periodicity bias, 167
Pilot study, 19–21
Placebo control, 92–93
Placebo effect, 92
Point estimate, 163
Points (measurement instrument), 232
Polychotomous classification, 195
Population, 9–11, 159 (box)
Population estimates, 177–179
Population size, 10, 159 (box)
Positive relationship, 52, 53f
Posttest observation point, 96–98
Posttest-only control group design, 143–144
Precoded question, 273
Predictive criterion validity, 213
Prenotification letter, 320
Prenotification strategy, 40, 41 (box)
Pretest observation point, 96
Pretest-posttest control group design, 84, 143, 144 (box)
Prevailing conditions, 89
Primacy response effects, 293
Principle investigator, 32
Privacy, 39

Privacy Rule of HIPPA (1996), 39
Private information, 39
Probabilities proportionate to size (PPS), 174–175
Probability sampling, 158
Probability theory, 158
Probing question, 248, 328–329
Problem statement, 12–13
Process evaluation, 97
Proportionate allocation, 171
Protocol, 6
Proximal outcomes, 67–68
Publication bias, 384
Purposeful sampling, 359–360
Purposive allocation, 172–173
Purposive sampling, 359–360
P value, 406

Qualitative data, 8
Qualitative data analysis:
    characteristics of, 409–410
    coding process, 410–411
    conceptual map for, 412–413
    conclusions, 412–413
    confirmability, 413
    credibility, 413
    data preparation phase, 410
    dependability, 413
    software programs for, 410
    study exercise, 414
    themes, 412–413
    transferability, 413
    trustworthiness, 413
Qualitative data sources, 378
Qualitative research methods:
    atypical case sample, 360
    basic concepts, 340–342
    chain referral sample, 361
    characteristics of, 340–341
    complete participant observation, 352, 353 (box)
    convenience sample, 361–362
    covert observation, 356–357
    descriptive notes, 357–359
    field notes, 352, 357–359
    focus group, 343t, 345–348
    going-native approach, 352–353
    heterogeneous sample, 360
    homogeneous sample, 360
    in-depth interview, 342–343
    inductive approach, 340
    interview guide, 343–344
    interviews, 342–351
    jottings, 359
    key informants sample, 361
    limitations of, 341
    limited participant observation, 352
    nonparticipant observation, 351, 352t, 354–355, 356 (box)
    observation, 351–359
    open-ended interview, 342, 343t, 344, 345 (box)
    open-response format, 342
    participant observation, 351–353, 354 (box)
    participating observer, 352–353, 354 (box)
    purposive sampling, 359–360
    quota sample, 360
    reactivity in observation, 356–357
    referral sample, 361
    reflective notes, 357–359
    respondent-driven sample (RDS), 361
    sample size, 362
    sampling, 359–362
    saturation point, 362
    semistructured interview, 343–344
    snowball sample, 361
    software programs, 340
    structured open-ended interview, 343t, 344, 345 (box)
    study exercise, 342, 349, 351, 357, 362, 368–369
    typical case sample, 360
    unstructured interview, 342–343
    See also Mixed methods research designs
Quantitative data, 8
Quantitative data analysis:
    alpha, 406
    alpha error, 408–409
    assessing differences, 405
    beta error, 408–409
    bivariate regression analysis, 405
    central tendency measures, 403
    characteristics of, 400–401
    contingency analysis, 404
    correlation analysis, 404–405
    critical value, 406
    decision errors, 408–409
    dispersion measures, 403–404
    hypothesis, 405
    hypothesis testing, 405–409
    mean, 403
    median, 403
    mode, 403
    multiple regression analysis, 405
    null hypothesis, 406–408
    Pearson's r, 404
    percentages, 402
    p value, 406
    range, 403
    regression analysis, 405
    research hypothesis, 405–406
    Spearman's rank-order coefficient, 405
    squared correlation coefficient, 404–405

Index **459**

    standard deviation, 403–404
    statistical significance, 406
    study exercise, 409
    substantive significance assessment, 409
    tables, 401–402
    type I error, 408–409
    type II error, 408–409
    validity assessment, 409
    variance, 403–404
Quasi-experimental design, 146–150
Question-by-question review, 251
Questionnaires:
    basic concepts, 244–246
    behavior coding, 250, 252
    closed-response format, 244
    cognitive interview, 247–248, 249 (box)
    data collection mode, 252–258
    debriefing interview, 250–251
    defined, 244
    design strategies, 252–258
    development process, 246–252
    double-banking format, 260–261
    drafting phase, 247
    field pretest, 248–252
    filter question, 253, 266, 267 (box)
    format of, 258–263
    funnel sequence, 264–266
    in-person interview, 253–258
    interviewer/staff debriefing, 250, 251
    inverted funnel sequence, 264–266
    layout guidelines, 259–262
    look-back, 266
    mailed questionnaire, 253–258
    monitored questionnaire, 253–258
    navigation guides, 266
    nondifferentiation bias, 246
    opening questions, 263–264
    open questions, 257–258
    optimizing behavior, 245–246
    outline phase, 246, 247 (box)
    question-by-question review, 251
    question complexity, 255
    question comprehension, 253
    questionnaire complexity, 255–256
    questionnaire length, 256
    question numbering, 266
    question order, 253–254, 263–266
    question stem, 265
    radio buttons, 262, 263 (box)
    recorded response quality, 255
    records referral, 257
    respondent, 244
    respondent debriefing, 250
    response instructions, 262
    response process, 244–245
    response review, 250, 251–252
    response-situation control, 254–255
    rostering, 256
    satisficing, 245–246
    satisficing theory, 245–246
    self-administered questionnaire (SAQ), 253–258
    self-report, 244–245
    sensitive topics, 257
    skip pattern, 255–256, 266, 267 (box)
    standardized approach, 244
    structured questionnaire, 244
    structure of, 263–267
    study exercise, 246, 252, 258, 263, 267, 269
    telephone interview, 253–258
    topic questions, 264–266
    typeface guidelines, 259
    visual aids, 256–257
    Web questionnaire, 253–258, 262, 263 (box)
    white-space format, 259
    See also Survey methods; Survey questions
Question stem, 265
Quota sample, 360

Radio buttons, 262, 263 (box)
Random assignment:
    block randomization, 181, 182–183, 184t
    frequency matching, 183
    matched pairs, 183
    matching strategy, 181, 183
    pairwise matching, 183
    research design diagrams, 85
    research design validity, 113–114
    separate random samples, 181, 182
    simple random assignment, 181, 182
    stratified random assignment, 181, 182
Random-digit dialing (RDD), 324
Random error, 199–200
Randomization, 181–183, 184t
Randomization check, 96
Randomized controlled trial (RCT), 84, 143
Random number selection, 165
Random sample, 158
Random sampling:
    basic concepts, 159–163
    basic random selection, 165
    block randomization, 181, 182–183, 184t
    central limit theorem, 162
    certainty cluster, 175
    characteristics of, 158
    cluster, 173
    cluster random sampling, 173–177
    cluster size, 174
    confidence interval (CI), 163

confidence level, 163
coverage, 164
design effect, 176–177
disproportionate allocation, 171–173
dual frame sample, 164
duplicate elements, 164–165
element, 159 (box)
equal allocation, 171–172
Equal Probability Selection Method, 160
expected value, 162
field sample size (FSS), 180
finite population correction, 178
frequency matching, 183
ineligible elements, 165
Internet resources, 165, 179
interval estimate, 163
margin of error (MOE), 178
matched pairs, 183
matching strategy, 181, 183
measure of size (MOS), 174–175
noncoverage bias, 164
nonprobability sampling, 158
nonrandom sample, 158
nonrandom sampling, 158
normal distribution, 162
notation, 159
null hypothesis, 179
objectives of, 158–159
pairwise matching, 183
parameter, 159 (box)
periodicity, 167–168
periodicity bias, 167
point estimate, 163
population, 159 (box)
population estimates, 177–179
population size, 159 (box)
probabilities proportionate to size (PPS), 174–175
probability sampling, 158
probability theory, 158
procedures, 164–168
proportionate allocation, 171
purposive allocation, 172–173
random assignment, 181–183, 184*t*
randomization, 181–183, 184*t*
random number selection, 165
random sample, 158
random selection methods, 160, 165–168
random starting point, 166
Research Randomizer, 165
sample, 159 (box)
sample size, 159 (box), 177–181
sampling distribution, 160–162
sampling error, 162
sampling fraction, 160
sampling frame, 164–165
sampling unit, 159 (box)
selection bias, 158
selection interval, 166
separate random samples, 181, 182
simple random assignment, 181, 182
simple random sampling (SRS), 160–163
simple random sampling without replacement, 160, 161 (box)
simple random sampling with replacement, 160, 161 (box)
software programs, 179
standard error (SE), 162
statistic, 159 (box)
statistical power analysis, 179
stratified random assignment, 181, 182
stratified random sampling, 169–173
stratum, 169–173
stratum weight, 172–173
study exercise, 163, 168, 173, 177, 181, 183, 187–188
systematic random sample, 165–168
terminology, 159 (box)
unbiased sample, 162
within-cluster homogeneity, 176–177
Random selection methods, 160, 165–168
Random starting point, 166
Range, 403
Ranking, 197
Ranking survey question, 294–295, 296 (box)
Rating, 197
Rating scale, 227–238, 294, 295 (box)
Reactivity in observation, 356–357
Reasoning, 8–9
Recall errors, 98
Recency response effects, 293
Reciprocal causality, 64–66
Records, 378
Refereed publication, 5
Reference category comparison, 196–197
Referral sample, 361
Reflective notes, 357–359
Refusal-conversion case, 324
Regression analysis, 112, 405
Regression-toward-the-norm:
  strategy for, 118
  as validity threat, 107 (box), 112, 113*f*
Reliability:
  in data analysis, 397
  of measurement, 200, 202–208, 216 (box)
Repeated-measures design, 88
Replication approach, 6–7
Research:
  advisory panel, 4
  blinding strategy, 4–5

conceptual framework, 7–8
control condition, 4
control group, 4
control of conditions, 6
deductive reasoning, 8–9
defined, 26, 29–30
double blind protocol, 5
elements of population, 9–10
empirical assessment, 5
exploratory research, 2
full blind strategy, 4
full disclosure, 5
holistic perspective, 9
independent monitoring, 4
inductive reasoning, 8, 9f
inference process, 9–11
interviewer bias, 5
monitoring research, 4
objectives, 2, 3 (box)
objectivity, 3–5
parameters of population, 9–11
partial blind strategy, 4–5
peer review, 5
population, 9–11
population size, 10
protocols, 6
qualitative data, 8
quantitative data, 8
reasoning, 8–9
refereed publication, 5
replication approach, 6–7
researcher bias, 3–4
researcher blind, 4
research validity, 11–12
sample size, 10
sampling unit, 10
scientific approach, 2–7
self-monitoring approach, 4
sequential replications studies, 6–7
simultaneous replication studies, 7
single-blind situation, 5
statistics, 10–11
study exercise, 12
subject-blind strategy, 5
subsample, 7
theory role, 7–8
treatment group, 4
Research design:
 case-control design, 149
 causal design, 140–152
 cohort study, 149–150
 counterbalancing design, 152
 crossover design, 151–152
 cross-sectional design, 136–137
 defined, 14
 design variations, 150–152
 experimental design, 143–146
 interrupted time-series design, 147–149
 longitudinal design, 137–139
 multiple-group cross-sectional design, 136–137
 nonequivalent-groups posttest-only design, 142
 nonequivalent pretest-posttest control group design, 146–147
 nonexperimental design, 140–142
 observational design, 136–139
 one-group cross-sectional design, 136
 one-group posttest-only design, 140–141
 one-group pretest-posttest design, 141–142
 panel conditioning, 139
 panel maintenance, 139
 panel study, 138–139
 posttest-only control group design, 143–144
 pretest-posttest control group design, 143, 144 (box)
 quasi-experimental design, 146–150
 separate-sample design, 145–146
 separate-sample three-group design, 145–146
 separate-sample two-group design, 145
 sequential cross-sectional design, 137–138
 Solomon four-group design, 144–145
 staggered-starts design, 150, 151 (box)
 study exercise, 139, 142, 146, 150, 152, 154
 switching-replications design, 151–152
 trend study, 137–138
Research design diagrams:
 attention-placebo condition, 92
 attrition, 96, 98–99
 components, 83–99
 conditions, 84–85, 89–95
 control conditions, 91–93
 control group contamination, 98
 control group model, 90, 91 (box)
 counterfactual condition, 90
 counterfactual model, 90
 cross-sectional design, 87–88
 deferred-treatment control condition, 91–92
 defined, 83
 difference-in-differences analysis, 97
 factorial design, 94–95
 false negative, 93
 false positive, 92
 groups, 83–85, 87–89
 history effect, 87
 informational-control condition, 92
 intact groups, 89
 internal validity, 90
 manipulated conditions, 89
 model illustration, 84 (box)
 multiple-group design, 88, 89, 90–95

no-treatment control condition, 85, 91–92
observational design, 89, 98–99
observation points, 84–85, 95–99
one-group design, 87–89
panel, 88
panel design, 88
placebo control, 92–93
posttest observation point, 96–98
pretest observation point, 96
pretest-posttest control group design, 84
prevailing conditions, 89
process evaluation, 97
random assignment, 85
randomization check, 96
randomized controlled trial (RCT), 84
recall errors, 98
repeated-measures design, 88
sample, 89
standard-treatment control condition, 93
study exercise, 85, 87, 89, 95, 99–100
time frame, 83–85, 86–87
timing, 86
treatment, 84
treatment condition, 90, 93–95
wait-list control condition, 91–92
waves, 98

Research design validity:
attrition bias, 110
attrition strategy, 116–117
attrition threat, 107 (box), 109–110
causal design, 104–105, 106 (box)
compensatory equalization strategy, 122
compensatory equalization threat, 120
compensatory rivalry strategy, 122
compensatory rivalry threat, 120
control group contamination, 114, 119, 121
demoralization strategy, 122
demoralization threat, 120
design strategies, 106, 113–118
design threats, 106–113
direct effect, 113
effectiveness of treatment, 129
effectiveness trials, 129, 130f
efficacy of treatment, 129
efficacy trials, 129, 130f
equivalent groups, 107
external validity, 105, 106 (box)
external validity threats, 123–129
history strategy, 114–115
history threat, 107 (box), 108–109
instrumentation bias, 111–112
instrumentation effect, 111–112
instrumentation strategy, 118
instrumentation threat, 107 (box), 111–112
internal-external validity balance, 129, 130f
internal validity, 104–105
internal validity threats, 106–123
maturation strategy, 115–116
maturation threat, 107 (box), 109
nondesign strategies, 120–122
nondesign threats, 119–120
nonequivalent groups, 114
nonequivalent groups strategy, 113–114
nonequivalent groups threat, 106–108
observational design, 104
observer drift, 112
participant reactivity strategy, 122
participant reactivity threat, 120
random assignment, 113–114
regression analysis, 112
regression-toward-the-norm strategy, 118
regression-toward-the-norm threat, 107 (box), 112, 113f
self-assignment, 114
self-selection bias, 114
statistically equivalent groups, 113
study exercise, 104, 106, 123, 129, 130, 132
testing effect, 110–111
testing strategy, 117–118
testing threat, 107 (box), 110–111
treatment diffusion strategy, 121
treatment diffusion threat, 119
treatment imitation strategy, 121
treatment imitation threat, 119–120
unobtrusive measurement, 117
unrepresentative outcome strategy, 128
unrepresentative outcome threat, 123 (box), 127–128
unrepresentative setting strategy, 125
unrepresentative setting threat, 123 (box), 125
unrepresentative treatment strategy, 126–127
unrepresentative treatment threat, 123 (box), 126
unrepresentative units strategy, 124–125
unrepresentative units threat, 123–124
Researcher bias, 3–4
Researcher blind, 4
Research hypothesis, 405–406
Research process:
conceptual approach, 14
conclusions of research, 18
data analysis, 18
data collection, 17–18
defined, 12
exclusion criteria, 16, 17 (box)
inclusion criteria, 16, 17 (box)
literature review, 12–13
model illustration, 13f
next-study focus, 18–19
pilot study, 19–21
problem statement, 12–13

    research design, 14
    research question, 13–14
    sample size, 17
    study exercise, 21
    subjects, 15–17
    target population, 15–16
    units of study, 16
Research question, 13–14
Research Randomizer, 165
Research report:
    abstract, 415–416
    acknowledgments, 420
    appendix, 419–420
    authorship, 421
    background, 416–417
    conflict-of-interest disclosure, 420–421
    data analysis, 418
    data collection, 418
    discussion, 419
    executive summary, 416
    funding support, 420
    general report format, 415–421
    human subjects protection, 420
    Internet resources, 415, 416, 420–421
    introduction, 416
    literature review, 416–417
    measurements/instrumentation, 418
    methods, 417–418
    presentation formats, 414
    references, 419
    research design, 417
    results/findings, 418–419
    study exercise, 421
    subjects/participants, 417
Research validity, 11–12
    See also External validity; Internal validity;
        Research design validity; Validity
Resentful demoralization, 120
Respect for persons, 26–27, 33
Respondent, 244
Respondent debriefing, 250
Respondent-driven sample (RDS), 361
Response heaping, 298
Response review, 250, 251–252
Reverse coding, 395
Risk factor:
    in research, 28
    in variables, 57
Rostering, 256

Sample, 89, 159 (box)
Sample size, 10, 17, 159 (box), 177–181, 362
Sampling, 359–362
Sampling distribution, 160–162

Sampling error, 162
Sampling fraction, 160
Sampling frame, 164–165
Sampling unit, 10, 159 (box)
Satisficing, 233, 245–246
Satisficing theory, 245–246
Saturation point, 362
Scientific approach:
    control, 6
    objectivity, 3–5
    replication, 6–7
Secondary data analysis:
    advantages of, 374–375
    analytic process, 373–374
    big data, 371–372, 379, 380 (box)
    data sources, 376–379, 380 (box)
    defined, 371, 372
    documents, 378
    ethical principles, 376
    gray literature, 384
    Internet resources, 372 (box), 377t, 378
    limitations of, 375–376
    longitudinal data, 375
    meta-analysis, 372, 384–385
    narrative review, 381
    observation points, 375
    publication bias, 384
    qualitative data sources, 378
    records, 378
    study exercise, 374, 376, 380, 386, 388
    synthesizing results, 381–385
    systematic review, 372, 381–384
    trend analysis, 375
Selection bias, 158
Selection interval, 166
Self-administered questionnaire (SAQ), 253–258, 309–322
Self-assignment, 114
Self-determination principle, 26–27
Self-monitoring approach, 4
Self-report, 244–245
Self-selection bias, 114
Semistructured interview, 343–344
Sensitive topics:
    ethical research, 35, 38
    questionnaires, 257
    survey questions, 285–287
Separate random sample, 181, 182
Separate-sample three-group design, 145–146
Separate-sample two-group design, 145
Sequential cross-sectional design, 137–138
Sequential multiple mediator model, 71
Sequential replications studies, 6–7
Sequential strategy, 314, 315 (box)
Serial multiple mediator model, 71

Silent-probe technique, 329
Simple random assignment, 181, 182
Simple random sampling (SRS), 160–163
Simple random sampling without replacement, 160, 161 (box)
Simple random sampling with replacement, 160, 161 (box)
Simultaneous multiple mediator model, 71
Simultaneous replication studies, 7
Simultaneous strategy, 314
Single-blind situation, 5
Single-item scale, 228–236, 237 (box)
Skip pattern, 255–256, 266, 267 (box)
Snowball sample, 361
Social Cognitive Theory, 7
Social desirability bias, 228
Social Ecological Model, 7
Software programs. See Computer software programs
Solomon four-group design, 144–145
Spearman's rank-order coefficient, 405
Special case sample, 360
Split-half reliability, 207
Spurious relationship, 58–60
Squared correlation coefficient, 404–405
Staggered-starts design, 150, 151 (box)
Standard deviation, 403–404
Standard error (SE), 162
Standard-treatment control condition, 93
Statistic, 10–11, 159 (box)
Statistically equivalent groups, 113
Statistical power analysis, 179
Statistical significance, 406
Straight, single-headed arrow, 55
Stratified random assignment, 181, 182
Stratified random sampling, 169–173
Stratum, 169–173
Stratum weight, 172–173
Strength of relationship, 54
Structured open-ended interview, 343t, 344, 345 (box)
Structured questionnaires. See Questionnaires
Study-specific codes, 43
Subject, 15–17, 28
Subject-blind strategy, 5
Subsample, 7
Substantive significance assessment, 409
Sufficient condition, 56–57
Supplementary mode, 314
Survey methods:
    address-based sampling (ABS), 321
    advantages of, 306–307
    anonymity, 310t, 311–312
    audio computer-assisted self-interview (ACASI), 316
    basic concepts, 306–309
    clarification of response, 329–330
    completeness of response, 330
    computer-assisted in-person interview (CAPI), 315–316
    computer-assisted self-interview (CASI), 316
    computer-assisted surveys, 315–317
    computer-assisted telephone interview (CATI), 315
    contact log, 323–324
    costs of, 310–311
    data collection comparisons, 310–313
    data collection mode, 309–317
    defined, 306
    disadvantages of, 307
    email survey, 310
    encouragement strategy, 329
    follow-up mode, 314
    geographic distribution, 310t, 311
    in-person interview, 310–313, 324–326
    Internet resources, 312
    Internet survey, 309–313, 322
    interviewer characteristics, 330, 331 (box)
    interviewer safety, 313–314
    interviewer supervision, 331–332
    interviewer training, 331
    interviewer variance, 313
    interview guidelines, 326–330
    item nonresponse, 310t, 312–313
    mail survey, 309–313, 317–321
    missing data, 312
    mixed-mode survey, 314–315
    mock interview, 331
    mode effects, 315
    monitored self-administered questionnaire, 309–313, 321–322
    nonresponse bias, 312
    prenotification letter, 320
    probing question, 328–329
    process for, 307–309, 317–326
    random-digit dialing (RDD), 324
    recording responses, 327–328
    refusal-conversion case, 324
    self-administered questionnaire (SAQ), 309–322
    sequential strategy, 314, 315 (box)
    silent-probe technique, 329
    simultaneous strategy, 314
    study exercise, 309, 314, 326, 332, 333–336
    supplementary mode, 314
    survey plan, 306, 307–309
    telephone interview, 310–313, 322–324
    time factor, 310t, 311
    unit response rate, 310t, 312
    Web survey, 309–313, 322
    See also Questionnaires
Survey plan, 306, 307–309
Survey questions:
    abbreviations, 277
    biased questions, 283–285

categories of, 272–275
closed question, 272, 273
completely open question, 274
complete sentences, 281
compound question, 281–282, 288–289
dichtomous-choice question, 292, 294
double-barreled question, 281–282, 288–289
double negatives, 282
fill-in-the-blank question, 291, 296
interval/ratio-level questions, 296–299
limited open question, 274
multiple-choice question, 292, 294, 297–299
multiple-response question, 275, 293
multiple responses, 275
nominal-level questions, 291–294
open question, 272, 274–275
ordinal-level questions, 294–296
precoded question, 273
primacy response effects, 293
problem words, 278–279
question structure, 279–287
question tone, 277
question wording, 275–279
ranking question, 294–295, 296 (box)
rating-scale question, 294, 295 (box)
recency response effects, 293
response choices, 287–299
response guidelines, 287–291
response heaping, 298
sensitive topics, 285–287
short/simple question, 279–281
specified response-conditions, 282–283
study exercise, 275, 279, 287, 299, 300–303
vocabulary guidelines, 276–277
Switching-replications design, 151–152
Systematic error, 200–201
Systematic random sample, 165–168
Systematic review, 372, 381–384

Target population, 15–16
Telephone interview, 253–258, 310–313, 322–324
Temporal precedence, 55, 61, 62
Testing:
    strategy for, 117–118
    as validity threat, 107 (box), 110–111
Testing effect, 110–111
Test-retest reliability, 204–205
Theory, 7–8
Theory of Planned Behavior, 7, 14, 15 (box), 72
Thinking aloud technique, 247
Time frame, 83–85, 86–87
Timing, 86
Total effect, 68, 69f
Transferability, 413

Treatment, 84
Treatment condition, 90, 93–95
Treatment diffusion:
    strategy for, 121
    as validity threat, 119
Treatment equality, 29
Treatment group, 4
Treatment imitation:
    strategy for, 121
    as validity threat, 119–120
Trend study, 137–138, 375
Triangulation, 364
True value, 199
Trustworthiness, 413
Tuskegee Study of Untreated Syphilis in the Negro Male (1932-1972), 26 (box)
Two-headed curved arrow, 58
Type I error, 408–409
Type II error, 408–409
Typical case sample, 360

UK Data Service QualiBank, 378
Unbiased sample, 162
Unfolding strategy, 231
Unipolar scale, 229–230, 233 (box), 237 (box)
Unit response rate, 310t, 312
Units of study, 16
Unobtrusive measurement, 117
Unrepresentative outcome:
    strategy for, 128
    as validity threat, 123 (box), 127–128
Unrepresentative setting:
    strategy for, 125
    as validity threat, 123 (box), 125
Unrepresentative treatment:
    strategy for, 126–127
    as validity threat, 123 (box), 126
Unrepresentative units:
    strategy for, 124–125
    as validity threat, 123–124
Unstructured interview, 342–343
U.S. Food and Drug Administration (FDA), 29
U.S. Office for Human Research Protections (OHRP), 29, 30

Validity:
    in data analysis, 397
    of measurement, 201, 202, 209–215, 216 (box)
    in quantitative data analysis, 409
    See also External validity; Internal validity; Research design validity
Value label, 394
Value neutrality, 3–4
Variable chart, 223, 224t
Variable label, 394

Variable list, 222, 223*t*
Variable name, 394
Variables:
   alternative causal explanations, 61, 62
   categories of, 50–51
   causal inference, 61–6361–63
   causal mechanisms, 61, 62–63
   causal relationships, 54–79
   cause, 54–55
   common cause, 57–58
   completely-mediated causal relationship, 68, 69*f*
   complex causal models, 77, 78f
   component causes, 56–57
   confounder variable, 59–60
   contingency analysis, 51
   contingency table, 51, 52*t*
   continuous variable, 50–51
   correlation coefficient computation, 54
   covariation, 61–62
   defined, 49–50
   dependent variable, 54–55
   direction of relationship, 52–53
   direct research effect, 66, 69*f*
   discrete variable, 50
   distal outcomes, 67–68
   ecological fallacy, 60, 61*f*
   effect, 54–55
   endogenous variable, 56
   exogenous variable, 55–56
   explanatory variable, 59–60
   extraneous variable, 59–60
   independent variable, 54–55
   indirect research effect, 66, 69*f*
   interaction effect, 73
   intermediate outcomes, 66–68
   Internet resources, 51
   interval/ratio-level measurement, 50
   level of measurement, 50
   linear relationship, 52, 53*f*
   longitudinal design research, 65–66
   manipulation, 62
   mediated causal relationships, 66–71
   mediated effect, 77
   mediated moderation model, 75, 76*f*, 77
   mediation model, 66–68
   mediator variable, 66
   mixed multiple mediator model, 72
   moderated causal relationships, 73–75
   moderated effect, 77
   moderated mediation model, 76, 77
   moderation model, 73–74
   moderator variable, 73
   multiple causes, 63–64
   multiple effects, 63–64
   multiple independent variable mediation, 72
   multiple mediator models, 71–72
   multiple moderator models, 75
   necessary condition, 56–57
   negative relationship, 52, 53*f*
   nominal-level measurement, 50
   noncausal relationships, 57–61
   nonlinear relationship, 52–53, 54*f*
   ordinal-level measurement, 50
   parallel multiple mediator model, 71
   partially-mediated causal relationship, 68, 69*f*
   path, 55
   path diagram, 55–56
   positive relationship, 52, 53*f*
   proximal outcomes, 67–68
   reciprocal causality, 64–66
   relationship attributes, 51–54
   risk factor, 57
   sequential multiple mediator model, 71
   serial multiple mediator model, 71
   simultaneous multiple mediator model, 71
   spurious relationship, 58–60
   straight,single-headed arrow, 55
   strength of relationship, 54
   study exercise, 51, 54, 57, 60, 63, 79, 80–81
   sufficient condition, 56–57
   temporal precedence, 55, 61, 62
   total effect, 68, 69*f*
   two-headed curved arrow, 58
Variance, 403–404
Verbal label, 234–236
Vulnerable population, 27

Wait-list control condition, 91–92
Waves, 98
Web questionnaire, 253–258, 262, 263 (box)
Web survey, 309–313, 322
Weighting procedures, 397
White-space format, 259
Within-cluster homogeneity, 176–177